# The Encyclopedia of
# ALTERNATIVE
# MEDICINE

*The Encyclopedia of AlternativeMedicine* reports information and opinions of medical and other professionals which may be of general interest to the reader. It is advisory only and is not intended to serve as a medical textbook or other procedural guidebook for either physicians or patients. The information and opinions contained herein, which should not be used or relied upon without consultation and advice of a physician, are those solely of the authors and not those of the publishers who disclaim any responsibility for the accuracy of such information and opinions and any responsibility for any consequences that may result from any use or reliance thereon by the reader.

First published in the United States of America in 1996 by
Journey Editions, an imprint of Charles E. Tuttle Co., Inc.
of Rutland, Vermont, and Tokyo, Japan, with editorial offices at
153 Milk Street, Boston, Massachusetts, 02109.

Library of Congress Cataloging-in-Publication Data

The encyclopedia of alternative medicine : a complete family guide to
     complementary therapies / by Jennifer Jacobs, consultant editor.
          p.     cm.
     Includes bibliographical references and index.
     ISBN 1-885203-36-5
     1. Alternative medicine—Encylopedias.     I. Jacobs, Jennifer.
     R733.E496     1996
     615.5—dc20                                              96–18786
                                                                   CIP

10 9 8 7 6 5 4 3 2 1     00 99 98 97 96

Project Editor: Heather Thomas
Art Editor: Rolando Ugolini
Production: Sarah Schuman

Printed and bound in Italy

# The Encyclopedia of
# ALTERNATIVE
# MEDICINE

## A COMPLETE FAMILY GUIDE TO COMPLEMENTARY THERAPIES

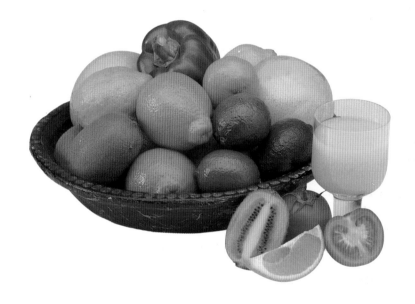

CONSULTANT EDITOR
JENNIFER JACOBS, MD, MPH

JOURNEY EDITIONS
BOSTON • TOKYO

# CONTENTS

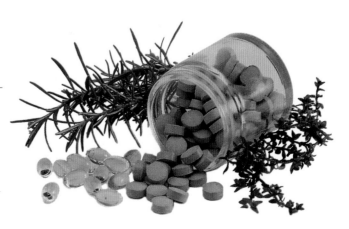

# FOREWORD

JENNIFER JACOBS, M.D., M.P.H.

In the United States, a Harvard University study demonstrated that nearly a third of the population had used complementary and alternative therapies during 1990. The Office of Alternative Medicine, at the National Institutes of Health in Bethesda, Maryland, was created by the U.S. Congress in 1992 to scientifically investigate the field. Insurance companies and managed care plans are beginning to incorporate alternative and complementary providers into their networks as public interest grows in these low-cost and non-invasive therapies. More and more physicians are attending training programs and discussing how to integrate these modalities into their practices.

There are several key concepts common to the therapies described in this book. The first is an underlying belief in the innate self-healing capacity of the body. Called "chi" in Chinese Medicine and the "vital force" by the founder of homeopathic medicine, Samuel Hahnemann, this ability of the body to heal itself was first recognized by the Greek physician Hippocrates as *vis medicatrix naturae*. Therapies are used to stimulate and enhance this healing life energy, either directly through therapies such as homeopathy and acupuncture, or indirectly through such practices as nutrition and herbs that promote optimal functioning of the body.

Another concept is that of holism—the idea that the physical, emotional, mental, and spiritual aspects of health are all interrelated. Rather than treat various symptoms or diseases as separate entities to be controlled by pharmaceutical agents or surgery, the human organism is seen as a whole system that interacts on various levels to create a state of health or disease. Therapeutic interventions in one or more of these spheres are thought to have an effect on the total being to enhance wellness.

Health is seen as a state of harmony or balance in the organism. Negative influences in one's life are thought to throw the body out of balance and create illness. Such factors as overwork, family stress, and excessive anger or grief can affect the mental/emotional levels of health, while poor eating habits, lack of exercise, exposure to harmful microorganisms, and hereditary tendencies can create illness in the physical sphere. The goal of treatment is to correct this imbalance, either by removing the negative influence, if possible, or by strengthening the self-healing capacity of the organism to overcome the stress.

As we approach the twenty-first century, it is clear that we are undergoing a revolution in our attitudes toward health and disease. Led primarily by consumer interest, the medical profession is reluctantly being pushed into a greater acceptance of any alternative and complementary therapies. Some of these, such as Traditional Chinese Medicine and Acupuncture, have been practiced for thousands of years while others, such as Polarity Therapy, Rolfing, and the Alexander Technique, are unique to the twentieth century. As alternative and complementary treatments move into the mainstream, it is important that consumers educate themselves about various modalities so that they can make intelligent choices about their health care. We hope this book will be helpful in that process.

# CONTRIBUTORS

## ACUPRESSURE

**Michael Reed Gach** is a Director of the Acupressure Institute in Berkeley, California, and has written several books on Acupressure, published by Bantam Books, Celestial Arts, Simon & Schuster and Warner Books.

## ACUPUNCTURE

**Christina Stemmler, M.D.** combines Eastern and Western medicine, providing multiple options and creative alternatives to adverse-effects ridden chemical treatments, unnecessary surgical procedures, and hazardous diagnostic and therapeutic modalities. She has been in private practice in Houston, Texas, since 1984 and holds Diplomate status with the American Academy of Pain Management, is the Immediate Past President of the American Academy of Medical Acupuncture (AAMA), is an Executive Director of the Institute for the Advancement of Medical Acupuncture, and Founding Editor-in-Chief of the AAMA Review.

## ALEXANDER TECHNIQUE

**Don Krim, M.S.,** is Chairman of the North American Society of Teachers of Alexander Technique. He holds a Master of Science degree in Physical Education and teaches at the California State University, Fullerton. He teaches the Alexander Technique in corporate settings, specifically to address worker safety related issues, such as stress, back injury and repetitive strain injury. He maintains his private teaching practice in Beverly Hills and Fullerton, California.

## AROMATHERAPY

**Jeanne Rose** is a leading pioneer in the revival of herbal and natural remedies and aromatherapy to maintain good health. She is also an international authority on the therapeutic uses of herbs, both medicinal and cosmetic, and a teacher of aromatherapy since 1972. She is President of the National Association for Holistic Aromatherapy (NAHA) and the author of 14 herbal books.

**Susan Earle** serves on the Executive Committee of the NAHA, and is a research author in the fields of herbalism and aromatherapy.

## AUTOGENIC TRAINING AND VISUALIZATION THERAPY

**Dr. Kai Kermani,** B.Sc., L.R.C.P., M.R.C.S., M.B.B.S., D.R.C.O.G., M.R.C.G.P., is a practicing medical doctor in the UK, and a member of several Royal Colleges. He also has a degree in science (physiology). He is a member of the Holistic Medical Association, the National Federation of Spiritual Healers and The Healing Foundation. He is a counselor, stress management consultant, Autogenic Trainer and therapist. He lectures internationally and has run workshops for both the British and European Houses of Parliament on the holistic management of catastrophic illness. He has written numerous articles and is the author of *Autogenic Training; the effective holistic way to better health.*

## CHINESE HERBAL MEDICINE

**Stephen Kippax** is a Member of the National Institute of Medical Herbalists; a Member of the Register of Chinese Herbal Medicine; a practitioner of Chinese Acupuncture; and a Homeopath. He regularly lectures and runs courses on his specialist modalities.

## CHIROPRACTIC

**Dr. George K. Herkert** is an American trained and licensed chiropractor, presently in practice at his clinic, The American Chiropractic Center in Buckinghamshire, England. He has a degree of Doctor of Chiropractic, from Columbia Institute of Chiropractic in New York. Amongst his many credentials are: Member of the International Chiropractic Association, Member of the American Chiropractic Association and of the Diplomatic American National Board of Chiropractic Examiners.

## COLOR THERAPY

**Bonney Whittington** has been working with color as an artist and a healer since 1969. She studied color healing with Theo Gimbel, director of research and principal of The Hygeia College of Color Therapy in England. She has been involved in energy work and healing with Rosalyn Bruyere and Dr. Dawn Markova, and essence work with Li Bette Porter. She works as a color therapist and runs her company, Lightwater Essences, producing a wide range of essential essences.

## CRANIAL OSTEOPATHY

**Dr. Robert P. Lee,** D.O., S.P.O.M.M., is a practicing osteopath in Durango, Colorado, and is a Member of the American Osteopathic Association, the American Academy of Osteopathy and the American Academy of Medical Acupuncture. He is also a Member of the International Issues Task Force of the Cranial Academy, and has written articles and contributions in many books and publications.

8

## DANCE THERAPY

**Claire Schmais,** Ph.D., A.D.T.R., C.M.A., is one of the founders and the coordinator of the Hunter College Dance/Movement Therapy Program, CUNY. She has published numerous articles and is a charter member of the American Dance Therapy Association. She lectures in the United States and abroad.

**Elissa Queyquep White,** A.D.T.R., C.M.A., is the chairperson of the Central Conference Committee of the Board of Directors of the American Dance Therapy Association. A charter member of the ADTA and one of the founders of the Hunter College Program, she is now in private practice.

## DIET THERAPIES

**Dr. Kurt Donsbach** D.C., N.D., Ph.D., graduated in chiropractic which then led him to the study of nutrition. He also has a naturopathic degree and Master of Science and Doctor of Philosphy degrees in nutrition. Dr Donsbach is the author of more than 50 books and booklets, and is the founder of the Donsbach University. He was Chairman of the Board of the National Health Federation for 15 years. He has established the two largest wholistic hospitals in the world specializing in cancer and degenerative diseases; Hospital Santa Monica in Rosarito Beach, Baja California, Mexico, and Institut Santa Monica in Kamien Pomorski, Poland. He is the editor of two magazines, *The HealthKeeper's Journal* and the *Official Journal of The American Naturopathic Medical Association* and *The American Association of Nutritional Consultants.*

## FLOWER THERAPY

**Patricia Kaminski** is co-director of the Flower Essence Society in Nevada City, California. She has been instrumental in designing and administrating the Society's research and practitioner training programs, and also maintains a private flower essence therapy practice. She has written articles and co-authored a book on flower essences, and has taught around the world on this subject for over 15 years.

## HERBAL MEDICINE

**Caroline Wheeler** has a degree in biochemistry from the University of Manchester. She spent several years working in orthodox laboratory science before taking a four-year course in Herbal Medicine and becoming a Member of the National Institute of Medical Herbalists. She combines her herbal practice with teaching biological and medical sciences.

## HOMEOPATHY

**Dr. William Shevin,** M.D., D.Ht. is a practicing medical doctor and homeopath. He is a past president of the National Center for Homeopathy, and serves on the Board of Directors of the Homeopathic Pharmacopoeia Convention of the United States.

## HYPNOTHERAPY

**Dr. William E. Kemery** is a leading hypnotherapist, psychotherapist and sex therapist who has been at the forefront of understanding hypnotherapy and professionalizing its practice. A fellow of the Academy of Scientific Hypnotherapy, a member of the American Mental Health Counselors Association and founding director of the California Hypnotists Examining Council, Dr. Kemery is a contributor to numerous professional journals.

## IRIDOLOGY

**Angela Bradbury,** D.Hom., F.G.N.I., M.R.N.T., trained as a homeopath. She subsequently studied iridology at the School of Natural Medicine. After five years of further studies in nutrition and naturopathy and fifteen years of practice and research, she and her husband established

The Holistic Health College in 1993.

## MASSAGE

**Elliot Greene** is the Immediate Past President of the American Massage Therapy Association and an expert in the field of massage therapy. He is nationally certified in Therapeutic Massage and Bodywork and has qualified as a Registered Massage Therapist, Sports Massage Therapist and Approved Continuing Education Instructor. While representing the AMTA he was invited to the White House to work with President Clinton's Task Force for Health Care Reform and has testified on massage therapy before the National Institutes of Health's Office of Alternative Medicine Ad Hoc Panel. He is on the Board of Directors of the National Wellness Coalition and is the author of many articles on massage therapy. He has extensive teaching experience and maintains a private practice in the Washington DC area.

## MEDITATION

**Amy Gage** is President Emeritus of the International Association of Yoga Therapists and has extensive experience since 1963 practicing and teaching stress awareness and control using traditional yoga practices as holistic therapy for various populations and physical conditions. Her interests focus primarily on the areas of lifestyle management and stress control, and she teaches and conducts workshops for a wide range of user groups.

## MUSIC THERAPY

**Michael J. Rohrbacher,** Ph.D., M.T.-B.C., is Director of Music Therapy at Shenandoah University in Winchester, Virginia. He holds a Bachelor of Music with a major in music therapy from East Carolina University, Master of Science in Education with a major in communicative disorders from Johns Hopkins University, and a Ph.D. in Ethnomusicology from the University of Maryland Baltimore County. He is a member of the National Association for Music Therapy, Inc., and holds the credential "Music Therapist-Board Certified" through the Certification Board for Music Therapists (C.B.M.T.). He served as consultant to "Music Therapy and Psychosocial Adjustment for Persons with Head Injury," a research award from the National Institutes of Health, Office of Alternative Medicine. He served on the Board of Directors for CBMT, 1992-1996.

## NATUROPATHY

Jared L Zeff, N.D., L.Ac., is a consultant in both Naturopathic Medicine and Acupuncture, the Chairman and Founder of the Institute for Advanced Studies in the Healing Arts in Portland and affiliated to the American Association of Naturopathic Physicians. He has enormous professional experience and expertise in naturopathic medicine and has acted in an executive capacity on the boards of a number of naturopathic associations. He is the author of a number of publications and articles on naturopathic medicine and was honored as "Naturopathic Physician of the Year" by the American Association of Naturopathic Physicians in 1989.

## OSTEOPATHY

Michael Kuchera, D.O., F.A.A.O., is Professor and Chairperson of the Department of Osteopathic Manipulative Medicine at Kirksville College of Osteopathic Medicine. He is Chairperson of the Postdoctoral Standards and Evaluation Committee of the American Academy of Osteopathy and a member of the Task Force and Steering Committee on Osteopathic Graduate Medical Education for the American Osteopathic Association. He is also Chairperson of the Educational Committee of the American Association of Orthopedic Medicine, and has written several articles and papers in medical journals.

## POLARITY THERAPY

John Chitty, R.P.P., is the President of the American Polarity Therapy Association and Director of the Polarity Center of Colorado. He is the author of the Polarity book, *Energy Exercises*.

## PSYCHOTHERAPY

Dr. Maureen O'Hara, B.Sc., Ph.D., is a past president of the Association for Humanistic Psychology. She is trained in Client-Centered Therapy, Gestalt Therapy, Emancipatory Therapy and Relational Therapy. A Distinguished Clinical member of the California Association for Marriage and Family Therapy, she also serves as Associate Editor of the *Journal of Humanistic Psychology*, and on the editorial boards of the *Humanistic Psychologist* and the *Journal of Constructivist Psychology*. A long-time colleague of Carl Rogers, she has conducted Person-Centered Approach community workshops and has trained psychotherapists in client-centered therapy and gestalt therapy worldwide. She is widely published in professional and popular publications and has been in private practice as a psychotherapist for over 20 years.

## REFLEXOLOGY

Carolyn Long is a writer, public speaker and certified reflexologist in Columbia, Maryland. She has studied the Ingham Method of Reflexology at workshops run by the International Institute of Reflexology throughout the United States and Canada, and conducts training programs on stress reduction.

## ROLFING

Christopher Amodeo is a Board member of the Rolf Institute and a practicing rolfer in private practice in Costa Mesa, California. While working in hospital and pursuing a graduate degree in psychology, he discovered rolfing and subsequently changed his course of study. He graduated from the International Rolf Institute in Boulder, Colorado, and is currently serving on the Rolf Institute's board of directors.

## SHIATSU

Nigel Dawes, M.A., C.Ac., Dipl. Ac., specializes in oriental medicine and is Academic Dean of The New Center in New York state, an educational institute specializing in treatment and research in wholistic medicine. He trained in Shiatsu in Tokyo under Master Takeo Suzuki, a Disciple of Shizuto Masunaga.

## T'AI CHI CH'UAN

Marvin Smalheiser is Editor and Publisher of *T'ai Chi Magazine*. He has practiced the Yang style for more than 25 years, and has met and interviewed many of the leading T'ai Chi Ch'uan masters in China and other countries.

## TRANSCENDENTAL MEDITATION

Robert Roth has lectured and taught transcendental meditation for over 25 years to tens of thousands of people in the U.S., Canada and Europe. He is a senior advisor to the Maharishi Corporate Development Program, and a founder of the Institute for Fitness and Athletic Excellence, which offers the technique to amateur and professional athletes.

## YOGA

Jnani Chapman trained as a nurse and then specialized in yoga, massage, acupressure and nutrition. She currently practices and teaches yoga, as well as working as a stress management instructor for the Preventive Medicine Research Institute in Sausalito. She holds the Sigma Theta Tau and Alpha Sigma Nu honours.

# INTRODUCTION

"The cure of the part should not be attempted without treatment of the whole. No attempt should be made to cure the body without the soul, and therefore, if the head and the body are to be healthy, you must begin by curing the mind. That is the first thing. Let no one persuade you to cure the head until he has first given you his soul to be cured. For this is the great error of our day in the treatment of the human body, that physicians first separate the soul from the body." Plato wrote this in 380B.C. in his book *The Republic*.

From earliest times, the concept of treating the physical and mental aspects of the patient in concert with the soul or spirit has been central to the medical services of the time. Plato knew well the importance of both because they are central elements in the ancient perception of the healing process although he was not the first to appreciate this concept. Understanding the way in which healing works still eludes much twentieth-century scientific thought but it is crucial to the concepts of traditional medicine that are currently practiced under its many names.

The Chinese believe that life and health are directly related to the flow of energy throughout the body: this is called "Chi." When the energy is blocked, disease is manifested. The Chinese also believe that Chi is found outside the body and is both the energy that governs the universe and which also has a direct relationship to astrological medicine. This is well documented in the *Nei Ching*, possibly the oldest Chinese book on medicine, said to have been written 4,500 years ago by Koai Yu Chu. He states that "... an essential primordial energy that gives birth to all the elements and is integrated into them ... this energy is only an abstract substance in the sky, whereas on earth it is transformed into a concrete physical substance."

Just as the Chinese have considered Chi as a form of healing energy, so other individuals have attempted to describe it throughout history. Pythagoras, born in Greece circa 580B.C., was a physician who considered healing to be a noble art. He integrated this thinking into his researches and suggested that it came from a central fire in the universe which gave each living being a spark of life.

Hippocrates, thought to have been born on the Greek island of Kos circa 460B.C., taught that to maintain good health it was necessary to keep all aspects of body chemistry in balance; phlegm, blood and bile (black and yellow) were seen as the basic elements governing individual health. When these fluids (humors) were out of balance and not blending correctly, disease would appear. The resulting fever would "cook" these juices and remove any unnecessary substances. Hippocrates believed that balance would automatically be restored by a natural healing mechanism which he called the *vis medicatrix naturae*. His guiding principle was not to interfere with symptoms so that nature could effectively heal the disease.

Paracelsus was born in Switzerland in 1493. He is best known for his understanding of venereal diseases, tumors and the healing of wounds together with an understanding that "what makes a man ill can also cure him." This was effectively an early concept of homeopathy and an idea that was not new to religions but was certainly new to health care. He considered that man has two bodies: one animal and one sidereal (astral). The animal body contained the lower instincts whilst the astral was the agent for the creation of wisdom and art. The idea that the higher body could also experience illness and could be treated formed the basis of his thinking. Paracelsus called the healing energy the *archaeus*.

Samuel Hahnemann (1755-1843) developed homeopathy as we know it today. He recognized the healing energy which he called vital force. The discovery of healing energies was not confined to these names alone and history is full of pioneers who sought to extend the natural healing process into more conventional methods of medical treatment. However, the scientific view rejected the concept in favour of treating the physical body and the mind alone. Even so, healing was continued in the churches as part of a specific religious practice.

Many of the following chapters contributed by specialist practitioners, describe the ancient roots of the various disciplines giving credit to both the holistic and the healing vision which are common to all. Practitioners talk about getting patients into "balance," "unblocking energy pathways,"

and "providing the correct nutrition and support." All this is part of helping patients to help themselves back to health by allowing the immune system to function at optimum levels and regaining a structural integrity of the physical body where this has been impaired.

Descriptions of the collective philosophy have varied and the most common names are as follows:

■ **Alternative medicine** was mainly used by those practitioners who wished to establish that they were an alternative to orthodox medicine.

■ **Holism** was used in the 1970s to indicate care of the whole person: body, mind and spirit.

■ **Complementary medicine** was first used in 1976 in the United Kingdom as a means of linking the most appropriate techniques to serve the patient at physical, mental, emotional and vitality or spiritual dimensions. Complementary medicine is holism in practice.

Whereas "fringe" described a political relationship with the doctor, "alternative" and "complementary" allowed all health

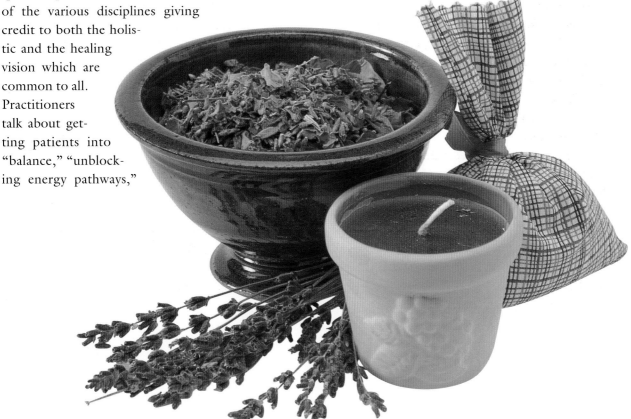

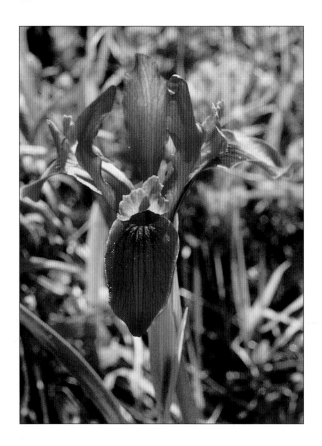

those grants that have been made have limited the protocols to double blind placebo trials. The problem for healers using any form of physical or mental approach has been the requirement to offer correct treatments to some and sham treatments to others. Many felt such an approach was unethical.

The situation is further complicated by the attitude of the patient. An offer of any type of treatment may well stimulate the healing intention within the patient and allow progress to be made. This placebo effect is well known and should be more clearly recognized. It is as much a part of the healing mechanism as physical treatment even though science attempts to downgrade the placebo effect to explain unexpected results which cannot be readily understood in terms of current technology. In reality, the practitioners of traditional medicine know that belief is central to the healing process and without the effective co-operation of the patient successful treatments are rarely possible. The delicate line between giving hope and making extravagant claims is a problem for all health care practitioners.

It is clear that many scientists have found it difficult to accept the healing of any case unless it falls neatly into their preconceived notion of treatment. On the other hand, the media often present only the successful results of complementary treatments which may give a distorted picture. It is always so difficult to give an accurate prognosis in any case, and unexpected cures offer the most interesting copy. The success of these traditional medicines and their modern derivatives has not come about because the practitioners have financed some hugely expensive advertising campaign but because the public know, instinctively, that they must play an active part in their own health care. The complementary/alternative approach allows just this and provides a high percentage of successful treatments.

practitioners to seek to complement the needs of the patient. By placing the patients first, this effectively removed any implied competition between professionals and was directly in line with the modern counterpart of the Hippocratic Oath.

Whichever name is used, the principles are the same and the public is now responding to the services that offer new challenges to all patients.

"But there is no scientific evidence." There can be few practitioners who have not been challenged by this statement at some time, especially when there have been a number of successful treatments that have made headlines in the local press. One might think that disciplines and techniques that have had such a long history of successful use might attract research grants and capital investment. Generally this has not been so and even

Readers of this book should find not only the inspiration on the way in which these disciplines work but also the insight it will give them on the manner in which they work. Patients who use these traditional disciplines find that they become more aware of all aspects of their consciousness and the relationship with their family and the environment. This greater understanding has a continuing effect on all concerned which is why so many practitioners have trained as a result of overcoming their illness and wish to use their new-found health to serve humanity.

Excessive stress is one of the most common factors that can cause problems in the work-place, in sport and in the home. Many of the techniques that are described in this book can help everyone to understand their problems and learn to cope with life in a more effective way. Most people need to consider some change of attitude and/or lifestyle if the healing is to be successful. Of equal importance is the ability to focus on the future.

Many people blame themselves for their problems and believe their present illnesses have been brought about by their thoughts and actions in the past. Others see their future health as being dependent upon some pre-ordained program which cannot be changed. Both of these attitudes are reasonable but the responsibility for the future can be in our own hands. In the final analysis, all healing is achieved by the patient with the practitioner acting as a support for the time being. Each person has an opportunity to effect changes for themselves and it is always possible to expect some betterment even with the most daunting situations. In the final analysis, health and a sense of wellbeing are perhaps the most important factors in life and everyone needs the opportunity to have access to modern technology as well as understanding something of the ancient traditions of healing.

Complementary/alternative medicine encompasses systems of health care which add another dimension to health care. All recognize the healing energy and the crucial part that the patient must play if the full benefits are to be received. W.H. Henley put it so well:

*It matters not how strait the gate*
*How charged with punishment the scroll*
*I am the master of my fate*
*I am the captain of my soul.*

(Oxford Book of English Verse)

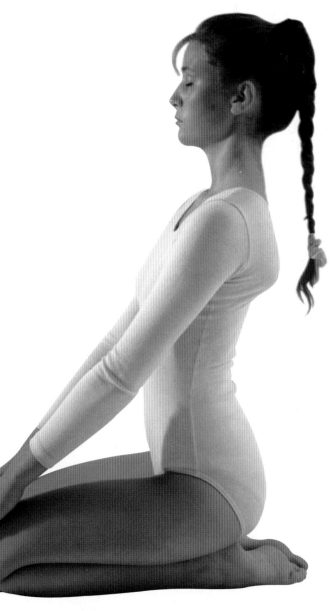

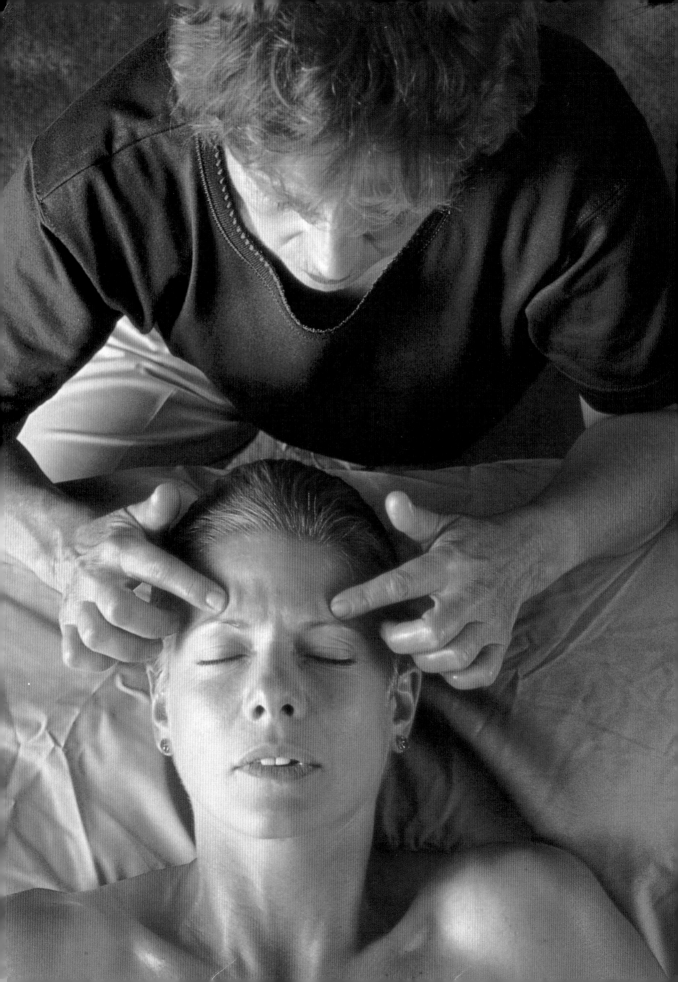

# FINDING THE RIGHT THERAPY

As more people realize that alternative medicine has a positive contribution to make to meeting our healthcare requirements, they want to select a suitable therapy which will suit their individual needs. Selecting a therapy is a matter for the patient but it is usually best to seek advice so that he or she can make an informed choice.

A common way of making this decision is to choose a therapy that has been recommended by a friend for whom it has been beneficial. Alternatively, you may feel intuitively that a specific therapy will be "right" for you. You personal health is your own responsibility and ultimately it is your decision as to which therapy you choose.

It is sometimes helpful to go to an alternative health clinic where a wide range of different therapies and treatments are available and to have an advisory session with a member of staff who, after discussing your problem and general health and condition with you, will be able to advise you as to which therapy is going to be best for you. The decision made should take into account not only your complaint or problem, be it physical, mental or emotional, but also you as a whole person. Be sure to ask lots of questions to ascertain which approach feels right for you. Because alternative practitioners complement the work of your orthodox medical doctor, it is a good idea to discuss what you are intending to do with your doctor and to seek his advice.

Here is some broad advice for selecting the right therapy and finding a practitioner:

■ Decide on a therapy or form of alternative medicine with which you feel comfortable.

■ Contact a reputable clinic or one of the professional registers and governing bodies to find a therapist (see Useful Addresses at the back of this book).

■ Check out the practitioner's qualifications, training and membership of professional bodies.

■ Check out the clinic and ensure that you are happy with the general atmosphere, the professional attitude of the staff, and the level of hygiene.

■ Ask the practitioner whether he has treated the condition in question before and whether he thinks he can help.

■ Get him to explain the treatment to you, what is involved, how long it will take and the likely effects of treatment.

Overleaf you will find some charts to help you. They are not definitive and are for reference purposes only. However, they might serve to point you in the right direction so that you can make further enquiries about specific therapies and forms of treatment.

# RESPIRATORY AND CARDIOVASCULAR DISEASES

| | Anemia | Arteriosclerosis | Asthma | Blood pressure (hyper) | Bronchitis | Circulation (poor) | Colds | Coughs | Hay fever | Sinusitis | Sore throats | Varicose veins |
|---|---|---|---|---|---|---|---|---|---|---|---|---|
| ACUPRESSURE | | | ✔ | ✔ | ✔ | | | ✔ | ✔ | | ✔ | |
| ACUPUNCTURE | | | ✔ | ✔ | ✔ | ✔ | ✔ | ✔ | ✔ | ✔ | ✔ | |
| ALEXANDER TECHNIQUE | | | ✔ | | | | | | | | | |
| AROMATHERAPY | | | ✔ | ✔ | ✔ | ✔ | ✔ | ✔ | | ✔ | ✔ | |
| AUTOGENIC TRAINING | | | ✔ | ✔ | ✔ | | | | | | | |
| CHIROPRACTIC | | | ✔ | | | | | | | | | |
| COLOR THERAPY | | | ✔ | | | | | | | | | |
| CRANIAL OSTEOPATHY | | | | | | | | | | | | |
| DANCE MOVEMENT THERAPY | | | | | | | | | | | | |
| DIET THERAPIES | ✔ | | ✔ | ✔ | ✔ | ✔ | | ✔ | ✔ | | | |
| FLOWER REMEDIES | | | ✔ | | | | | | | | | |
| HERBAL MEDICINE | ✔ | ✔ | ✔ | | ✔ | ✔ | ✔ | ✔ | ✔ | ✔ | ✔ | ✔ |
| CHINESE HERBAL | | | ✔ | ✔ | ✔ | | ✔ | | | | | |
| HOMEOPATHY | ✔ | ✔ | ✔ | | ✔ | ✔ | ✔ | ✔ | ✔ | ✔ | ✔ | ✔ |
| HYPNOTHERAPY | | | ✔ | ✔ | | | | ✔ | | | | |
| IRIDOLOGY | ✔ | ✔ | | | | | | | | ✔ | | |
| MASSAGE THERAPY | | | ✔ | ✔ | ✔ | | | | ✔ | | ✔ | |
| MEDITATION | | | ✔ | ✔ | ✔ | ✔ | | | | | | |
| MUSIC THERAPY | | | | | | | | | | | | |
| NATUROPATHY | ✔ | | ✔ | ✔ | ✔ | ✔ | | ✔ | ✔ | | | |
| OSTEOPATHY | | | ✔ | ✔ | ✔ | | | | | | | ✔ |
| POLARITY THERAPY | | | ✔ | ✔ | ✔ | | | | | | | |
| PSYCHOTHERAPY | | | ✔ | | | | | | | | | |
| REFLEXOLOGY | | | ✔ | | ✔ | ✔ | ✔ | | ✔ | ✔ | | |
| ROLFING | | | ✔ | | | | | | | | | |
| SHIATSU | | | ✔ | ✔ | | ✔ | ✔ | | | | | |
| T'AI CHI CH'UAN | | | | | | | | | | | | |
| VISUALIZATION THERAPY | | | ✔ | | | | | | | | | |
| YOGA | | | ✔ | ✔ | ✔ | | | | | | ✔ | |

# DIGESTIVE AND URINARY DISORDERS

| | Colic | Constipation | Cystitis | Diverticulitis | Fluid retention | Gastroenteritis | Hemorrhoids | Indigestion | Irritable bowel | Nausea | Ulcers | Vomiting |
|---|---|---|---|---|---|---|---|---|---|---|---|---|
| ACUPRESSURE | ✓ | ✓ | | | ✓ | | ✓ | | | | | |
| ACUPUNCTURE | ✓ | ✓ | ✓ | ✓ | ✓ | ✓ | ✓ | ✓ | ✓ | ✓ | ✓ | |
| ALEXANDER TECHNIQUE | | | | | | | | ✓ | | ✓ | | |
| AROMATHERAPY | ✓ | ✓ | ✓ | | ✓ | ✓ | ✓ | ✓ | ✓ | ✓ | | |
| AUTOGENIC TRAINING | | | | | | | | ✓ | ✓ | ✓ | | |
| CHIROPRACTIC | | ✓ | | | | ✓ | | | | | | |
| COLOR THERAPY | ✓ | ✓ | | ✓ | | | | | | | | |
| CRANIAL OSTEOPATHY | | | | | | | | | | | | |
| DANCE MOVEMENT THERAPY | | | | | | | | | | | | |
| DIET THERAPIES | ✓ | ✓ | ✓ | ✓ | ✓ | ✓ | | ✓ | ✓ | ✓ | ✓ | |
| FLOWER REMEDIES | | | | | | | | ✓ | | | | |
| HERBAL MEDICINE | ✓ | ✓ | ✓ | ✓ | ✓ | ✓ | ✓ | ✓ | ✓ | ✓ | ✓ | |
| CHINESE HERBAL | | ✓ | | | | ✓ | ✓ | | | ✓ | | |
| HOMEOPATHY | ✓ | ✓ | ✓ | ✓ | ✓ | ✓ | ✓ | ✓ | | ✓ | ✓ | ✓ |
| HYPNOTHERAPY | | | | | | | | | ✓ | | | |
| IRIDOLOGY | | | | | ✓ | | ✓ | ✓ | | | | |
| MASSAGE THERAPY | | ✓ | | | ✓ | | | | | | | |
| MEDITATION | | | | | | | | | | | | |
| MUSIC THERAPY | | | | | | | | | | | | |
| NATUROPATHY | ✓ | ✓ | ✓ | ✓ | ✓ | ✓ | ✓ | ✓ | ✓ | ✓ | ✓ | ✓ |
| OSTEOPATHY | | ✓ | | ✓ | | ✓ | | | | | | |
| POLARITY THERAPY | ✓ | ✓ | ✓ | ✓ | | ✓ | | ✓ | ✓ | ✓ | | |
| PSYCHOTHERAPY | | | | | | | | | ✓ | | | |
| REFLEXOLOGY | ✓ | ✓ | ✓ | ✓ | ✓ | ✓ | ✓ | ✓ | ✓ | ✓ | ✓ | |
| ROLFING | | ✓ | | | | | ✓ | ✓ | | | | |
| SHIATSU | ✓ | ✓ | | | ✓ | | ✓ | | | | | |
| T'AI CHI CH'UAN | | | | | | | | | | | | |
| VISUALIZATION THERAPY | | | | | | | | | | | | |
| YOGA | | | | | | | | | | | | |

# REPRODUCTIVE SYSTEM DISEASES AND PROBLEMS

| | Candida | Endometriosis | Fibroids | Genital herpes | Impotence | Infertility | Mastitis | Menopause | Menstrual problems | Pregnancy | Prostate | Vaginitis |
|---|---|---|---|---|---|---|---|---|---|---|---|---|
| ACUPRESSURE | | | ✓ | | ✓ | | | ✓ | | | | |
| ACUPUNCTURE | ✓ | ✓ | ✓ | ✓ | ✓ | ✓ | ✓ | ✓ | ✓ | ✓ | ✓ | |
| ALEXANDER TECHNIQUE | | | | | | | | ✓ | | | | |
| AROMATHERAPY | ✓ | ✓ | | ✓ | ✓ | ✓ | ✓ | ✓ | | ✓ | ✓ | ✓ |
| AUTOGENIC TRAINING | | | | | | | | | | | | |
| CHIROPRACTIC | | | | | | | | | | | | |
| COLOR THERAPY | | | | ✓ | ✓ | | ✓ | ✓ | ✓ | | | |
| CRANIAL OSTEOPATHY | | | | | | | | | | | | |
| DANCE MOVEMENT THERAPY | | | | | | | | | | | | |
| DIET THERAPIES | ✓ | | | | | | ✓ | ✓ | ✓ | | | |
| FLOWER REMEDIES | | | | ✓ | ✓ | | ✓ | ✓ | ✓ | | | |
| HERBAL MEDICINE | ✓ | ✓ | ✓ | ✓ | ✓ | ✓ | ✓ | ✓ | ✓ | ✓ | ✓ | ✓ |
| CHINESE HERBAL | | ✓ | | ✓ | ✓ | | ✓ | ✓ | | | | ✓ |
| HOMEOPATHY | ✓ | ✓ | ✓ | ✓ | ✓ | ✓ | ✓ | ✓ | | ✓ | ✓ | ✓ |
| HYPNOTHERAPY | | | | | ✓ | | ✓ | | | ✓ | | |
| IRIDOLOGY | | | ✓ | | ✓ | ✓ | | ✓ | ✓ | | | |
| MASSAGE THERAPY | | | ✓ | | | | | ✓ | ✓ | | | |
| MEDITATION | | | | | | | | | | | | |
| MUSIC THERAPY | | | | | | | | | | | | |
| NATUROPATHY | ✓ | | | | | | ✓ | ✓ | ✓ | | | |
| OSTEOPATHY | | | | | | | | | | | | |
| POLARITY THERAPY | ✓ | | ✓ | | ✓ | ✓ | | ✓ | ✓ | | | |
| PSYCHOTHERAPY | | | | | ✓ | ✓ | ✓ | | | | | |
| REFLEXOLOGY | ✓ | ✓ | ✓ | | | ✓ | ✓ | ✓ | ✓ | | | |
| ROLFING | | | | | | | | | | | | |
| SHIATSU | | | ✓ | | | | | ✓ | ✓ | | | |
| T'AI CHI CH'UAN | | | | | | | | | | | | |
| VISUALIZATION THERAPY | | | | | | | | | | | | |
| YOGA | | | | | | | | | | | | |

## Musculo-skeletal problems

| | Arthritis | Back problems | Cramp | Disk problems | Fibrositis | Lumbago | Muscle strains | Osteoporosis | Rheumatism | Sciatica | Tenosynovitis | Trapped nerve |
|---|---|---|---|---|---|---|---|---|---|---|---|---|
| ACUPRESSURE | ✓ | ✓ | ✓ | ✓ | | ✓ | ✓ | | ✓ | ✓ | ✓ | ✓ |
| ACUPUNCTURE | ✓ | ✓ | ✓ | ✓ | ✓ | ✓ | ✓ | | ✓ | ✓ | ✓ | ✓ |
| ALEXANDER TECHNIQUE | | ✓ | | ✓ | | ✓ | ✓ | | ✓ | ✓ | | ✓ |
| AROMATHERAPY | ✓ | ✓ | ✓ | | ✓ | | ✓ | | ✓ | ✓ | | |
| AUTOGENIC TRAINING | | ✓ | ✓ | | | ✓ | | | ✓ | | | |
| CHIROPRACTIC | ✓ | ✓ | ✓ | ✓ | ✓ | ✓ | ✓ | | ✓ | ✓ | ✓ | ✓ |
| COLOR THERAPY | | | | | | | | | | | | |
| CRANIAL OSTEOPATHY | | | | | | | | | | | | |
| DANCE MOVEMENT THERAPY | | | | | | | | | | | | |
| DIET THERAPIES | ✓ | | ✓ | | | | | | | | | |
| FLOWER REMEDIES | | | | | | | | | | | | |
| HERBAL MEDICINE | ✓ | | ✓ | | ✓ | ✓ | ✓ | ✓ | ✓ | | | |
| CHINESE HERBAL | ✓ | | ✓ | | | ✓ | ✓ | | ✓ | | | |
| HOMEOPATHY | ✓ | | ✓ | | ✓ | ✓ | ✓ | | ✓ | ✓ | | |
| HYPNOTHERAPY | ✓ | | ✓ | | | ✓ | | | ✓ | | | |
| IRIDOLOGY | | | | | | | | | | | | |
| MASSAGE THERAPY | ✓ | ✓ | ✓ | ✓ | ✓ | ✓ | | ✓ | ✓ | | | |
| MEDITATION | | | | | | | | | | | | |
| MUSIC THERAPY | | | | | | | | | | | | |
| NATUROPATHY | ✓ | | ✓ | | | | | | | | | |
| OSTEOPATHY | ✓ | ✓ | ✓ | ✓ | ✓ | ✓ | ✓ | ✓ | ✓ | ✓ | ✓ | |
| POLARITY THERAPY | ✓ | ✓ | ✓ | | | | | | | | | |
| PSYCHOTHERAPY | | | | | | | | | | | | |
| REFLEXOLOGY | | ✓ | | | | ✓ | | | | | | |
| ROLFING | | ✓ | ✓ | ✓ | ✓ | ✓ | ✓ | | ✓ | ✓ | ✓ | ✓ |
| SHIATSU | ✓ | ✓ | ✓ | ✓ | ✓ | ✓ | ✓ | | ✓ | ✓ | ✓ | ✓ |
| T'AI CHI CH'UAN | ✓ | | | | | | | | | | | |
| VISUALIZATION THERAPY | | | | | | | | | | | | |
| YOGA | ✓ | ✓ | | | | | ✓ | ✓ | | | | |

# EMOTIONAL AND NERVOUS DISORDERS

| | Addictions | Anorexia and bulimia | Anxiety | Depression | Fainting | Grief | Headaches | Insomnia | Neuralgia | Phobias | Stress | Trauma |
|---|---|---|---|---|---|---|---|---|---|---|---|---|
| ACUPRESSURE | | | ✔ | ✔ | ✔ | ✔ | ✔ | | ✔ | ✔ | | |
| ACUPUNCTURE | ✔ | ✔ | ✔ | ✔ | ✔ | ✔ | ✔ | ✔ | ✔ | ✔ | ✔ | |
| ALEXANDER TECHNIQUE | | | ✔ | | | | ✔ | | | ✔ | | |
| AROMATHERAPY | | | ✔ | ✔ | | ✔ | ✔ | ✔ | ✔ | ✔ | ✔ | |
| AUTOGENIC TRAINING | ✔ | ✔ | ✔ | ✔ | | ✔ | ✔ | | | ✔ | ✔ | |
| CHIROPRACTIC | ✔ | | | | | ✔ | ✔ | ✔ | | | ✔ | ✔ |
| COLOR THERAPY | | | ✔ | ✔ | | ✔ | ✔ | | | | ✔ | ✔ |
| CRANIAL OSTEOPATHY | | | | | | | | | | | | |
| DANCE MOVEMENT THERAPY | | ✔ | | | | | | | | ✔ | | |
| DIET THERAPIES | | ✔ | | ✔ | ✔ | ✔ | | | | | | |
| FLOWER REMEDIES | ✔ | ✔ | ✔ | ✔ | ✔ | ✔ | ✔ | | ✔ | ✔ | ✔ | |
| HERBAL MEDICINE | ✔ | ✔ | ✔ | ✔ | ✔ | ✔ | ✔ | ✔ | | ✔ | ✔ | |
| CHINESE HERBAL | | | ✔ | ✔ | | | ✔ | | | ✔ | | |
| HOMEOPATHY | ✔ | ✔ | ✔ | ✔ | ✔ | ✔ | ✔ | ✔ | ✔ | ✔ | ✔ | |
| HYPNOTHERAPY | ✔ | ✔ | ✔ | | | ✔ | ✔ | | | ✔ | ✔ | |
| IRIDOLOGY | | | | ✔ | | ✔ | | | | | | |
| MASSAGE THERAPY | | | ✔ | ✔ | | ✔ | ✔ | ✔ | | ✔ | | |
| MEDITATION | | | ✔ | | | | | | ✔ | ✔ | | |
| MUSIC THERAPY | | | | | | | | | | | | |
| NATUROPATHY | ✔ | ✔ | | ✔ | | ✔ | | ✔ | | | | |
| OSTEOPATHY | | | | ✔ | | ✔ | | ✔ | | | ✔ | ✔ |
| POLARITY THERAPY | | ✔ | ✔ | ✔ | | ✔ | ✔ | | | | ✔ | ✔ |
| PSYCHOTHERAPY | ✔ | ✔ | ✔ | ✔ | | ✔ | | | | ✔ | ✔ | ✔ |
| REFLEXOLOGY | | | | | | ✔ | ✔ | ✔ | | | ✔ | |
| ROLFING | | | | | | ✔ | ✔ | | | | ✔ | |
| SHIATSU | | ✔ | | | | ✔ | ✔ | | | | ✔ | |
| T'AI CHI CH'UAN | | | | | | | | | | ✔ | | |
| VISUALIZATION THERAPY | | | | | | | | | ✔ | ✔ | | |
| YOGA | | | ✔ | | | | ✔ | | | ✔ | | |

# SKIN DISORDERS

| | Abscesses | Acne | Alopecia | Athletes foot | Boils | Chilblains | Cold sores | Eczema | Oily skin | Psoriasis | Ulcers | Warts |
|---|---|---|---|---|---|---|---|---|---|---|---|---|
| ACUPRESSURE | | | | | ✔ | | | | | ✔ | | |
| ACUPUNCTURE | | ✔ | ✔ | | ✔ | ✔ | ✔ | ✔ | ✔ | ✔ | ✔ | |
| ALEXANDER TECHNIQUE | | | | | | | | | | | | |
| AROMATHERAPY | ✔ | ✔ | ✔ | ✔ | ✔ | ✔ | ✔ | ✔ | ✔ | ✔ | ✔ | |
| AUTOGENIC TRAINING | | | | | | | ✔ | | | | | |
| CHIROPRACTIC | | | | | | | | | | | | |
| COLOR THERAPY | | ✔ | | | | | | | | | | |
| CRANIAL OSTEOPATHY | | | | | | | | | | | | |
| DANCE MOVEMENT THERAPY | | | | | | | | | | | | |
| DIET THERAPIES | ✔ | ✔ | ✔ | ✔ | ✔ | ✔ | ✔ | ✔ | ✔ | ✔ | ✔ | ✔ |
| FLOWER REMEDIES | | ✔ | | | | | ✔ | | ✔ | | | |
| HERBAL MEDICINE | ✔ | ✔ | ✔ | ✔ | ✔ | ✔ | ✔ | ✔ | ✔ | | ✔ | ✔ |
| CHINESE HERBAL | ✔ | ✔ | | | | | ✔ | | | ✔ | | |
| HOMEOPATHY | ✔ | ✔ | ✔ | ✔ | ✔ | ✔ | ✔ | ✔ | ✔ | ✔ | | ✔ |
| HYPNOTHERAPY | | ✔ | ✔ | | | | | ✔ | ✔ | ✔ | | |
| IRIDOLOGY | ✔ | | ✔ | | ✔ | ✔ | ✔ | | ✔ | ✔ | | |
| MASSAGE THERAPY | | ✔ | | | ✔ | | | | | ✔ | | |
| MEDITATION | | | | | | | | | | | | |
| MUSIC THERAPY | | | | | | | | | | | | |
| NATUROPATHY | ✔ | ✔ | ✔ | ✔ | ✔ | ✔ | ✔ | ✔ | ✔ | ✔ | ✔ | ✔ |
| OSTEOPATHY | | | | | | | | | | | | |
| POLARITY THERAPY | ✔ | | ✔ | ✔ | ✔ | ✔ | ✔ | ✔ | ✔ | ✔ | ✔ | ✔ |
| PSYCHOTHERAPY | | ✔ | | | | | | | | | | |
| REFLEXOLOGY | ✔ | | ✔ | ✔ | ✔ | ✔ | ✔ | ✔ | ✔ | ✔ | | |
| ROLFING | | | | | | | | | | | | |
| SHIATSU | | | | | ✔ | | | | | | | |
| T'AI CHI CH'UAN | | | | | | | | | | | | |
| VISUALIZATION THERAPY | | | | | | | | | | | | |
| YOGA | | | | | | | | | | | | |

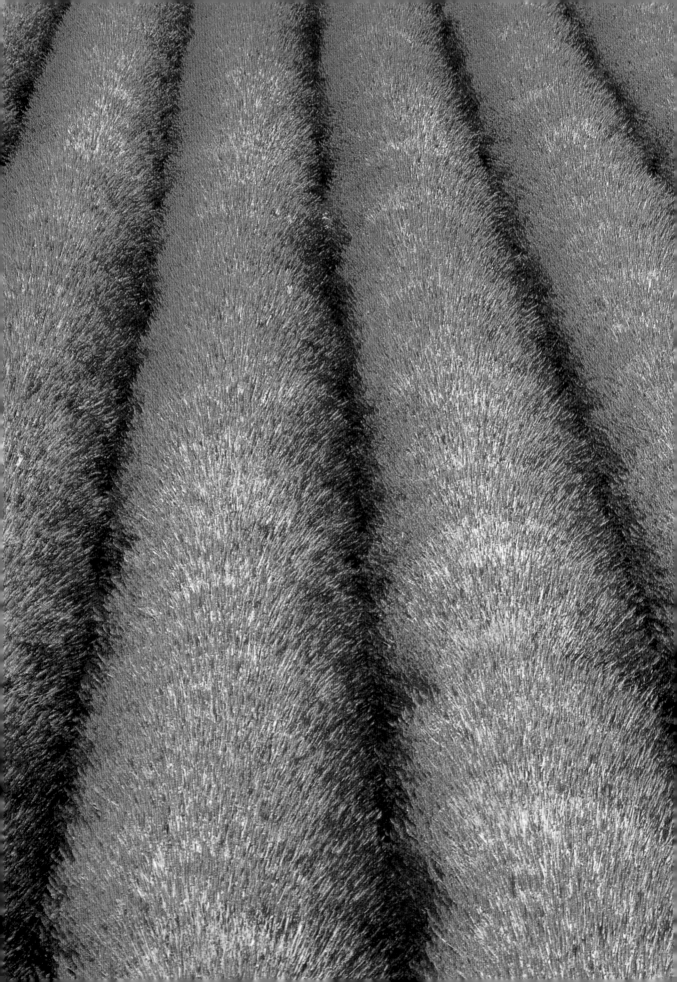

# NATURAL HEALING

## PART ONE

*T*his section focuses on gentle non-invasive systems of healing and diagnosis. Color therapy has been practiced since ancient times and people have long recognized the healing properties of color. Homeopathy is a complete system of healing whereby minute amounts of natural substances are used to stimulate the body's natural defenses and aid the patient's recovery. Iridology is a diagnostic method for determining disease, while polarity therapy is a comprehensive health system incorporating bodywork, diet, exercise and counseling.

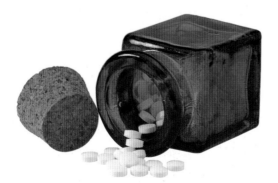

# COLOR THERAPY

CHAPTER ONE

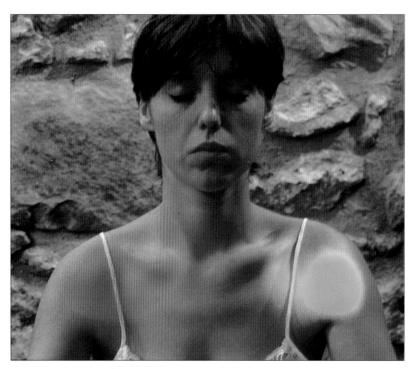

*W*hen we see a bright yellow daffodil blooming above the new purple violets in the spring sun, our hearts open to the day and we feel more alive. As we sit and watch the sun setting into the sea, the yellow turning to orange, then rose and purple as the light begins to fade, we feel peaceful and ready for rest. Yellow and purple by day, and yellow and purple at the beginning of night. These are examples of the complementary colors that our bodies appreciate and use to maintain our health and a positive outlook on life.

*Our way to health is always given to us in nature if we have the eyes to see. With color, nature gives us one of our most powerful tools for health, wellbeing and joy—the food all around us to sustain our bodies and our souls. Think of how you feel when you are arrested from your thoughts by your neighbor's rose, blooming along the hedge. The rose is red and vibrant. Its petals form in a beautiful spiral pattern. It brings to mind the first rose given to you by someone you love very much. Its aroma heightens and blesses your senses. All this is possible because your attention was caught by the red of the rose.*

*This is what color can do for us. It captures us and throws us into the dance of beauty happening all around us on this planet. Its vibration draws us to it, and resonates with vibrations in our own bodies. It feeds us its vibration if we need it to balance our energies, perhaps lacking in that particular color at that specific time. The whole world of color is there, waiting to play with our energies and our spirits. We have only to open our eyes to its possibilities, to notice and to love.*

# A DYNAMIC BALANCE

Nature thrives on dynamic balance, in whichever of the myriad forms it is expressed; a fern opening its tight spiral to the sun, a chambered nautilus resting on the shore, a sunflower standing tall and radiant, are all expressing the same proportional relationship in nature. That "golden mean" relationship is exhibited in plants, animals, the human body and, some believe, in universal consciousness. It acts as a tone or a filament of connection throughout the universe. It shows the interrelationships of all forms of energy, visible and invisible. Color is one of the ambassadors of this universal knowledge in nature. It can bring us to our joy, to our health and our life.

## COLOR IN ANCIENT TIMES

Healing with color, or color therapy, has been practiced from the time of the ancients. From Heliopolis in Egypt, to Iran, to India and China, people recognized the healing properties of color, and expressed it in various ways. In the temple at Heliopolis, rooms were specially designed so that the sun's rays were broken up into the seven colors of the spectrum in order to be used for healing. In Iran, glazed ceramic tiles of different colors and geometric shapes were used architecturally in mosques for the upliftment and cleansing of the spirit, and the teaching of natural law and consciousness. All these cultures, to varying degrees, used color in architecture, solarized water, the shining of light through crystals, and the grinding up and

# THE CHAKRAS

The chakras have been recognized as major components of the human energy system for over two thousand years. Many traditions have historically recognized seven, and now eight are commonly acknowledged, with some evidence of possibly twelve, and beyond. Chakras are centers of energy that lie along the axis of our spines, just outside our physical bodies, in what is called the etheric sheath. In different traditions they have been referred to as wheels of spinning light, lotus blossoms, roses, or lens-like structures, to name a few. These centers act in complementary fashion with our auras to maintain us in a healthy fashion. Each chakra has its corresponding color.

| The Chakras | Color | Function |
| --- | --- | --- |
| Base | Red | Connects to life energy, sexuality, and creative power. |
| Sacral | Orange | Connects with physical movement, and our emotions. |
| Solar Plexus | Yellow | Connects with feelings of self-worth. |
| Heart | Green | Center of love, harmony. |
| Thymus | Turquoise | Generosity, compassion, the "High Heart." |
| Throat | Blue | Center of creative expression through sound, speaking one's truth. |
| Brow | Violet | The Third Eye. Center of visualization and intuition. |
| Crown | Magenta | The Eternal, Spiritual Self |

ingesting of powered gems. Natural pigments were made from ground minerals and beetles for body ornamentation.

## OUR COLOR VOCABULARY

The visible spectrum, part of the electromagnetic spectrum containing energies from cosmic rays to radio waves, is what we observe in our daily world. Sunlight, or what we now call full-spectrum light, holds all the wavelengths of color from ultra violet through the visible spectrum, and including infrared. The well-documented effect of the lack of sunlight in northern climates in winter, causing conditions such as "Seasonal Affective Disorder," is a simple demonstration of the role of color on our health.

People talk about painters having different palettes, or of using varied ranges of color to convey that which they wish to express. In ancient Greece in the fourth and fifth centuries B.C., documents refer to the four primary colors of white, black, red and yellow. For many centuries, the visible spectrum has been known to have seven colors: red, orange, yellow, green, blue, indigo and violet. These colors corresponded to the seven chakras in the human body. Today, the colors turquoise and magenta have been added to the healing spectrum, and eight chakras rather than seven are now accepted by many. It seems as we evolve in consciousness, our abilities to perceive numbers and qualities of colors increase.

## THE HUMAN AURA

The word "aura" is fairly common in our vocabulary today. We often hear someone say, "Oh, I don't know, she just had a certain aura about her." In actual fact, each of us has a particular and unique aura which is a manifestation of who we are and how we are feeling. The aura consists of the layers of color around the human body, each layer or band being one color. All these together make up the auric field, sometimes referred to as the rainbow body. When we are healthy, the eight colors in the auric field are clear and luminous. When our bodies are out of balance, particular colors may appear darker or paler, less substantial. You can experience the quality of auric color by the trick of after-imaging that our eyes do so well.

Take a square of bright turquoise and stare at it intently for three or four minutes. Then immediately

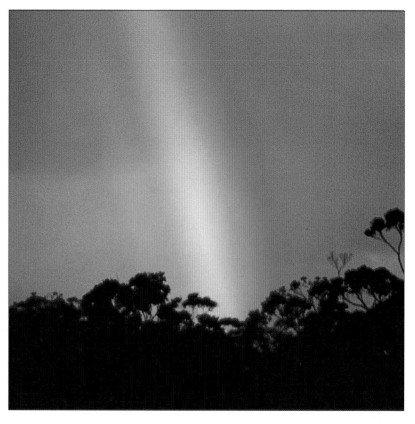

shift your gaze to a clean sheet of white paper next to you. In a few moments you should see a softly glowing red square on the white paper. This glowing color is similar to the quality of auric color.

## USING COLOR IN OUR DAILY LIVES

How can we take this wonderful energy that is part of our everyday experience, and more consciously use it to enrich our lives and promote healing? The first thing to remember is that Nature loves balance, and that is why the complementary principle is often applied in healing. If you use one color, you also use its complement. A healthy body contains complementary colors in equal proportion to each other.

While practicing the following exercises, remember that Nature loves richness and balance.

## COLOR MEDITATION

Remember a favorite place of yours in nature—a place where you can relax, feel safe, and at home. Lie on your back, get comfortable, and then start breathing naturally and easily. Take yourself to that place in your mind. Remember a time there when you felt happy and relaxed. If a place and time do not easily come to mind, then tell yourself a story about a place where you would feel happy and relaxed. See yourself walking gently to that place, lying down comfortably on the ground, or sitting peacefully in a chair. Notice the colors around you. Breathe them in, in all their richness as you see them in your mind's eye. The bright blue sky, the azure lake in the distance, the green grass all around you, the oranges, reds, yellows, and violets of the flowers in the nearby beds in full bloom. Breathe in the colors. Increase their richness and variety in your mind. Do this for ten minutes. Then gently come back to the present, newly refreshed and relaxed. As you practice this, so your ability to bring more detail and variety in color and scene will increase.

## VISITING A COLOR THERAPY PRACTITIONER

It is now commonly acknowledged in the healing professions that the emotions play a big role in influencing our state of health. Being aware of our feelings is not always as easy as it sounds, especially in today's fast-paced world.

A good practitioner will listen to you carefully, see with an open mind and heart, and, using the diagnostic tools available today, will be able to suggest a course of treatment to assist in dissolving blockages to bring the body's energies back into dynamic balance.

Color therapy uses a variety of measures for diagnosis and treatment. Some practitioners read your auric field in order to diagnose the state of color balance in the body. Others dowse to read the balance of color energies in the spine, and then with the use of a chart, will set up a program to rebalance the color energies if needed.

Psychological tests which involve color may be used. For instance, the Luscher color test uses both the client's conscious and unconscious mind to provide physiological information. Art therapy looks at paintings to see how they express a patient's attitudes toward life at that time.

Colored light represents the most subtle and powerful way to use color in healing. These treatments should be done only by skilled and trained color practitioners.

Water, solarized in bottles covered with filters for the different colors of the spectrum, and colored oils, made from natural plant materials, are options to work with at home to support the healing process between sessions with a trained color practitioner. The colors in your home environment, clothes, food, and the use of colored silk cloths as body wraps are also good tools.

Color therapy is being used today in complementary medicine, to treat spiritual, mental, emotional, and physical ailments. The key is to bring the body back into balance, and color is a very good tool for this process. It works well in conjunction with other therapies, including acupuncture, acupressure, essence and herbal work, and visualization. The most important thing to remember is that it is a joyful part of our world and of ourselves.

## COLOR BREATHING

Sit, or lie down comfortably with your spine relaxed. Breathe naturally. You can either breathe through the whole spectrum of colors, or choose one for its particular healing qualities. The following chart will offer suggestions.

| | |
|---|---|
| **Red** | Breathe in red for vitality. Breathe out turquoise. |
| **Orange** | Breathe in orange for joy. Breathe out blue. |
| **Yellow** | Breathe in yellow for increased objectivity and intellectual powers. Breathe out violet. |
| **Green** | Breathe in green to cleanse and balance. Breathe out magenta. |
| **Turquoise** | Breathe in turquoise to strengthen the immune system. Breathe out red. |
| **Blue** | Breathe in blue for relaxation, peace. Breathe out orange. |
| **Violet** | Breathe in violet to increase self-respect, to connect with feelings of dignity and beauty. Breathe out yellow. |
| **Magenta** | Breathe in magenta to release obsessional images and thoughts. Breathe out green. |

You will find as you practice this simple technique of color breathing, that you will feel more energy and balance in your whole system.

# HOMEOPATHY

## CHAPTER TWO

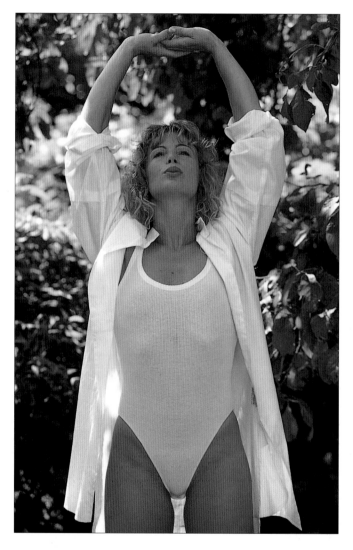

*I*n the mid 1700s, medicine in Europe was characterized by practices now considered barbaric: poisonous doses of mercury and other heavy metals, and the extensive use of blood-letting etc. A German physician named Samuel Hahnemann, born in 1755, gave up the practice of medicine out of concern for the harm being done to sick people by these practices. While translating a work by Cullen, a Scottish herbalist, he came upon a theory concerning the curative action of "Peruvian bark," also known as Cinchona. This medicine, which was effective against malaria (a scourge in Europe at that time), had been brought back to Europe from South America by Spanish explorers. Cullen's theory was that the extreme bitterness of the bark acted as a "tonic" to the stomach and hence drove out the fever.

Hahnemann rejected this theory, since he knew of several substances equally, if not more, bitter that did not cure malaria. However, he did note that the medicine was effective, and so was intensely interested. As an experiment, he started taking the medicine himself, even though he was not sick. The result was that he developed many of the symptoms of malaria, but without the fever. The symptoms cleared when he stopped taking the bark preparation and reappeared on taking it again. From this experiment, he formed the theory that the curative action of the medicine on the disease was related to the medicine's ability to cause similar symptoms in healthy persons taking the medicine (law of similars).

Homeopathy is a medical therapy using natural substances to stimulate the body's natural defenses. In health, these natural defenses are effective and efficient. To understand what this means, consider the following example: five different people, at different levels of health, are exposed to influenza.

■ **Person "A"** is very healthy and vital. The flu virus enters the body through the nose, attaches itself to the lining of the lung, and then attempts to enter the cell in order for it to reproduce. Recognizing the attempt, the immune system quickly attacks the virus, and renders it harmless. Person "A" never notices anything (silent healing).

■ **Person "B"** is fairly healthy, but does tend to get flu and other illnesses that "go around." The flu virus enters the body, attaches itself to the lining of the lung, enters the cells, and is then able to start to reproduce. Recognizing this, "B's" immune system mounts a defense, but not as effectively as "A's." The virus is able to reproduce, and "B" must work harder. The energy it takes to defend is therefore greater than in the case of "A." Fever is needed, and fatigue and muscle aches are felt. After a couple of days, the symptoms subside, and "B" feels fine within a few more days.

■ **Person "C"** is not so healthy as "A" or "B." The fever needs to be even higher so that the body can fight, and the battle rages for a longer period. The level of fatigue is greater. Finally, after several days, the fever breaks and it takes another week to

recover, and perhaps a few weeks to feel normal again.

■ **Person "D"** is even less healthy. There simply isn't enough vitality (energy) in the system to mount an effective defense. There is a low-grade fever, but it drags on for weeks. "D" feels quite unwell and just can't get over it.

■ **Person "E"** is in very poor health. Unable to mount any kind of effective defense, pneumonia and death follow in a relatively short time.

The object of homeopathic therapy in the above instances is not to kill the flu virus with the medicine itself, but rather to make the sick person's defenses more effective at a lower volume of effort. This enhanced defensive effort results in the death of the virus and recovery from the illness.

In the case of "A," vitality is so high that "A" defends with so little effort that no symptoms are felt. "B" needs a more vigorous defense and just notes some discomfort. Everything noticeable by the sick person is, in homeopathy, considered to be a symptom. Fever, muscle aches, cough, sputum, headache etc., all result from the body's defensive effort. Since the objective in homeopathy is to render the defensive effort more effective, a medicine is given that could cause the same symptoms if given to a healthy person. Consider the following example.

### ENHANCING THE BODY'S NATURAL DEFENSES

A person moderately allergic to bee stings is stung on the arm. The result is a large area of swelling and redness, with burning or stinging pain. The pain feels better from the application of an ice-pack. These are the "symptoms" caused by bee venom.

"C," in the attack of influenza, develops a very sore throat. The pain is burning or stinging, and "C"

## LAW OF SIMILARS

A medicine may cure an illness in a sick person if it can cause a similar set of symptoms when it is given to a healthy person.

To test this theory, Hahnemann did similar experiments (called provings, from the German word for "test") using other medicines, the use of which had been passed down in folk-lore. He found that each medicine produced a unique set of symptoms ("symptom picture").

■ **Belladonna**, in provings, produced symptoms of agitation, flushing of the face, throbbing pains, enlargement of the pupil and aversion to light, sore throat, and many other symptoms. This picture closely resembled that of scarlet fever, another epidemic scourge of the times. Belladonna proved curative in many cases of scarlet fever, and was also noted to protect those exposed but not yet sick.

■ **Arnica montana**, used in mountainous regions of Europe for generations for its beneficial effects in relieving bruising pains from falling down, produced bruised, sore tenderness in provings.

notices that cold drinks, especially ice-cold ones, relieve the pain. On examination, the homeopath notes that the throat is very red, and there is considerable swelling. It is as if "C's" symptoms were caused by a bee sting of the throat, but actually they are the result of "C's" defense against the flu. *Apis mellifica* (a homeopathic remedy prepared from the honeybee) is administered and, within a short time, "C's" sore throat pain and swelling diminish, and he feels much better.

In this example, the homeopath recognizes that the body is trying to defend itself, and assumes that this defense is the best that can be mounted at this time. It is not, however, ideally effective. Rather than substitute another defensive effort, the homeopath respects the wisdom of the body and seeks to enhance the effectiveness of the natural defense. If you are struggling to climb a mountain, a steady push

## PROVINGS

An experiment in which one or more healthy people take a medicine repetitively until it causes them to feel symptoms. The changes noticed by the "provers" are collected in journals and are later evaluated and combined to form a "symptom picture" of the medicine.

In his lifetime, Hahnemann and a group of colleagues experimented with 99 different medicines, laboriously compiling lists of the symptoms brought out in such provings. These lists were published in books known as *materia medicae*, latin for "medical materials." Homeopathy proved very popular with the common people, as it was highly effective in treating scarlet fever, cholera, influenza, and other infectious diseases. Over the remainder of Hahnemann's life, he constantly experimented with his methods, refining them and proving new medicines. Unfortunately, he was an angry and scornful man who alienated the medical profession with his often scathing attacks. Toward the end of his life, he settled in Paris where he died in 1843.

from behind is much more helpful than a steady push from the side, or in front. If the body mounts a fever to fight a disease, aspirin or other anti-inflammatory drugs which block the body's ability to produce fever would seem to undercut the defense, rather than support it.

**ACUTE AND CHRONIC DISEASES**
The early example, that of influenza, is an "acute" disease. This generally means an illness that arises over a short period of time, runs its course, and subsides. People also suffer from "chronic" diseases, such as arthritis, migraine, colitis, asthma etc., which can flare up from time to time but which, basically, continue to develop over the years and may gradually worsen. The homeopathic analysis of these illnesses is fundamentally no different from that of the case of influenza which was presented above. The symptoms of the sick person are evaluated, and a medicine is given that could cause similar symptoms if given to a healthy person. If a correct choice of medicine is made, the defensive effort becomes more effective at a lower volume of effort and the healing begins.

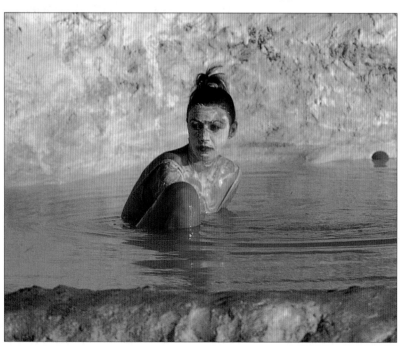

*Left: some homeopathic medicines are made from minerals, such as sulfur. The beneficial health effects of sulfur have long been recognized as in sulfur springs.*

# THE MEDICINES

Homeopathic medicines are made almost exclusively from three sources:

■ **Minerals**, such as Phosphorus, Gold, and Sulfur, or mineral salts, such as Sodium Chloride, Potassium Carbonate and Calcium Phosphate.

■ **Vegetable substances**, such as *Pulsatilla* (wind flower), *Staphysagria* (stavesacre), Chamomilla (Chamomile), and *Ruta graveolens* (bittersweet) etc.

■ **Animal substances,** such as *Tarentula* (the spider), *Lac caninum* (the breast milk of the female dog) and *Lachesis* (the venom of the Bushmaster snake) etc.

All of the medicines are known by their Latin names. This ensures that homeopaths the world over can communicate their results. Most of the medicines have provings that define their use. The manufacture of the medicines is regulated in each country and the standards are published in documents called *Pharmacopoeia* (e.g. the *Homeopathic Pharmocopoeia of the United States*).

Hahnemann found that the medicines worked best if they were given in small amounts. Contrary to what one might expect, the correct medicine acts more gently and for a longer time if it is given in a smaller dose. Today homeopaths think this is so because the sick person is more sensitive in general just because he or she is sick, and especially sensitive to a medicine that could cause the very same symptoms in healthy people.

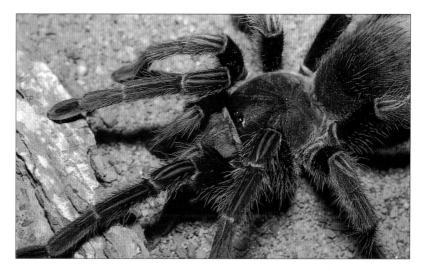

## PREPARATION OF MEDICINES

To make smaller doses, Hahnemann devised a method of dispersing the medicine in a neutral substance by grinding or shaking it in either milk sugar or alcohol, and then diluting that mixture again in milk sugar or alcohol, then grinding or shaking again, and so on.

Commonly, the dilution is done as a mixture of one part medicine to 99 parts neutral substance, giving a 1:100 dilution, called a centessimal, or "C" dilution.

The number of subsequent dilutions and dispersions is used to indicate the "strength" of the medicine (e.g. a 30C has been through this process 30 times using a 1:100 dilution). If the medicine is diluted 1:10, an "X" is used instead of a "C." In some European countries, a "D" is used (for

*Right: minerals such as sodium and phosphorus are used in some homeopathic medicines. Phosphorus is an essential constituent of our bodies as well as being a very important homeopathic remedy. It may be used in the treatment of digestive problems.*

*Above: homeopathic medicines are also derived from animal sources, including the Tarentula spider. Problems that can be helped by Tarentula include abscesses, boils and skin eruptions.*

"decimal") instead of an "X."

When the medicines are prepared

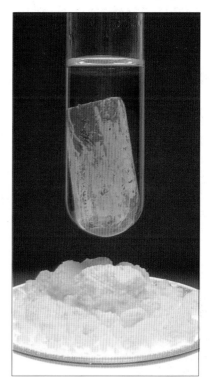

in this way, they can be given in any number of ways. Most commonly, the resulting liquid is mixed with either sucrose granules or lactose tablets, and is then allowed to dry. Homeopathic medicines prepared in this way have an extremely long shelf life—medicines that Hahnemann made in the eighteenth century are still active today! Homeopathic medicines can also be dispensed as liquids, sprays, ointments, suppositories, and also as injections.

## HOW HOMEOPATHY WORKS

Unfortunately, we do not yet understand the mechanism of action of homeopathic medicines. Scientific studies, published recently, conclusively prove that they do work and are not simply placebos (that is, an inactive substance which works through the power of suggestion).

Because of the observations made when treating patients, homeopaths conjecture that the correct homeopathic medicine stimulates the inner, natural defenses of the human organism. In the case of

a bladder infection, for example, where the invading bacteria is *E. Coli*, the medicine does not directly kill the *E. Coli* but rather causes the body's own natural infection-fighting defenses to do the job that they had not quite been able to perform before the medicine.

In the case of relieving an acute migraine headache, the action of the medicine must result in correcting the imbalance in the nervous system which causes the painful constriction of the blood vessels. In the case of depression, the action of the medicine must result in restoring balance to the brain's chemistry. These results do not appear to come from a direct action of the medicine on the blood vessels, or brain chemistry, but rather from some other effect of the medicine, as yet undetermined.

### HOMEOPATHIC AND ORTHODOX MEDICINE

There is certainly a physical basis to life, and in orthodox medicine the "mechanism" of the body seems to be considered the most important thing to understand and to control. Although one can certainly understand an automobile by understanding the engine, transmission, brakes, electrical system etc., a car is simply an unmoving object unless there is a driver in it. One

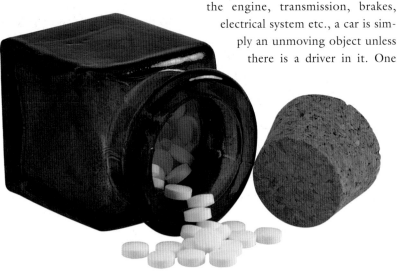

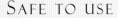

## SAFE TO USE

Homeopathic medicines are very safe. Even highly toxic substances, such as mercury, arsenic, snake venoms etc., can be safely stored in the house for as long as the dilution factor is at least 6X. In such a preparation, there is one part of actual medicine to a million parts of the sugar! One would have to ingest an improbably huge amount of granules or tablets in order to get any toxic effects. Even children playing with the bottles and taking the medicines are not in danger from them. A child could do a "proving" by taking the medicine repetitively, but this might require days or weeks of taking the medicine, and the symptoms would gradually clear after stopping the medicine.

might put the best fuel in the car, keep the tires perfectly inflated, keep the spark plugs cleaned etc., but no matter how well one takes care of the car, if it is driven with the emergency brake on, or the gears are not shifted properly, it will break down.

Homeopathy seems to work as a "tune up" and with the "driver" of the human organism. Hahnemann referred to this as the "vital force" and considered that disease resulted from an "imbalance" of the vital force. Stress seems to throw the system out of balance. Today, medical researchers are starting to document the negative effects of many forms of stress on our health. Hahnemann was simply ahead of his time by recognizing the negative effects on health that come from a variety of stresses, including emotional factors.

# PRACTICAL APPLICATION

## VISITING A HOMEOPATH

A visit to a homeopathic practitioner is essentially a medical visit. You will be expected to describe the problem or problems you are having, in as much detail as possible. In general, the homeopath will be interested in the following:

■ How the problem started—were there any special stresses that were present when it started?

■ How the problem developed—the sequence of events.

■ How you feel "in yourself" with the problem—both physically, emotionally, and mentally. Examples of this might include the physical symptoms of fatigue, restlessness, low appetite; emotional symptoms of sadness, anxiety, irritability; and mental symptoms of memory loss, difficulty concentrating, unusual ideas about the body (e.g. that the body is fragile and might break in two) etc.

■ The particulars of the problem— in general, symptoms have four main characteristics, as detailed below.

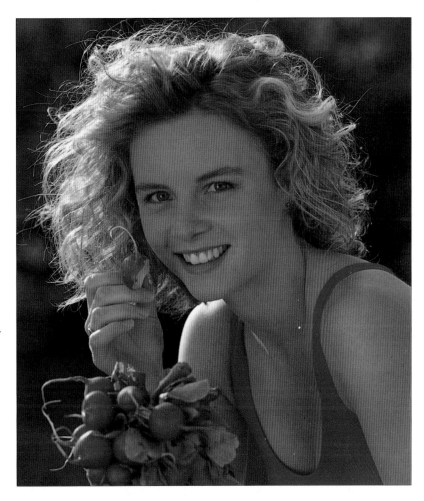

## CHARACTERISTICS OF SYMPTOMS

### 1 The nature of any "sensations"

Pains can have many qualities, such as throbbing, burning, tearing, stitching etc. There can be feelings of fullness, pressure, crawling, stinging, itching, movement etc. Any sensation should be described as accurately as possible.

### 2 The "location" of a problem

Headaches can be in the forehead, the temples, the back of the head, the ears, the jaw etc. Furthermore, pains and other sensations often "extend" to other parts: for example, pain in the neck muscles which radiates up to the back of the head and from there to the forehead over the eyes. Another example is pain in the lower spine which extends into the buttocks and from there to the back of the thigh.

### 3 What makes the problem better or worse

In homeopathy we call these "modalities" and consider them to be quite important, as they are expressions of the uniqueness of the person. Pains, for example, can be made better or worse from applying ice or heat, from standing, lying, sitting, or moving, from eating, at certain times of day, in certain types of weather, from sleeping or not sleeping, from perspiring or not perspiring etc. There are many things that make problems better or worse. People often feel better or worse at certain times of day, in certain types of weather, from eating or fasting, from certain foods, from being indoors or outdoors, from exercise or from rest etc.

### 4 Anything that happens before, during or after the problem

In homeopathy, these are known as "concommitant" symptoms. Migraine, for example, is often accompanied by nausea. Menstruation is often preceded by certain food cravings, certain emotional states etc.

## MEDICAL HISTORY

There are other aspects to describing symptoms, but the trained homeopath will help take the "case" through questioning and discussion. In addition, the homeopath will generally want to understand the family medical history, the illnesses you have had in the past, any medications you are using, your allergies etc., as would any other medical practitioner.

In one case, the correct remedy was finally found when the patient described a trivial but very peculiar pain in the foot which often occurred when he was troubled with his main complaints of indigestion and heart palpitations.

### A HOLISTIC APPROACH

Once the questioning is finished, the homeopath should have a sense not only of the problem you are having, but also of you as a unique person. This is quite important since treatment is aimed at stimulating your defenses in general, rather than eliminating a particular problem. By strengthening you, your health improves, and in the future there are fewer problems that will need to be helped. Eliminating particular problems without helping you at a deeper level will not produce the same result.

*Right: homeopathic medicines in the form of tablets (as shown here), ointments, liquids and sprays, can be used to treat a wide range of conditions.*

# THE "SYMPTOM PICTURE"

The homeopath may or may not do a complete physical examination depending on his or her training and the nature of the problem which you present for treatment. The understanding that the homeopath develops is called the "symptom picture." Some of the symptoms will be considered to be more important than others. However, in general, symptoms are more important if:

■ They are unusual for the problem you are having. For example, with a fever, there should be increased thirst ordinarily so as to replenish the body's water supply which is being lost to perspiration. Thirstlessness during fever, therefore, is unusual. Another example is a sore throat in which the pain is worse from swallowing liquids or saliva but is made better by swallowing solid food.

■ They are "characteristic" symptoms, i.e. they can be described in terms of sensation, location, modality and concommitant. The complaint of "headache" is useless without any further description. The complaint of a severe, throbbing pain located in the ear made much worse by anyone bumping the bed on which you lie, and accompanied by high fevers and a red face, is quite characteristic of Belladonna.

■ They are "strange, rare and peculiar," symptoms that are striking because they are only very rarely described.

■ They are symptoms that frequently arise when you are sick. If you have throbbing pains, for example, with headaches, or earaches, or sore throats, then "throbbing" becomes an important point.

■ They are true of you in general rather than of a particular part of the body. Headache, for example, is a "local" symptom of the head. A feeling of being "drained" when hungry, is considered a "general" symptom of

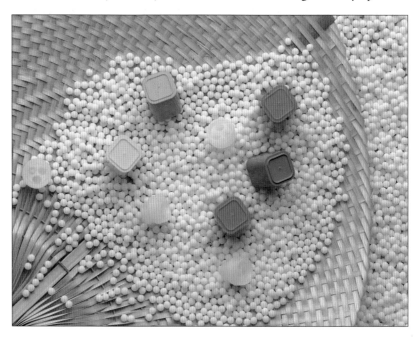

the person as a whole. The local symptoms might point to a few remedies, but the correct remedy must cover the "general" symptom.

## SELECTING A REMEDY

The next step in treatment is to determine which remedy could cause, in a proving, the important symptoms of the sick person. To do this, the *homeopathic materia medica* is consulted. Many practitioners use an index of this, called a "repertory," to begin the process. A repertory shows the symptoms, and the medicines that cause them. For example, the symptom "Throat, pain, stinging" has 13 medicines listed, with *Apis mellifica* being the most prominent one of these.

The medicines that appear for most of the important symptoms must be considered by the homeopath, who may consult the actual *materia medica* itself (each medicine is described according to all the symptoms, in all parts of the body, which it can cause in a proving). Two hundred years of homeopathic experience has taught us that each medicine has its own individual characteristics, just as each person is unique. The homeopath tries to select the most appropriate medicine based upon this understanding.

## ASSESSING THE PATIENT'S "VITALITY"

There are many ways to assess the "vitality" of the patient. This includes the person's level of "energy" but it is not limited to this. In fact, some people who are very tired have good underlying vitality, and some people who appear very energetic have actually used up much of their

---

# DETERMINING THE STRENGTH

Having selected the medicine, the next step is to determine the proper strength to use. There are many different styles of practise that may be employed. Each practitioner will have one or two styles with which he is most experienced and comfortable. Some will use low potencies and repeat them often, even several times a day. Others favor higher potencies given once and then observed over a period of time. It is necessary to be flexible in one's approach according to the problem being presented. A person with a very high fever and severe pain needs fast relief and one might give the medicine quite often, even every few minutes. Being a homeopath can be compared to being an astronaut in the space shuttle, sent up to retrieve and repair a satellite.

You have to get into the same orbit as the satellite (find the correct medicine) and then you have to be going around the Earth at the same speed as the satellite, otherwise you cannot stay next to it to work on it (find the correct strength of the medicine). The strength of the medicine needs to match the vitality of the patient. If the medicine is too weak, not very much effect will follow. If the medicine is too strong, there can be an intensification of the symptoms (the so-called "homeopathic aggravation"). If the medicine is given way too strongly, there may be no effect at all. It is important, then, to give the correct medicine in the correct strength, although giving the correct medicine itself is the most important consideration.

---

reserve energy and may be about to collapse! From a medical standpoint, vitality and the potency selection are linked in this way (schema of Ananda Zaren).

If the person is very sensitive, vitality is considered low and the potency should be correspondingly low. Sensitivity can take the form of allergy to pollens, dusts, foods etc., or may be more extreme as in people who cannot tolerate auto-exhaust fumes, the smell of newsprint or of flowers, cleaning fluids etc.

Sensitivity can also be related to emotions—some people are very easily offended and have strong reactions; some seem more thick-skinned and tolerant. In health, they are solidly grounded and not so easily pushed off center. In illness, they

are more precariously poised and have to work harder to stay in balance, and are more easily pushed off balance (like a tightrope walker).

The more that past medical treatment has "suppressed" the problem, the lower the vitality and the lower the potency that should be used. The classic example of this is in eczema, where cortisone creams have been used. Cortisone does not "cure" eczema, but it does block the inflammatory reaction that produces the rash. In some patients, long use of cortisone creams results in the disappearance of the eczema, with the creation of a new problem, asthma. When a homeopath treats the person successfully, the asthma should clear and the eczema reappear. When the eczema reappears, if the homeopathic

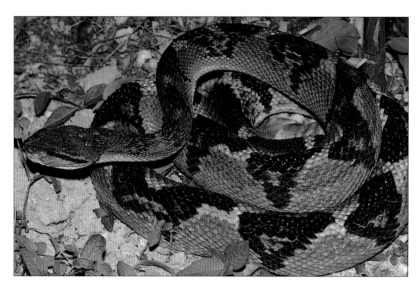

*Left: Lachesis is prepared from the venom of the Bushmaster snake, found in Central and South America. Lachesis is used for treating throat infections and some premenstrual problems.*

medicine was used in too high a potency the rash may be more intense than necessary. It is good to go slowly and gently in cases like this.

The "deeper" the illness, the weaker the vitality, and the lower the potency indicated to treat it. Multiple sclerosis, for example,

being a disease of the nervous system, is "deeper" in the body than arthritis, or skin problems.

The nature of the family history can also be important here. The more the problems appear in the family history, the more "deeply rooted" they are. One surmises, in a

case like this, that vitality is lower and therefore a lower potency is needed. Strong, clearly presented symptoms indicate a high vitality. The energy to produce these symptoms comes from vitality. In such a case, a higher potency is indicated.

Having made these decisions, the medicine is generally administered as globules, which dissolve in the mouth. Depending on the nature of the case and the style of practise the homeopath follows, the medicine may be given as a single dose or as multiple doses, one or more times a day.

## REACTION TO MEDICINES

### Good reaction

It is very desirable that, in some general way, the person feels better following the prescription. This means an increased sense of wellbeing, perhaps better mood, better sleep and appetite etc. Even if the particular symptoms of a chronic case have not changed at all, but the person is better in himself, this usually means a good reaction and that watchful waiting is indicated.

### Negative reaction

If the particular symptoms of a case are better following the medicine, but the person feels worse in their energy, mood etc., this may mean a negative reaction to the medicine. This is rare, but possible. In a case where there has been emotional suppression, it is often a good sign when the suppressed feelings come up. However, it can, on occasion, be "stormy"—because the vitality is improved the feelings should be more easily handled than in the past. Adjunctive therapy, such as counseling, can be extremely helpful.

### No reaction

If, by four to six weeks there is no reaction at all, or just a short reaction to the medicine, this usually means that the prescription was incorrect. This can be a difficult judgement to make. In long-standing chronic cases, improvement can be very slow. Even if minor changes are all that is noted at the first follow-up visit, this may be enough—watchful waiting should be the order of the day. If the homeopath determines that there has been no reaction to the medicine in a reasonable period of time, it is necessary to consider the following possibilities:

■ The choice of medicine was incorrect, and a more suitable one needs to be chosen.
■ The choice of medicine was correct, but the potency unsuitable, and a more suitable one needs to be chosen.
■ The choice of medicine was correct but it was "antidoted" in some way.

## SUBSEQUENT VISITS

A follow-up appointment will be scheduled to evaluate the reaction to the medicine. The time between the initial visit and the follow up will depend on the nature of the problem; an acute sickness should respond rapidly to treatment, whereas a chronic long-standing problem will change more slowly. In chronic cases, four to six weeks may be required to evaluate the action of the medicine.

At the second visit, the key question is whether or not the underlying vitality of the person has improved. This is evaluated primarily by considering what types of stresses throw the person off balance (symptoms from the original case, such as weather changes or types of weather, eating or not eating, loss of sleep, emotions etc.) and the reactions that the person has to those stresses. Generally speaking, the more intense the reactions the lower the vitality (until, as discussed above, vitality falls too low to "fuel" the reactions).

After the remedy, ideally the person will handle a given degree of stress more effectively with less effort. For example, if a light rain is enough to bring on a cold, then following treatment, there should be greater resistance to light rain; perhaps a heavier rain will be necessary to cause a cold. Ultimately, there should be no colds despite a heavy downpour.

## ANTIDOTING

Antidoting (negating the effect) of homeopathic medicines can occur from the following:

**1 Extreme psychological stress**—

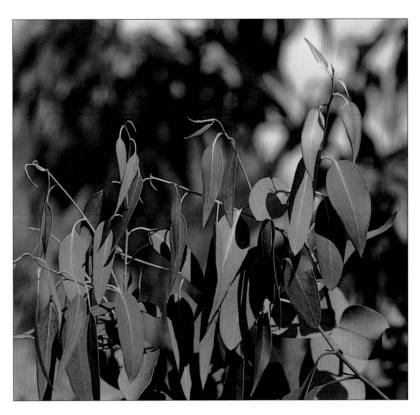

*Above: eucalyptus is an extremely volatile substance, often used in treating colds, and most homeopaths believe it should be avoided while on homeopathic treatment.*

although the treatment will help the person to tolerate stress more effectively, early on in the course of treatment the effect of the remedy can be overcome by stress.

**2 Dental work**—in general, dental work should either be completed before beginning homeopathic treatment, or deferred, if possible, until the improvement from treatment is well established. If in doubt, consult your homeopath and seek his advice.

**3 Volatile substances**, such as eucalyptus, menthol, camphor etc.—most homeopaths believe that these should be avoided while on homeopathic treatment.

**4 Mint tends to antidote** the following remedies: *Natrum muriaticum* and the other natrum salts, *Ignatia*, and Phosphorus.

**5 Coffee antidotes many remedies,** and is generally best avoided during homeopathic treatment. Black tea is acceptable as it is not caffeine that is problematic, but rather some other component of the coffee.

**6 Recreational drugs** generally act against homeopathic treatment and should be avoided.

**7 Orthodox medical drugs** that change or mask symptoms can make selecting the remedy and evaluating its action difficult. They should be avoided if possible.

**8 Any substance to which the sick person is very sensitive** can antidote the remedy.

## CONDITIONS THAT CAN BE TREATED

In theory, homeopathy can treat any medical condition, provided that:

■ The sick person has, or can, develop sufficient vitality to energize the healing process.

■ The body is capable of repairing or regenerating any physical damage already done (this is certainly not always possible).

### ■ ACUTE ILLNESSES, INFECTIONS AND OTHER ACUTE PROBLEMS

Homeopathy is quite effective against all kinds of infections and other acute illnesses—bacterial, viral, parasitic, fungal etc. This includes recurrent problems, such as ear infections, sinus problems, bronchitis, bladder infections etc. It is also good for injuries and first aid situations, burns, insect bites, food poisoning, skin rashes and toothache.

### ■ CHRONIC ILLNESSES

Many forms of arthritis can be helped by homeopathy. Again, the longer the illness has been present and the more damage already done to the joints, the less effective it will be. Other chronic illnesses such as migraine headaches, tension headaches, irritable bowel syndromes, asthma are very treatable, as are allergies, ulcers, skin problems, menstrual disorders, menopausal symptoms and chronic sinusitis.

### ■ CANCER

Cancer is not well treated by homeopathy, as there is usually severe damage already done by the time of diagnosis, and the vitality of the sick person is quite low. The homeopathic literature does contain reports of cures of patients with cancer. Homeopathy is used to relieve symptoms associated with chemotherapy and alleviate pain.

### HIGH BLOOD PRESSURE

High blood pressure is lowered in about one-third of cases, and generally not when it has been present for a long time. High blood cholesterol also does not generally respond to homeopathic treatment alone.

### MENTAL AND EMOTIONAL PROBLEMS

Mental and emotional problems, such as depression, anxiety disorders, premenstrual syndrome etc., respond well to homeopathy. More serious problems, such as manic depressive illness, should only be treated by an experienced practitioner. The prognosis in schizophrenia is quite guarded, and requires superb homeopathic evaluation and management.

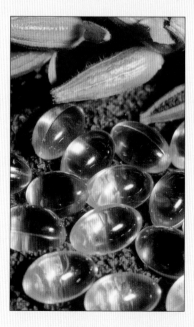

## EXAMPLES OF HOMEOPATHIC TREATMENT

As discussed above, homeopathic remedies are prescribed on the individualizing symptoms presented by the patient and not for specific conditions. It is helpful, however, in understanding homeopathy, to relate the medicines to conditions with which people are familiar. In this section, therefore, some common conditions are described in terms of typical pictures of certain homeopathic remedies.

### ASTHMA

This common condition occurs when there is an excessive "irritability" or "reactivity" of the bronchial tubes, causing constriction of the bronchial muscles and therefore wheezing and difficulty in breathing. Often related to allergy, and also precipitated by infection, this can be a very serious disorder. Conventional treatments are aimed at controlling the "irritability" with cortisone-like drugs, and blocking the constriction by using bronchodilator drugs. Homeopathic remedies which are often used for treating asthma include the following examples:

■ *Arsenicum album* (White oxide of arsenic)—the attack occurs in the few hours following midnight, especially at 2am. The patient is anxious and fearful to a very high degree. They must have someone near them. There is typically fatigue and weakness, but also a restlessness which may drive them from the bed to the chair, then to the couch, then back to bed etc.

■ *Kali carbonicum* (Potassium carbonate)—the attack typically

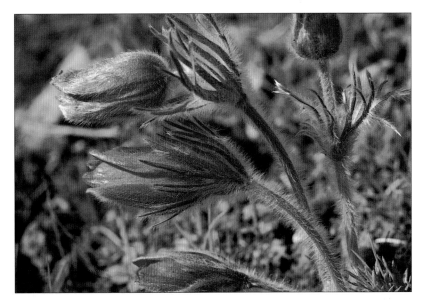

*Rhus toxicodendron*

*Left: Pulsatilla is a remedy derived from the wind flower (Pasque flower).*

occurs between 2am and 4am. Lying down is impossible; the person must sit up and possibly bend forward. They do not move, and are better while still. They do not like drafts of air, and are generally chilly. There is not so much fear and anxiety as with Arsenicum.

■ *Natrum sulphuricum* (Sodium sulphate)—the attack comes on around 4 or 5am. It is typically worse in the warm wet weather of summer or in winter with a change to warmer, moister air. The cough tends to be loose and accompanied by expectoration which may be greenish.

■ *Cuprum metallicum* (Copper)— spasmodic attacks, violent and sudden. Suffocating cough. This is often accompanied by grinding of the teeth, clenching of the thumbs, and cramping of the fingers and other muscles.

■ *Sambucus niger* (Black elder)— sudden attacks in the night while asleep, must spring out of bed, may be grasping at the throat. May turn blue (cyanosis), gasping for breath. The attack subsides, but reoccurs during the next sleep, and so on.

## CHICKEN-POX
A very common disease of childhood, accompanied by a typical rash consisting of groups of blisters which fill with yellowish fluid. There can be a lot of itching. It often starts out just looking like a cold.

■ *Rhus toxicodendron* (Poison ivy)— this is the classic remedy for chicken pox when there is intense itching relieved by a warm or hot bath or shower. There is great physical restlessness causing the person to change position constantly.

■ *Pulsatilla* (Wind flower) As in all conditions needing *Pulsatilla*, the patient is generally better from cool air, worse in a warm room (though with a fever they may be chilly, want to be bundled up but breathing cool-

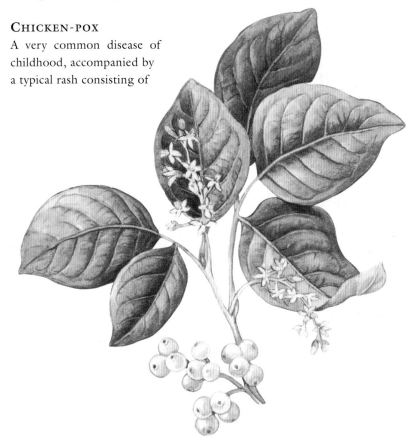

er air). They are emotionally fragile, tearful, needing support and comfort. They may whimper and moan.

■ *Mercurius* (Mercury)—in more advanced cases, with prolonged fever with sweating and debility. The rash becomes infected, containing pus instead of clear yellow fluid.

## TEETHING

The eruption of the teeth in babies may be accompanied by behavioral problems, fever, red ears, congestion of the nose and throat, and more or less pain.

■ *Chamomilla* (Chamomile)—the pain seems intense and the child intolerant of it. They are restless and angry, and find nothing makes them happy. They may only be quieted by

being carried about.

■ *Coffea* (Coffee)—they are overexcited, awake, sleepless. Not so much in severe pain, may even be happy and playful.

■ *Belladonna* (Deadly nightshade)— the child is over-sensitive to light and jar, and may have a high fever with a flushed face and glassy eyes. The gums are very red and swollen.

## BLADDER INFECTIONS

When bacteria grow in the urine the bladder becomes "irritable," urination becomes frequent and often painful. There may be blood in the urine. If the infection goes to the kidneys it is a much more serious problem, and high fevers, chills and nausea result, perhaps with back

pain. Kidney infections should not be self-treated.

■ *Cantharis* (Spanish fly)—the pain is very intense, and usually of a burning nature, much worse during urination. There can be cutting and stabbing pains in the bladder or urethra. Urging to urinate is almost constant, and painful. The whole person feels very agitated and distressed.

■ *Sarsaparilla* (wild licorice)—the pain is severe and felt especially at the very end of urination. It may be difficult to pass urine while sitting but it flows freely while standing.

■ *Staphysagria* (Stavesacre)—pain is of a burning nature, persists after urination. Often the remedy for "honeymoon cystitis", the problem comes on after sexual intercourse, especially after a period of abstinence.

## ACUTE GRIEF

The loss of a loved one can be expected to cause very intense feelings. Sometimes, the aggrieved person can become overwhelmed. Homeopathic treatment can enable the person to bear the grief and more effectively work through it.

■ *Ignatia amara* (St. Ignatius bean) —grief may be "silent" and the person uncommunicative and avoiding interaction with others. Much sighing. Moods can be very changeable. Can't stand criticism or contradiction, can manifest a lot of anger. Especially vulnerable to the break-up of a romantic relationship.

■ *Pulsatilla* (Wind flower)—very mild and tends to weep. The grief may be silent but they will usually want company, want consolation and

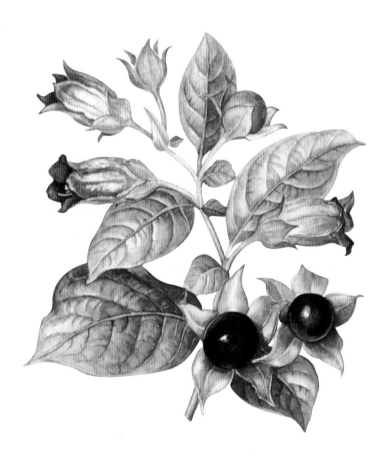

*Belladonna*

support. Very soft, perhaps moaning or lamenting in voice. Generally warm blooded and craves cool open air. Thirst may be quite low.

■ *Aurum metallicum* (Gold)—severe depression, when there seems to be no light in the world, suffering is extreme, and death is welcome as relief from the pain. Can be strongly suicidal. Brooding, morose and depressed, not inclined to talk. Can be very angry.

■ *Natrum muriaticum* (common salt)—sensitive, conscientious individuals who do not easily share their feelings. They tend to reject support and consolation, although deep inside they long for it. They are often the "strong ones" during a family crisis who take care of everyone else but don't let anyone take care of them.

## PANIC ATTACKS

Sudden attacks of intense anxiety in which the person may not be able to function. Attacks seem to come out of nowhere, and can become a chronic recurring problem. This should be treated by an experienced practitioner. The acute attack itself may respond to one of several remedies. Among them are:

■ *Aconitum napellus* (Monkshood) —intense fear and even hysteria is very prominent. The person is convinced that they will die, and may even profess to know exactly when death will occur. Hysteria may present with paralysis, rapid breathing, intense restlessness. Typically worse around midnight, but can occur at any time.

■ *Arsenicum album*—this remedy

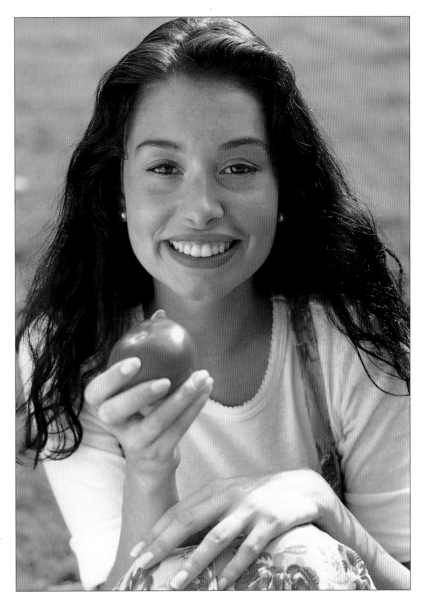

picture can appear much like *Aconitum*, but the restlessness is even more profound, driving them from place to place with no relief. They are demanding and need to have people around. Things must be put in order (fastidious) in order for them to control the panic and chaos that they feel inside.

■ *Opium*—people needing opium

can appear quite frightened and characteristically may become dazed, sleepy, or even stuporous. The pupils of the eyes are likely to be constricted.

■ *Belladonna*—the picture may be one of intense fear, appearing even delirious. The person is red, flushed, agitated, and may be in a frenzy to run away, to escape, to hide. The pupils are likely to be dilated.

# IRIDOLOGY

## CHAPTER THREE

*I* ridology is a method of diagnosis. By studying the iris of the eye, the colored part, one is looking at over 28,000 nerve endings, all of which are connected to the brain via the hypothalamus. Apart from those related to the brain zone, most of the neurological pathways extend down the spine and out, through to the various parts of the body. Rather like a reflexologist working on the nerve endings in the feet, an iridologist is studying the exposed nerve endings in the irides, all directly connected to the brain on the iris stalk. Indeed, the irides are part of the brain at the fetus stage of life.

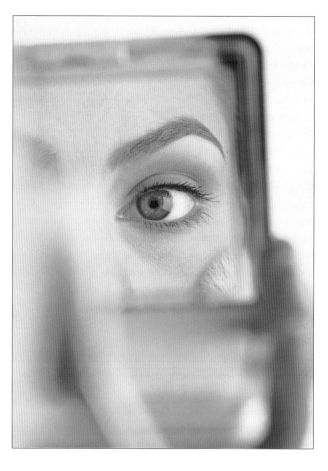

Under a microscope, the abnormalities in the iris read rather like a map and you look at a veritable microchip of information. An iris analysis reveals genetic strengths and weaknesses, congested or irritated zones and the interactions between the various bodily systems, from the digestive system, to the hormonal, neurological, eliminative and structural organisms. Modern medicine is developing magnificently in finding pathological diseases. On the other hand, iridology reveals non-pathological states that modern medicine is not really geared to find. To quote Dr. Henry Edward Lane, who carried out most of his research, practice and teaching in America: "The morbid changes going on in the system are making themselves noticeable in the eye, and the possibility exists to disclose the inner condition of man by careful observation of his eye, and consequently to make a diagnosis which is reliable in every respect." Insidious conditions, such as chronic lymphatic congestion, venous congestion and poor kidney detoxification, when combined, can lead to life-spoiling conditions, such as edema, skin eruptions, rheumatism and arthritis. A qualified iridologist is able to pin-point the root cause, or causes, of most conditions.

# HISTORY AND ORIGINS

Iridology is an ancient science which has gained more recent resurrection through scientific and medical research, particularly in Russia, Germany and America. In 1000B.C. the Chaldeans of Babylonia were carving depictions of the iris into stone slabs, along with its relationship to the rest of the body. Records show that Hippocrates, Philostratus and the Medical School of Salerno practiced iridology. More recently, in 1670, the physician Philippus Meyens published his book *Chiromatica Medica* in Dresden, within which he described the neurological reflex reactions of the iris as follows: "The right side of the eyes show as the liver, the right thorax and the blood vessels. The left side of the eyes can show all organs which lie on the left side, therefore the heart, left thorax, spleen and the small blood vessels."

Further writings on the iris and its signs were published thereafter, but it is the works of the Hungarian Dr. Ignatz von Peczely (1826-1911) that are most widely credited with the resurrection of this diagnostic tool. Dr. von Peczely produced one of the earliest European Iris Charts linked with the modern revival. It all began with the well recorded drama which occurred when he was 11 years old, involving breaking the leg of an owl whilst struggling to free it from a bush in his garden and subsequently noticing a black mark appear at 6 o'clock in its iris. As he nursed the owl and its injury back to recovery, he noticed the mark lighten and it was this event which led him on to study the eyes of his patients, first whilst working as a homeopath and later, after qualifying as a doctor of allopathic medicine. This gave him the opportunity to correlate his findings with patients studied before and after operations, along with the many autopsies he performed. His book, *Discoveries in the Realms of Nature and Art of Healing* was published in Budapest in 1880, recording his discoveries and research in diagnosing from the irides of the eye.

Soon afterwards, in 1893, the comprehensive research and findings by the Swedish homeopath Nils Liljequist were published. Though twenty-five years younger than von Peczely, and virtually a continent apart, these two, working totally independently, produced charts and used medical terminology which surprised many with their similarities. And yet it should not be so surprizing, human anatomy being what it is the world over.

As a boy, Liljequist was expected to study medicine, but by the time he was fifteen he had been reduced from a robust young man to a chronic sufferer of malaria, influenza, swollen lymph glands, nasal polyps and suffered pains in his limbs, all of which developed during the course of twelve months following a vaccination. Constant use of quinine led to him noticing that his blue eyes changed color and, by the time he was twenty, he published a paper called *Quinine and Iodine Change the Color of the Iris.* He wrote: "Formerly I had blue eyes, now they are greenish with red spots in them." Eventually he became disenchanted with medicine, discovering that without constant drugging, he would at least have had periods of remission instead of several years of constant headaches, vomiting and tinnitus. By the time he was thirty he decided to study homeopathy and the works of Professor Jaeger, never forgetting "that our sufferings should remind us to guard our fellow men against similar misery, and if they become afflicted with sickness to help them as much as possible."

## RESEARCH AND REFERENCE

Further research by such great masters of the subject as the German Pastor Felke (1856-1926), published in a book by A. Muller entitled *The Eye-diagnosis based upon the Principles of Pastor Felke*; the Austrian Dr. H. E. Lane, mentioned previously, and Dr. Henry Lindlahr, a student of Dr. Lane's, all helped to inspire today's world-renowned iridologists. Dr. Lindlahr was the first physician to create order out of the chaos of numerous treatments by correlating the best ones within one mammoth source of reference, *Nature Cure Philosophy and Practice*, published in 1913. By 1919 this had grown into six volumes, the last being *Iridiagnosis and Other Diagnostic Methods.* Today, a set of four volumes of his works is readily available and makes inspiring reading to all those interested in natural medicine and self help.

# THE IRIS CONSTITUTIONS

Modern medical research has helped us to develop the basic charts and knowledge we have today. Our contemporary masters of Iridology number the Germans Josef Deck and Joseph Angerer.

Iridology is a safe, non-invasive and inexpensive method of analysis which can be integrated with both orthodox and complementary medicine. It monitors the movement towards disease states and towards health. As bodily tissues become inflamed or toxic, white inflammatory or congestive discolorations are apparent in the relevant zones.

The genetic make-up, or constitution, is revealed at a glance. There are three main iris color types;

- Brown
- Blue
- Gray

There is also the exception to these basic types, known as a mixed or biliary type, which is part blue and part brown. This type has a combination of factors or tendencies which are to be found in both the blue and brown-eyed types. For the purpose of

# EYE COLOR

Blue eyes are known as lymphatic constitutions and are divided into several subgroupings, the main three being the neurogenic, the hydrogenic and the mesenchymal-pathological (sometimes called connective tissue) constitutions. Brown eyes come under the hematogenic constitution, and the mixed, hazel eyes, as previously mentioned, are known as biliary types. These terms are used medically and by homeopaths and other alternative medicine practitioners. In view of much of the research over the centuries having been carried out under medical influences, this is not surprising. However, it is more simple than it might appear to the uninitiated.

The hematogenic constitution revealed by the true brown iris appears, on close inspection, to have few features and to be of a velvet-like texture. Under magnification, however, the iridologist can detect zones of lighter shadings with a sandpaper appearance indicating that area is inflamed or irritated. A creamy film appearing in the outer, circulatory zone indicates raised cholesterol of blood fats; a bluish ring around the outer edge of the iris, known as an anemia ring, signifies poor iron metabolism, and radials or furrows emerging from the center of the iris, map the course of toxic overflow from the gastro-intestinal zone.

this introduction to Iridology, we will incorporate the gray eyes within the blue-eyed group because the constitutional differences are so slight as to be negligible.

- **The hematogenic constitution** is prone to anemia; blood diseases such as jaundice or hepatitis; arthritis; digestive disorders with lowered enzymatic production which can frequently manifest as an intolerance to cow's milk, amongst other things; constipation; ulcers; liver, gall-bladder or pancreatic malfunction; diabetes; circulatory disorders and auto-intoxification. These are predispositions and one hopes that few of these tendencies will develop, let alone all of them, but self abuse, poor dietary disciplines or disease is more likely to manifest along the above pathways than in other ways.

- **The lymphatic constitution** contrasts dramatically, not just in color but in tendencies. It is thus named because of a genetic inclination towards an over-production of lymphatic cells which react to irritations, inflammations and a build-up of excess mucous and catarrh in the system. This, in turn, makes this type

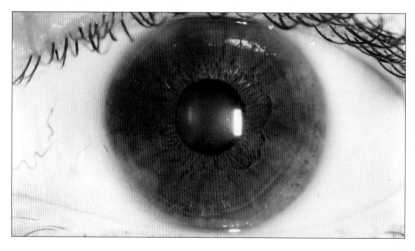

*Left: the hematogenic constitution is prone to anemia and blood diseases.*

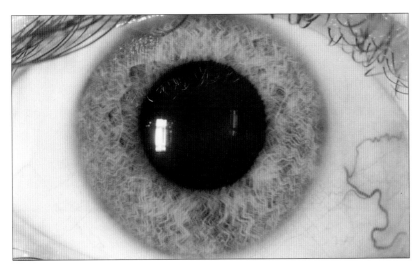

*Above: the lymphatic constitution is prone to skin and respiratory disorders.*

more prone to inflammatory conditions of the joints, allergies, respiratory and skin disorders.

The loose, wavy fibers, like combed hair in a blue or gray iris are indicative of a pure lymphatic constitution. The aforementioned hyper-reactivity tends to manifest along the lymphatic pathway with tonsil and adenoid irritations; splenitis; swollen lymph glands; irritated appendix; eczema; acne; flaky, dry skin; dandruff; asthma; chronic coughs; bronchitis; sinusitis; diarrhea; arthritis; eye irritations; fluid retention and vaginal discharge.

■ **The neurogenic constitution**, on the other hand, just as its name suggests, puts the emphasis on the nervous system. There are two types of neurogenic constitutions, the neurogenic sensitive and the neurogenic robust. The latter has coarser iris fibers than pictured and this type generally has nerves of steel and a daredevil attitude with an enviable resilience. However, they are more

prone to the lymphatic constitutional-type problems, mainly catarrh and inflammation, gastro-intestinal fermentation and serious fibrinous inflammations (tuberculosis, pleurisy, pericarditis, colitis, peritonitis and certain joint inflammations).

However, with regard to the neurogenic sensitive, the fine, silk-like fibers reflect a marked sensitivity of the central and autonomic nervous systems. This type is prone to overtax their natural strength. Their senses are usually hyperacute and, underneath an assertive, industrious, high-achiever, we find a nervous disposition being pushed to exhaustion and prone to nervous disorders. Though mentally hyperactive and strong willed, the sensitive nervous system may not be able to match the excessive demands laid upon it. When over-taxed, they can develop multiple functional disorders of the vital organs, such as heart and circulatory disorders, stomach ulcers and digestive problems, intestinal disorders such as colitis or constipation, and hormonal disorders such

*Right: the neurogenic constitution puts emphasis on the nervous system.*

as hyperactivity of the thyroid, parathyroids or adrenals. They are also more vulnerable to the effects of geopathic and electromagnetic stresses, noise and radiation.

■ **The hydrogenic constitution** is similar to the lymphatic constitution but white puff balls, known as tophi, are formed around the periphery of the iris. They stand out distinctly against the basic blue iris background color. The white flakes, or tophi, are considered to arise from deposits of endogenous toxins formed from a miasmic, or genetic influence of a previous, but inactive tuberculosis. This type of constitution is prone to all tendencies and conditions listed under the pure lymphatic but with an added emphasis on more chronic, lymphatic congestion, lowering resistance or immunity and toxically affecting the mucous and synovial membranes, thus reducing their function. The hydrogenic is more prone to acute rheumatism, bacterial infections, poor kidney detoxification with the subsequent fluid retention and toxin retention. The rheumatic tendency is exacerbated by latent streptococci increasing the antigen-antibody responses. This can set off histamine, acetycholine and other substances which, in diseases such as eczema and psoriasis, can be triggered as the endogenous toxins of

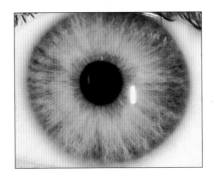

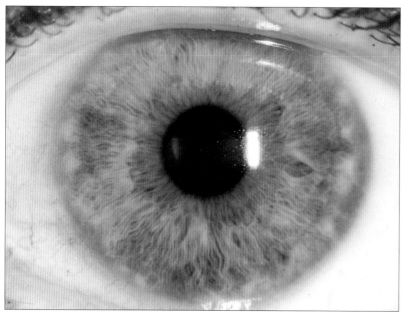

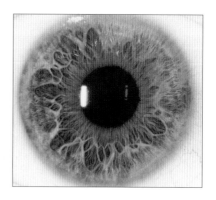

*The hydrogenic constitution (left) is prone to rheumatism and skin diseases, while the mesenchymal pathological iris (above) is prone to poor circulation.*

the tubercular bacillus release irritants not efficiently excreted by the lungs and kidneys.

The mesenchymal pathological iris contrasts with the other irides noticeably even to the most inexperienced examiner. The petal-like arrangement of the large lesions extending out to the periphery of the iris is sometimes described as a daisy iris. The loose, widened iris fibers, forming lesions over the various zones, indicate connective tissue weaknesses. This type is prone to varicose veins; hemorrhoids; hernias; prolapse; postural problems and spinal weaknesses; poor circulation;

strokes; slow recuperation from injuries; ligament and tendon weaknesses; reduced resistance and adrenal weakness of a genetic nature. On the positive side, they have a flexibility and we find such subjects more adaptable to altitude changes, less prone to stress (they let things go through them) and a tendency to "bounce" if they fall, which is fortunate in view of the "slow recuperation should they break a bone!"

■ **The biliary constitution,** of the mixed iris, has a basically blue background which often appears brown, or greenish brown, due to an overlay of pigmentation. This iris may appear as the "hazel" eye or even look uniformly brown. However, closer inspection removes confusion with the hematogenic type because the blueygreen iris fibers will show through in

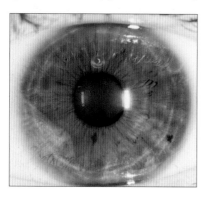

*Left: the biliary constitution, or the mixed iris, is prone to liver and pancreatic disorders, blood disease, diabetes, digestive problems and gall stones.*

varying degrees of contrast to the upper, brown pigmentation.

This constitutional type is prone to liver, gall-bladder, bile duct and pancreatic disorders, not dissimilar to the influences from the true brown hematogenic type. Similarly, they too are prone to blood disease, diabetes, constipation, colitis, flatulence and gallstones. However, the lymphatic influences are also present, as listed under the pure lymphatic eye.

## IRIS ANALYSIS

The majority of people seeking an iris diagnosis have already had pathology tests without being able to pin-point the root cause of their problems. Because the iris reveals so many nonpathological conditions, it provides highly comprehensive information on the activities and interactions with the systems. This veritable blueprint provides a key to the root causes of patients' problems, no matter what symptoms or disease has manifested. It also provides the key to preventive medicine, to correct living habits in mind, body and spirit. Through iridology we can work more effectively, meeting our own, highly individualized needs, in an effort to avoid the full repercussions of continued imbalance and disease states. However, it is not practical to attempt a full iris analysis for a child below the age of six, partly because the iris details are not fully established, and partly because they cannot keep their eyes still long enough.

## A DIAGNOSTIC TOOL

Iridology is not a therapy. However, as a highly detailed, diagnostic tool, revealing the status of neurological, chemical, organic and structural criteria, once an iris analysis is completed, the therapeutic pathway to take becomes obvious. For example, a person suffering from chronic headaches may find the main contributory factors are intercranial pressure from a previous cranial trauma, combined with a misalignment of the first cervical vertebra. The iridologist may not be a chiropractor or cranial osteopath, but at least the patient knows the next step to take. On the other hand, chronic sinus congestion might prove to be the main exacerbator and that would indicate a cleansing programme requiring possible herbal and nutritional approaches. Another common cause often proves to be gastric or liver toxicity. The iridologist will save the patient from the frustration of trying irrelevant treatments and thus be the guide towards the appropriate therapy.

## CONSULTING AN IRIDOLOGIST

When seeking an iridologist one should always check that they have

---

## VARIATIONS OF THE IRIS CONSTITUTION

There are approximately 25 variations of the iris constitutions. A well-trained iridologist will be able to provide very precise details in each individual's genetic and acquired strengths and weaknesses. In some instances, further laboratory or medical tests might be recommended where the specific naming of the disease, such as cancer, prompts medical attention.

The majority of doctors are most cooperative, probably in view of the fact that the patient's wellbeing is paramount. In fact, a lot of doctors in the Eastern European countries and Germany, not to mention graduates of the Bobigy Faculty of Medicine at the University of Paris Nord, where it is taught, use iridology themselves as a diagnostic tool.

---

had full, formal training. Do not expect them to diagnose in allopathic terms. Indeed, under the very strict Code of Ethics established by the Guild of Naturopathic Iridologists International, based in London, England, it is clearly stated that: "The complementary practitioner will need to assess the case from different criteria and no attempt should be made to describe a complementary diagnosis in allopathic terms unless the practitioner is so qualified. For example, an iridologist is qualified to make a medical diagnosis which might indicate inflammation or morbid congestion in certain areas, but it may be outside their competence to put an allopathic medical name to the condition."

It takes about an hour to complete and explain a thorough iris analysis. The iridologist will first take the details from the irides using a torch and magnifier, or, better still, a bioscope, much like a visit to the optician. Others may just home in on what they consider to be relevant to the patient's symptoms. This is frowned upon by the more eminent, iridology faculties.

In order to avoid depending on the practitioner's limited experiences, an overall, thorough analysis should be completed first, before the iridologist is given the symptoms. This is because the iris reveals previous traumas and conditions, as well as states which may not yet have manifested. The iris does not lie. However, the patient may be locked into certain symptoms and not aware of other equally revealing factors. Once the iridologist has done an unbiased analysis, he or she is able to explain to the patient specifically why the problems have arisen. To tell a patient that his right testicle has a trauma mark, when he has come about lower back pain and failed to mention he has a previously kicked, and now very tender, right testis, is highly conducive to winning confidence, and, in this example, is not irrelevant.

Most iridologists have qualifications in at least one therapeutic science and it is useful to find one who can also treat you. Most registers will include such details or you can contact the ruling body to discuss your needs, especially if you are fortunate enough to have more than one iridologist in your neighborhood.

# POLARITY THERAPY

CHAPTER FOUR

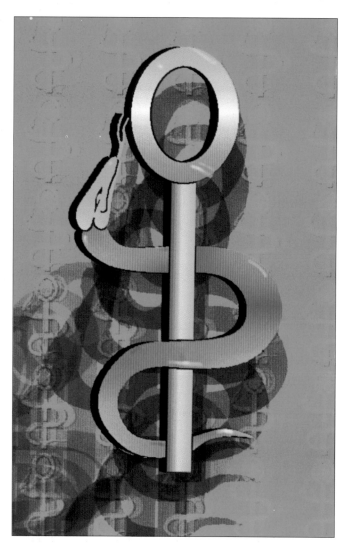

*P*olarity therapy is a comprehensive health system, which incorporates bodywork, diet, exercise and counseling. It is based on the concept of the Human Energy Field (see opposite): electromagnetic patterns which are expressed in terms of our mental, emotional and physical experience. In polarity therapy, health conditions are viewed as reflections of the condition of the energy field, and therapies are designed to stimulate and balance the field in order to achieve benefits for health.

Basic characteristics of the Human Energy Field are described in many sources, and polarity has strong links to many other holistic health systems. For example, the term "polarity" refers to the universal pulsation of expansion/ contraction or attraction/repulsion, which are known as Yang and Yin in Oriental therapies.

# THE HISTORY OF POLARITY THERAPY

Polarity therapy was developed by Randolph Stone, D.O., D.C., N.D. (1890-1981). As a young physician in the 1920s, he learned that the simple bodywork technique of chiropractic proved to be extremely valuable: chiropractic treatments were more effective, with patients experiencing deeper levels of awareness, and profound relaxation and healing were achieved. Fascinated by these consistent results that had no explanation in terms of conventional anatomy, Randolph Stone began a lifelong search for understanding of the deeper causes of health and disease. His quest led to the Aryuvedis and Oriental idea of the Human Energy Field, and to a thorough investigation of this revolutionary yet ancient approach to the healing arts.

Dr. Stone published his findings in the late 1940s. He chose the word "polarity" to describe the basic nature of the electromagnetic force-field of the body. He taught that polarized energy currents precede physical form and are primary factors in wellbeing.

He found that the Human Energy Field is affected by touch, by diet, by movement and sound, by attitudes, by relationships and by environmental factors. Polarity therapy sheds light on all these subjects; the scope of polarity practice can therefore be very broad, with implications for health professionals in many therapeutic disciplines.

Dr. Stone treated patients and conducted research at his office in Chicago for over 50 years. When he retired in 1974, many of his students continued to develop the system, using his books and pamphlets as a basis for their work.

## THE ENERGY FIELD

The shape of the energy field was depicted long ago by ancient Greeks and Egyptians as the Caduceus, or Staff of Hermes, which is commonly known today as the symbol of allopathic medicine.

The parts of the symbol correspond to the four distinct but interdependent parts of the Human Energy Field.

▥ The globe at the top and staff in the center are the core of Primary Energy, found in the Cranio-Sacral structures and functions.

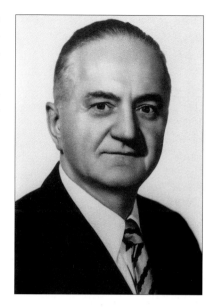

*Dr. Randolph Stone*

▥ The intertwining snakes are the Three Principles of attraction, repulsion and transitional stillness.
▥ The five intersections along the central core are the Five Elements.
▥ The wings represent Consciousness, which is humanity's potential to transcend materialism and reunite with its Source.

## THE TOTALITY OF HUMAN EXPERIENCE

Polarity therapy asserts that these four parts underlie the totality of human experience, preceding and determining spirit, mind, feelings and body. Understanding these four dimensions of the Human Energy Field and their applications is the scope of polarity therapy.

In the polarity model, good health is experienced when these systems are functioning normally:
▥ Energy flows smoothly without significant blockage or fixation on any level.

## RECENT DEVELOPMENTS AND PROGRESS

In recent years, polarity therapy has gained increased recognition, partially through the leadership of the American Polarity Therapy Association (APTA), the largest professional organization in the field. It has accomplished significant progress since 1987 with the creation of the Standards for Practice, a consensus document, which has been co-created by all three groups, and which defines concisely the scope and practice of polarity therapy. This very important document is the basis for polarity therapy professional certification from APTA.

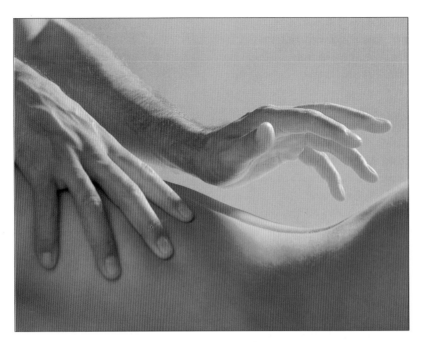

■ Disease and pain occur when energy is blocked, fixed or unbalanced.
■ Blockages occur due to stress and trauma, generally crystallizing from the subtle to the gross levels of the field.
■ Therapy is about finding the blockages, releasing energy to normal flow patterns, and maintaining the Energy Field in an open, flexible condition.

## BODYWORK TECHNIQUE

Polarity therapy is best known for its bodywork. The basic premise is that touch affects the Human Energy Field. The body is like a bar magnet, with a (+) pole at the top and a (-) pole at the bottom. Similarly, the hands have a charge, which tends to be (+) on the right and (-) on the left. Think of what happens when the (+) and (-) ends of two magnets are placed near each other, and what happens when the

end of one is reversed: one positioning (opposite poles) attracts; the other (like poles) repels.

Similarly, placing the hands on the body affects energy flow, with one placement stimulating and the reverse placement sedating energy flow. By knowing the major flow patterns and key intersections of any of the four dimensions of the Human Energy Field, and using appropriate hand placements, the practitioner can facilitate profound changes in the body/mind. In addition, the conscious intention of the practitioner affects energy flow, so instruction on "conscious touch," "mindfulness," "boundaries" and related topics is an important part of polarity therapy training.

In polarity therapy bodywork, healing is generally seen to come from within the client. The practitioner is a facilitator or helper, and not an external curative force. Emphasis is placed on awareness and sensitivity rather than medical correction.

## THE FOUR DIMENSIONS

Within each of the four dimensions of the Human Energy Field, bodywork techniques are based on specific considerations, locations and therapeutic intentions.

■ **For Primary Energy,** techniques center on the cranio-sacral system. The subtle movements and functions of the cranium, spine and sacrum are studied, focusing on the energy potency and free movement of the cerebrospinal fluid (CSF). CSF is considered to be a conveyor of the most subtle and most powerful energy flow in the body.

■ **For the Three Principles,** basic qualities of Yin and Yang are studied. These are the polarized forces which are well-described in traditional Aryuvedic and Oriental

## THE FIVE ELEMENTS

These relate to five stages of density in the form and function of the body. They are also known as Five Chakras (from Sanskrit, meaning "wheels" of energy). From gross to subtle, the Five Elements are:
■ Earth (solids)
■ Water (liquids)
■ Fire (heat)
■ Air (gases)
■ Ether (space which contains all the others)
These functions are associated with specific body areas and specific types of emotional and/or physical problems.

## RESULTS OF POLARITY THERAPY

The polarity practitioner is trained to recognize indicators relating to all of these dimensions of the Human Energy Field, and to provide touch and other guidance to balance the field. The results can be remarkable: deep relaxation, new insight into causes and patterns, and a sense of calm power are often reported.

medical systems. All tissues and functions, all microcosmic and macrocosmic relationships, can be understood in terms of charged energy, categorized in polarity as positive (+), negative (-) and neutral (0). These three are in constant dynamic tension with each other, creating the basis for physical manifestation. In physics, this is most clearly seen in the structure of the atom, with proton (+), electron (-) and neutron (0) in constantly self-adjusting interrelationship with each other.

In polarity bodywork, understanding of the Three Principles is applied in terms of location and quality of touch, in methods for balancing the nervous systems, and in numerous other ways.

### COGNITIVE AND NON-COGNITIVE METHODS

▓ Consciousness is affected by techniques for releasing old trauma and establishing new blueprint-level attitudes and expectations about self and others. Polarity therapy involves both cognitive (becoming more aware of factors affecting consciousness) and also non-cognitive methods (when energy is released, new behaviors arise spontaneously, without conscious effort).

## OTHER POLARITY THERAPY TECHNIQUES

Polarity also incorporates diet, exercise and other dimensions of healing.

▓ **In diet,** Dr. Stone taught the value of a vegetarian diet with no meat, fish, fowl or eggs. He also advocated the periodic use of a "cleansing diet," consisting of fresh and cooked vegetables, in addition to herbal cleansing practices and formulas.

▓ **In exercise,** Dr. Stone recognized that the Human Energy Field was affected by movement, posture, sound and other self-applied therapeutic possibilities. Drawing from Hatha Yoga and the Oriental martial arts, he developed what he called "Easy Stretching Postures" or "Polarity Yoga" as adaptations that affected energy flow but did not require the extensive training needed by the traditional exercise systems.

▓ **A way of life** is often a term used for describing polarity therapy. Dr. Stone's writings contain some wide-ranging references to the full spectrum of human experience, particularly spiritual development.

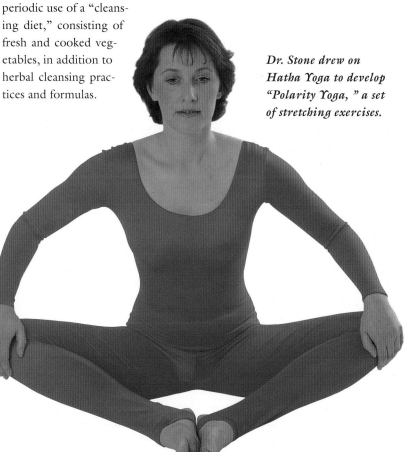

*Dr. Stone drew on Hatha Yoga to develop "Polarity Yoga," a set of stretching exercises.*

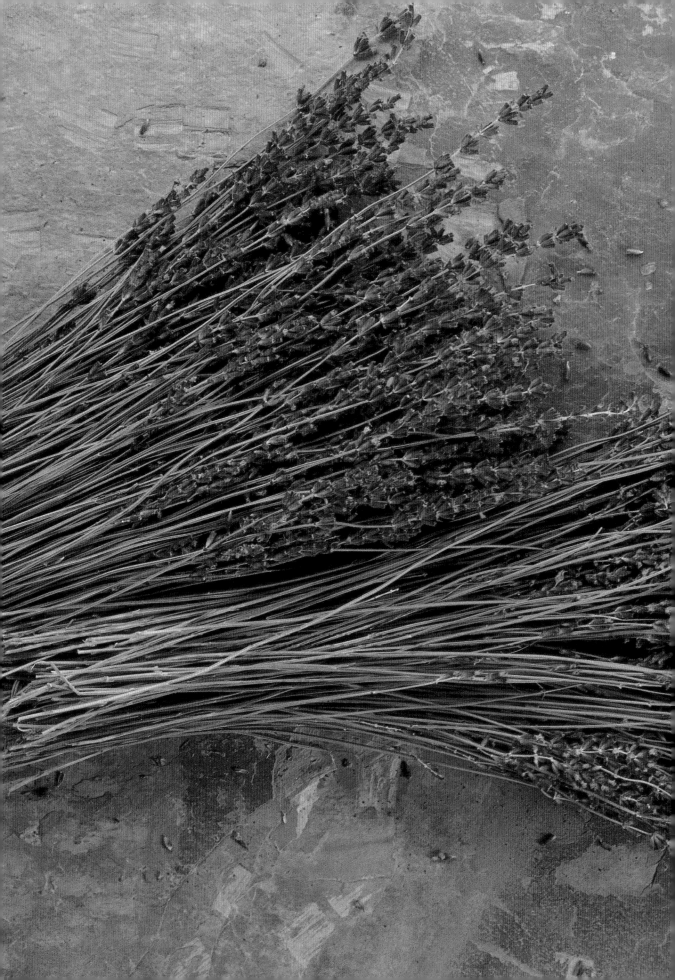

# THE POWER OF PLANTS

## PART TWO

*M*an has long recognized the healing properties of therapeutic plants and herbs, and their use dates back to ancient times. Herbalists and many alternative health practitioners believe that natural plant preparations can support the body's natural healing processes, restoring balance and helping the body to heal itself. Flower essence therapy is a unique system based on plant essences in liquid form, which work to restore balance and good health, interweaving the mind and the body.

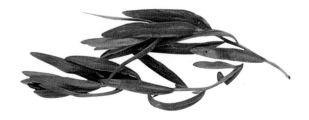

# FLOWER 5 ESSENCE THERAPY

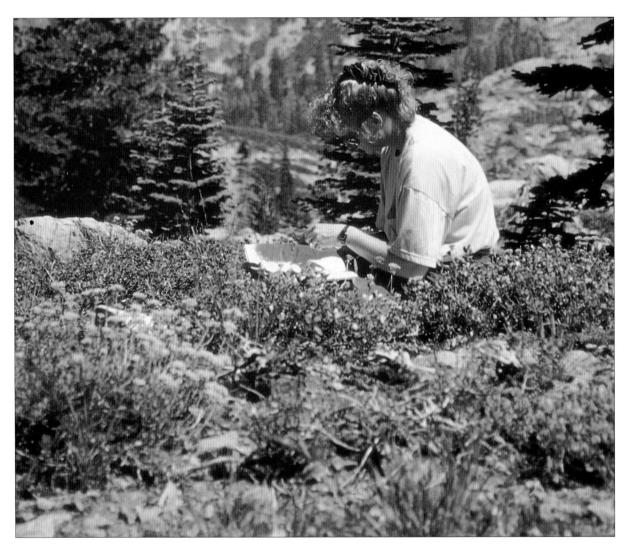

## CHAPTER FIVE

*H*ealing with flowers is both ancient and universal. All cultures, including our own contemporary one, intuitively sense that flowers express a soul language which is far more profound than words. Flowers are used to convey our deepest feelings of joy, grief, love or tribute at a range of family events such as births, weddings, funerals and numerous other celebrations and commemorations in human culture.

# FLOWER ESSENCE THERAPY: VISION AND VALUES

Modern flower essence therapy has evolved from the work of Dr. Edward Bach (see below). The stages in his medical career mirror the spectrum of development within our modern culture as we seek to understand what creates wellness, wholeness and health within the human being. The model that is now emerging is one that incorporates many different aspects of human wellness, from standard medicine and surgical intervention to preventative measures which seek to bolster healthy immune responses in the human body.

As our understanding of the human energy field becomes more refined, we are beginning to perceive and treat the larger energetic structures which surround the physical body itself. We are recognizing that the body and soul cannot be regarded as an opposing duality, but rather as one interweaving reality.

Especially since World War II, researchers have correlated distinct personality traits with specific diseases. One of the most famous of these studies was conducted by Drs. Meyer Reidman and Raymond Rosenman who coined the term "Type A behavior" for the impatient, hostile attitude connected with the greater risk of heart disease.

Since then numerous studies have pinpointed the decisive role of emotional factors such as anger, grief, depression or self-esteem on the outcome of specific diseases as well as overall immunity. A whole

## DR. EDWARD BACH

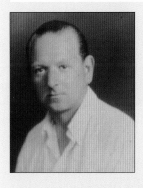

It was in England in the 1930s that Dr. Edward Bach, a well-known medical doctor and homeopathic physician, formulated the first precise system of soul healing based on medicines extracted from the flowering parts of plants. He was an early advocate for the kind of holistic healing that is finally receiving more widespread attention in the latter part of our century.

Bach completed his undergraduate training at Birmingham University and then graduated from University College Hospital in London in 1919. He assumed the post of Casualty Medical Officer for this same hospital and was in charge of over 400 beds during World War I. It was here that he clearly observed the effects of stress and trauma in relationship to the recovery potential of his patients. He believed that surgery and standard medicine did not hold all of the answers and he became interested in the field of immunology, assuming the role of Chief Bacteriologist at the hospital. Bach went on to develop a number of bacterial vaccines which were credited with saving many thousands of lives when he inoculated war troops during a virulent influenza epidemic. These clinical results were so impressive that they were recorded in several medical journals of the

time, including the prestigious Proceedings of the Royal Society of Medicine.

Bach felt that these vaccines were still too crude and when he accepted a post at the London Homeopathic Hospital he developed a series of bacterial nosodes which were diluted and potentized in a manner similar to that used in homeopathy. More significantly, he was able to document clear archetypal personality traits correlated with each nosode, and he began to diagnose and treat according to these mental and emotional aspects, rather than outer physical symptoms. These nosodes were used by many homeopathic practitioners, both in the United States and Europe, and they are still included in the standard homeopathic pharmacopeia.

Yet, as Bach became increasingly sensitized to the emotional and mental issues presented by his patients, he continued to seek remedies that could act with even greater depth and harmony than the homeopathic nosodes. By 1930, he abandoned his prominent career in London and returned to the countryside of his Welsh ancestry to begin an intensive study of the native plants which he had esteemed so much in his youth. As he treated the patients in the small villages of the Welsh and English countryside where he traveled, he developed entirely new remedies from the flowering parts of plants which could beneficially address the emotional and mental conditions which undermined the health and well-being of his patients. By the time he died in 1936, he had developed a collection of 38 flower essences.

new field of medical research has been established, designated as Psychoneuroimmunology (PNI), which has identified biochemical messengers which transmit emotional responses to and from the glands in the body, documenting definitive and substantive changes in emotional and physical wellness.

Seen from this perspective, flower essence therapy may be viewed as being on the vanguard of holistic medicine. It is perceived as a unique, integrative therapy which employs highly refined qualities from flowering plants to act within the physical matrix of the body, yet stimulates very precise states of psychological consciousness.

### ■ HOMEOPATHY

Flower essences are closely aligned to the field of homeopathy, since both use potentized medicines that affect trans-physical levels of the human being. However, homeopathic medicine incorporates a broad range of

## HOW FLOWER ESSENCES WORK

Flower essences are thought to work in a way similar to our experience of music or art: through the vehicle of sound or light we perceive something that moves or inspires us. The essences operate through the medium of water, which holds an imprint of the color, form and beauty of the flower in a way that speaks to the feelings and thoughts within the individual. Thus flower essences reveal rather than conceal aspects of the Self, so that new choices can be made about life issues. Because they are potentized energetic medicines, they work in a manner which is gentle and life-affirming without danger of overdose or long-term dependency.

substances, including animal and mineral sources as well as different parts of plants.

### ■ SOLAR EXTRACTION

By contrast, the flower essences are made specifically from fresh flowers collected from pristine habitats at the precise moment of flowering. The solar extraction methods which are thought to have been developed by Bach have brought forth a new genre of medicines which are uniquely capable of addressing more delicate and subtle aspects within the emotional and mental field of the human being.

The flower essences are also distinguished from psychopharmaceutical agents.

Flower essences seem to work as catalysts. They do not suppress symptoms; rather they stimulate consciousness by introducing new information into the emotional and mental fields of the individual.

## VISITING A THERAPIST

The key to successful use of flower essences involves the ability to select appropriate remedies. Flower essences work by a principle of resonance; the remedy must match a similar pattern within an individual in order to evoke a healing response. An inappropriate remedy will not be harmful, but neither will it be helpful—it simply will not register a significant response within the individual. This means that efficacious selection of flower essences involves honing one's perception of mental and emotional imbalances. We are taught from childhood how to articulate pain or discomfort in the physical body; for example, the specific attributes of a headache or injured foot, or when or how we feel nauseated or fatigued. By contrast, our ability to identify and describe emotional or mental imbalance is usually far less developed.

For this reason, most individuals find it useful to visit a therapist when first using flower essences (although the flower remedies are used quite safely and successfully by many families for basic home care). Some therapists specialize exclusively in flower essences, although most incorporate them within a spectrum of options which are offered to the client.

Flower remedy portraits involve the interweaving of both the mind and the body; therefore an effective practitioner is one who has developed the ability to see these relationships. This has more to do with the practitioner's skill in observing and asking questions than any particular healing modality; flower essences are successfully used by a broad range of practitioners including medical doctors and nurses, psychotherapists and other counselors, energetic practitioners such as acupuncturists and homeopaths, art therapists, teachers, nutritionists and body workers.

## APPLICATION AND RESPONSE

Flower essences are generally taken in liquid form, several drops at a time, although some practitioners apply them directly to meridians or other energy points on the body during a therapeutic session. They can also be added to skin creams or bath water, or put in misting bottles to be sprayed around the body and the environment.

Typically, the response to the remedies is of a more general nature in the early stages. Individuals report feeling calmer, clearer, better able to cope, or less fatigued. Through counseling, working with dreams, keeping a journal or other ways of learning to observe and articulate levels of emotional and mental phenomena, much more specific responses can be documented. For instance, the following is an actual quotation from an individual who was being treated with flower essences by a family therapist: "My usual reaction whenever my daughter starts whining and crying, is that a I get a knot in my stomach and feel quite tense and irritable. Invariably, I then begin to yell or get angry with her. However, since using flower essences, I don't seem to react so strongly to her. Instead, I'm understanding why she's upset and gradually seem to be discovering more creative ways to address her discomfort."

### COMBINING FLOWER ESSENCES

Although single remedies are quite effective, flower essences can be skilfully combined to create synergistic formulas—a typical formula involves up to five or six remedies. These "dosage bottles" are used several times daily: just before and after sleep and before meals. The flower essence formulas are used in cycles—a typical rhythm is about one month. During this period, the emotional body, like the moon itself, has usually "waxed and waned" through a phase of inner development. Flower essence therapy usually involves seeing a client for several months, with new applications of remedies as the individual moves through successive stages or "layers" of change and unfoldment.

## NEW DEVELOPMENTS AND RESEARCH

Dr. Bach identified 38 remedies in the rural areas of England and Wales during the brief time span of eight years before his untimely death in 1936. Since then, other practitioners from many countries around the world have confirmed through their own observation and research, the unique healing benefits of flower essence therapy. In 1979, the Flower Essence Society (FES) was founded as a non-profit world-wide educational and research organization.

The Flower Essence Society has investigated and collected empirical

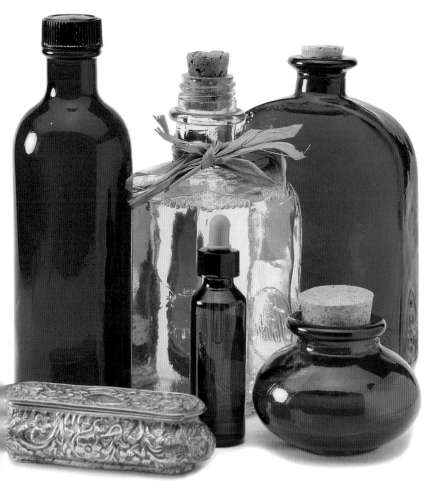

case studies not only for the original 38 English remedies, but also significant new essences derived from medicinal herbs and also North American wildflowers. The Society conducts an annual certification program for practitioners and publishes research. Its worldwide network of over 25,000 practitioners serves hundreds of thousands of clients.

## THE APPLICATION OF FLOWER ESSENCES

Cases have been collected that demonstrate the successful application of flower essences for a broad range of conditions and ailments including: learning disorders, child abandonment and abuse, family and personal relationships, work performance and career goals, envi-

ronmental sensitivities and allergies, depression and grief, body tension and general stress, nutritional and lifestyle choices, parenting, masculine and feminine identities, artistic expression, sexuality, coping with terminal illness or chronic disease, psychosomatic illness, overall immune response and a large number of specific diseases.

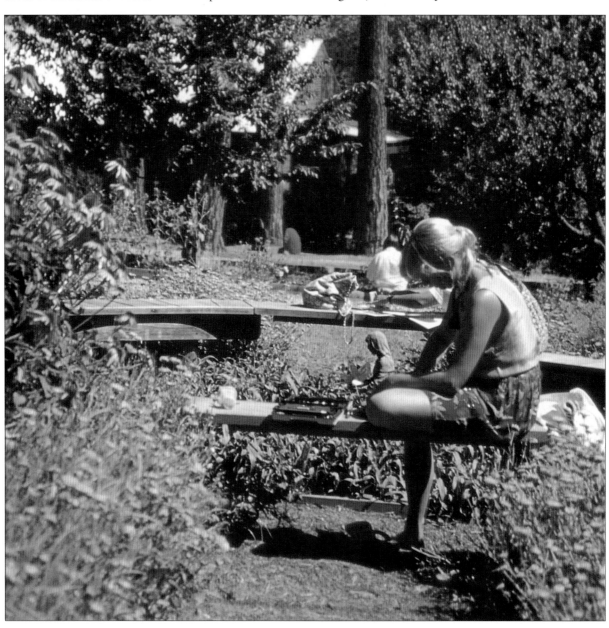

# SOME SAMPLE CASES

The following cases have been submitted by practitioners to the Flower Essence Society.

## BLEEDING HEART

A young girl of eight years old suddenly developed acute stomach pains and diarrhea, although there had been no prior history of such symptoms. A gastrointestinal expert conducted a full battery of tests and could find nothing wrong with the child. Finally her parents took her to a family counselor who also used flower essences.

In the opening diagnostic session, the child drew a large picture of a heart which was broken. The counselor used Bleeding Heart to help her address what was sensed as a deep source of grief within the child. The young girl began to share her sense of loss for a playmate who had been

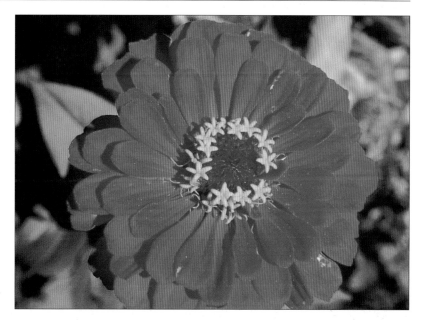

*Zinnia*

killed suddenly several months prior to the onset of her symptoms. Her family had no idea that she had been so profoundly affected by the death of her friend.

Within several days of taking the Bleeding Heart, the child's symptoms were drastically reduced and within several weeks they had completely disappeared and never returned again.

## IMPATIENS, ZINNIA AND BORAGE

An executive salesman, aged 58, contended with a great deal of stress in his daily lifestyle. He was diagnosed by his physician as having chronic high blood pressure and in the early stages of coronary heart disease.

The doctor asked him to make nutritional changes, and to incorporate exercise and stress reduction in his daily lifestyle. Despite enrolling in two different programs for reducing stress and teaching relaxation tech-

niques, the man made little progress. He still found himself anxious and irritable at the end of the day.

A flower essence therapist recommended a combination of the flower essences Impatiens, Zinnia and Borage. The man noticed an immediate effect using these remedies—he felt calmer and more centered. The

*Bleeding Heart*

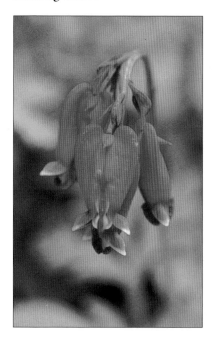

*Impatiens*

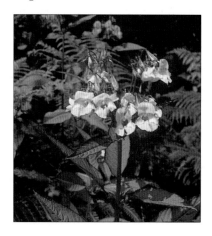

relaxation techniques that he had previously attempted seemed easier to incorporate. He noticed many situations at home and in the family that were changing due to his feeling of greater ease and self-control. When he went for his regular checkup six weeks later, the physician was amazed to discover that his blood pressure had dropped significantly and he wanted to know "what had changed" for his patient.

## MIMULUS

A woman in her seventies had gradually become a "shut-in" following the death of her husband. She was afraid to engage in household errands or go out alone, despite the fact that she was physically capable of doing so. Although she had a valid driver's license she had depended on her husband to drive and was reluctant to use her car. As her fear grew much more pronounced she became hypersensitive to many noises in her house and began to fear that her house would be broken into. Due to these fears she began to sleep very restlessly and also became increasingly fretful and agitated.

A flower essence counselor prescribed the single remedy of Mimulus. No clear changes were noted until about the third week of use. The woman then reported that she felt calmer and was getting more sleep at night. A week later she remarked to her daughter that she had been acting like a frightful child, and it was time to make some changes. Two weeks later she reported to her counselor that the time had come to get another life and to stop pretending that she was dead just because her husband was. She made

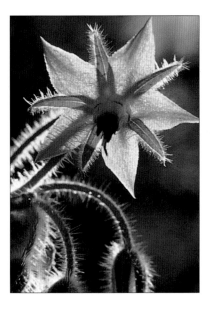

*Borage*

many incremental changes in her lifestyle, learning to drive her car and accepting many social invitations she had previously declined.

## CALIFORNIA WILD ROSE

This flower essence was used for a 16-year-old young woman who had become moody, dressed in dark colors and was emotionally distant from her own family. Furthermore, her grades had suddenly plunged from above average to barely passing. In a counseling session, the young woman stated she felt "bored" with life and didn't feel much interest or hope for her future. She had recently parted with a boyfriend and had also not been chosen for a part in a school play which she had wanted.

Her mother noticed a change within two weeks of taking the California Wild Rose. She was more willing

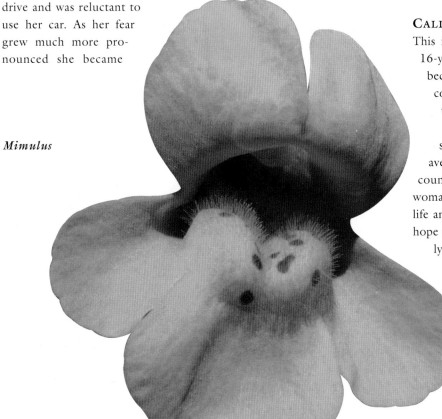

*Mimulus*

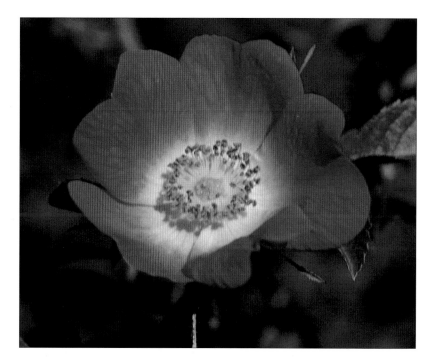

prior history of cervical dysplasia, she was now diagnosed with severe cervical dysplasia (CIN III) confirmed by tissue biopsies from five different areas of the cervical and vaginal tissue. Her physician recommended immediate surgical intervention, removing all of the affected tissue in the cervix and vagina, through a process called conization, requiring hospitalization, general anesthesia and a two-month recovery period. In his opinion, she was at high risk for cancer without these measures. Because this condition had developed so suddenly without any prior history, the woman sought psychotherapeutic counseling and nutritional counseling. She modified her diet to exclude foods that were irritating or difficult to digest.

Her counselor suggested a trine of Lily remedies, including Tiger Lily, Mariposa Lily and Alpine Lily, to address her feminine identity and its connection with her gynecological

to talk about her feelings of hurt and rejection and she found a new (girl)friend at school. Within several months her disposition was brighter and more cheerful and her grades at school had returned to their normal level.

## STAR OF BETHLEHEM

A young woman in her twenties had been violently attacked and raped and robbed at gunpoint. She had received counseling for these incidents and seemed to be in recovery. Six months later, she developed a severe eating disorder along with food allergies. Despite nutritional and psychotherapeutic counseling she continued to lose weight, and showed other signs of depression.

She was given Star of Bethlehem to address the shock and trauma of her violent attack. Through the use of the essence she began to re-live the original incident, but now acknowledging the tremendous feelings of

rage, grief and shame she felt about her attack. As she worked through and resolved these emotions, her eating disorder also subsided.

## TIGER LILY, MARIPOSA LILY, ALPINE LILY

A woman who had just turned 40 went for her regular check-up to her gynecologist. Although she had no

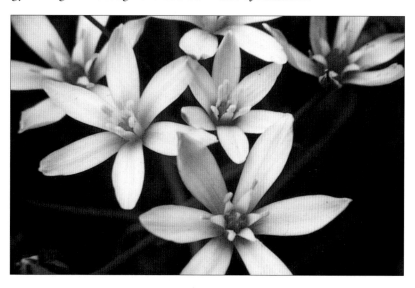

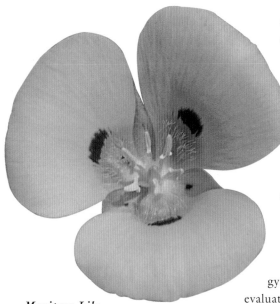

*Mariposa Lily*

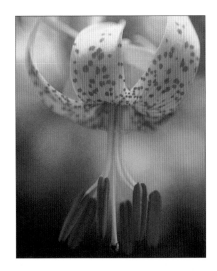

*Tiger Lily*

also realized she had ambivalent feelings about motherhood partly due to her own traumatized relationship with her mother. Her dream journal and daily life journal, and the sessions with her counselor revealed submerged emotional material which was now being revealed to her. After six months the woman returned to her gynecologist for another evaluation intending to allow surgery if her cell tissue was still disturbed. Tissue biopsies were taken of the original sites, and to the astonishment of her doctor the new tests showed absolutely no areas of

issues. During the next several months the woman did deep emotional work around her sense of grief about having never had a child; she

cervical dysplasia, even in a mild form; her tests were normal and have remained normal for five years.

*Alpine Lily*

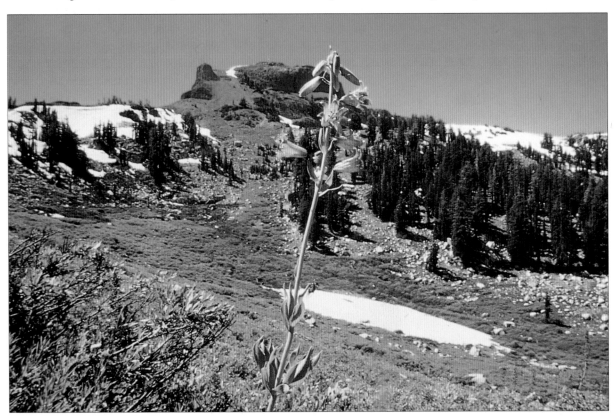

*Holly*

## HOLLY

A young boy of nine years of age was diagnosed as hyperactive. His parents sought help from a holistic doctor who also uses flower essences. In a diagnostic work-up for the boy, no significant nutritional or physiological problems were identified. However, the child showed clear emotional problems. His behavior was on edge, he was always irritated or hostile in his response to others. He seemed unable to be a part of his family system, or to be able to receive warmth and affection from other members of his family.

The single remedy of Holly was chosen. The parents reported amazement at the changes in their son. They commented to their doctor, "We can't thank you enough, whatever was in those drops has been so transforming to his personality; he's reintegrated himself into the warmth of our family."

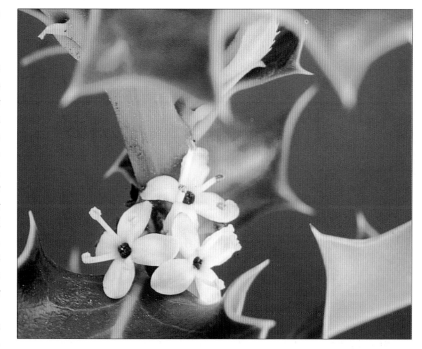

## ELM

A middle-aged man visited his chiropractic/naturopathic doctor presenting symptoms of severe, deep pain in his left shoulder joint. All typical protocols and tests were followed in evaluating this man's condition.

After six visits for chiropractic adjustments and soft tissue therapy, the agonizing pain continued unabated.

The doctor concluded that the cause of the pain was not of physical origin and prescribed Elm flower essence. After eight days the patient reported that his pain was completely gone. During this time he gained the insight that his discomfort came from his overwhelming sense of responsibility and burden, which had been manifested as a psychic "weight" on his left shoulder. With the help of the Elm flower essence this man made a permanent shift in his inner attitude about his life and work. The intense pain he felt in his left shoulder has never returned.

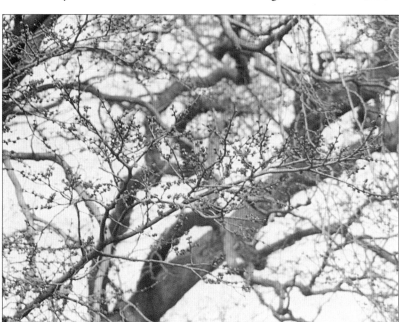

*Elm*

## NORTH AMERICAN FLOWER ESSENCES

The following essences are among the best-known flower remedies, used for many years by practitioners throughout the world. They are available individually, or in practitioner kits.

### ALOE VERA
*Aloe vera* (**yellow**)
*Positive qualities:* creative activity balanced and centered in vital life-energy.
*Patterns of imbalance:* overuse or misuse of fiery, creative forces; "burned-out" feeling.

### ANGELICA
*Angelica archangelica* (**white**)
*Positive qualities:* feeling protection and guidance from spiritual beings, especially at threshold experiences such as birth and death.
*Patterns of imbalance:* feeling cut off, bereft of spiritual guidance and protection.

### ARNICA
*Arnica mollis* (**yellow**)
*Positive qualities:* conscious embodiment, especially during shock or trauma; recovery from deep-seated shock or trauma.
*Patterns of imbalance:* disconnection of Higher Self from body during shock or trauma; disassociation, unconsciousness.

### BABY BLUE EYES
*Nemophila menziesii*
(**light blue**)
*Positive qualities:* childlike innocence and trust; feeling at home in the world and at ease with oneself, supported and loved; connected with the spiritual world.
*Patterns of imbalance:* defensiveness, insecurity, mistrust of others; estrangement from the spiritual world; lack of support from the father in childhood.

### BLEEDING HEART
*Dicentra formosa* (**pink**)
*Positive qualities:* loving others unconditionally, with an open heart; emotional freedom.
*Patterns of imbalance:* forming relationships which are based on fear or possessiveness; emotional co-dependence.

### BORAGE
*Borago officinalis* (**blue**)
*Positive qualities:* ebullient heart forces, buoyant courage and optimism.
*Patterns of imbalance:* heavy-heartedness, lack of confidence in facing difficult circumstances.

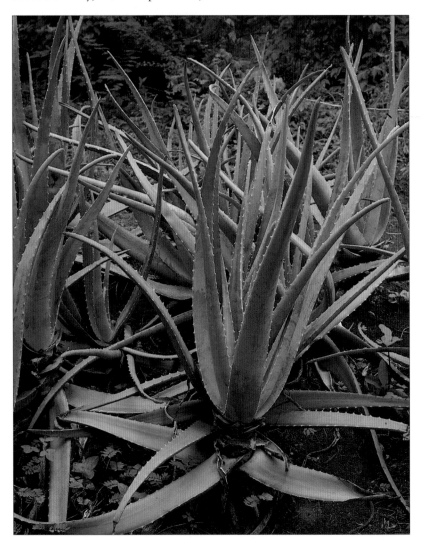

*Aloe*

## BUTTERCUP
*Ranunculus occidentalis* (yellow)
*Positive qualities:* radiant inner light, unattached to outer recognition or fame.
*Patterns of imbalance:* feelings of low self-worth, inability to acknowledge or experience one's inner light and uniqueness.

## CALIFORNIA POPPY
*Eschscholzia californica* (gold)
*Positive qualities:* finding spirituality within one's heart; balancing light and love; developing an inner center of knowing.
*Patterns of imbalance:* seeking outside oneself for false forms of light or a higher consciousness, especially through escapism or addiction.

## CALIFORNIA WILD ROSE
*Rosa californica* (pink)
*Positive qualities:* love for the Earth and for human life, enthusiasm for doing and serving.
*Patterns of imbalance:* apathy or resignation, inability to catalyze will forces through the heart.

## CHAMOMILE
*Matricaria recutita* (white/yellow center)
*Positive qualities:* serene, sun-like disposition, emotional balance.
*Patterns of imbalance:* easily upset, moody and irritable, inability to release emotional tension.

## DANDELION
*Taraxacum officinale* (yellow)
*Positive qualities:* dynamic, effortless energy; lively activity balanced with inner ease.
*Patterns of imbalance:* overly tense, especially in the musculature of the body, overstriving and hard-driving.

## ECHINACEA
*Echinacea purpurea* (pink/purple)
*Positive qualities:* core integrity, contacting and maintaining an integrated sense of Self, especially when severely challenged.
*Patterns of imbalance:* feeling shattered by severe trauma or abuse which has destroyed one's sense of Self; threatened by physical or emotional disintegration.

## GOLDEN YARROW
*Achillea filipendulina* (yellow)
*Positive qualities:* remaining open to others while still feeling inner protection; active social involvement which preserves the integrity of the Self.
*Patterns of imbalance:* for outgoing people who are overly influenced by their environment and by other people; protecting oneself from vulnerability to others by withdrawal and social isolation.

## GOLDENROD SOLIDAGO
*californica* (yellow)
*Positive qualities:* well-developed individuality, inner sense of Self balanced with group or social consciousness.
*Patterns of imbalance:* easily influenced by group or by family ties; an inability to be true to oneself, and subject to peer pressure or social expectations.

## INDIAN PAINTBRUSH
*Castilleja miniata* (red)
*Positive qualities:* lively, energetic creativity, exuberant artistic activity.
*Patterns of imbalance:* low vitality and exhaustion, difficulty rousing physical forces to sustain the intensity of creative work; inability to bring creative forces into physical expression.

## IRIS IRIS
*Douglasiana* (blue-violet)
*Positive qualities:* inspired artistry, deep soulfulness which is in touch with higher realms; radiant, iridescent vision and perspective.
*Patterns of imbalance:* lacking inspiration or creativity; feeling weighed down by the ordinariness of the world; dullness.

## LOTUS
*Nelumbo nucifera* (pink)
*Positive qualities:* open and expansive spirituality, meditative insight and synthesis.
*Patterns of imbalance:* spiritual pride, inflated spirituality.

## LOVE-LIES-BLEEDING
*Amaranthus caudatus* (red)
*Positive qualities:* transcendent consciousness, the ability to move beyond personal pain, suffering or mental anguish by finding larger, transpersonal meaning in such suffering; compassionate awareness of and attention to the meaning of pain or suffering.
*Patterns of imbalance:* intensification of pain and suffering due to isolation; profound melancholia due to the overpersonalization of one's pain.

## MANZANITA
*Arctostaphylos viscida* (white-pink)
*Positive qualities:* embodiment, integration of spiritual Self with the physical world.
*Patterns of imbalance:* estranged

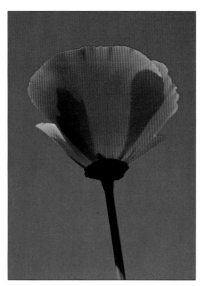

*California Poppy*

from the earthly world; aversion, disgust or revulsion toward the bodily Self and physical world.

## MARIPOSA LILY
*Calochortus leichtlinii* (white/yellow center/purple spots)
*Positive qualities:* maternal consciousness, warm, feminine and nurturing; mother-child bonding, healing of the inner child.
*Patterns of imbalance:* alienated from mother or from mothering, feelings of childhood abandonment or abuse.

## PINK YARROW
*Achillea millefolium var. rubra* (pink-purple)
*Positive qualities:* loving awareness of others from a self-contained consciousness; appropriate emotional boundaries.
*Patterns of imbalance:* unbalanced sympathetic forces, overly absorbent auric field, lack of emotional clarity, dysfunctional merging with others.

## POMEGRANATE
*Punica granatum* (red)
*Positive qualities:* warm-hearted feminine creativity, actively productive and nurturing at home or in the world.
*Patterns of imbalance:* ambivalent or confused about the focus of feminine creativity, especially between values of career and home, creative and procreative, personal and global.

## RED CLOVER
*Trifolium pratense* (pink-red)
*Positive qualities:* self-aware behavior, calm and steady presence, especially in emergency situations.
*Patterns of imbalance:* susceptible to mass hysteria and anxiety, easily influenced by panic or other forms of group thought.

## SAGEBRUSH ARTEMISIA
*Tridentata* (yellow)
*Positive qualities:* essential or "empty" consciousness, deep awareness of the inner Self, capable of transformation and change.
*Patterns of imbalance:* over-identification with the illusory parts of oneself; purifying and cleansing the Self to release dysfunctional aspects of one's personality or surroundings.

## SAINT JOHN'S WORT
*Hypericum perforatum* (yellow)
*Positive qualities:* illumined consciousness, light-filled awareness and strength.
*Patterns of imbalance:* an overly expanded state leading to psychic and physical vulnerability; deep fears, disturbed dreams.

## STAR TULIP
*Calochortus tolmiei* (white/purple)
*Positive qualities:* sensitive and receptive attunement; serene, inner listening to others and to higher worlds, especially in dreams and meditation.
*Patterns of imbalance:* feelings of being hardened or cut-off, inability to feel quiet inner presence or attunement, unable to meditate or pray.

## SUNFLOWER
*Helianthus annuus* (yellow)
*Positive qualities:* balanced sense of individuality, spiritualized ego forces, sun-radiant personality.
*Patterns of imbalance:* distorted sense of Self; inflation or self-effacement, low self-esteem or arrogance; poor relation to father or masculine aspect of Self.

## TIGER LILY *Lilium humboldtii* (orange/brown spots)
*Positive qualities:* cooperative service with others, extending feminine forces into social situations; inner peace and harmony as a foundation for outer relationships.
*Patterns of imbalance:* overly aggressive, competitive, hostile attitude; excessive "yang" forces, separatist tendencies.

## YARROW ACHILLEA
*Millefolium* (white)
*Positive qualities:* inner radiance and strength of aura, compassionate awareness, inclusive sensitivity, beneficent healing forces.
*Patterns of imbalance:* extreme vulnerability to others and to the environment; easily depleted, overly absorbent of negative influences and psychic toxicity.

**YARROW SPECIAL FORMULA** (flower essences of *Achillea millefolium* (white), *Arnica montana* and *Arnica mollis*, and *Echinacea purpurea*, with Yarrow, Arnica, and Echinacea tinctures, in a sea salt water base).
*Positive qualities:* enhancing integrity of etheric body, of vital formative forces.
*Patterns of imbalance:* disturbance of life-force and vitality by noxious radiation, pollution, or other geopathic stress; residual effects of past exposure.

**YERBA**
*Santa Eriodictyon californicum* (**violet**)
*Positive qualities:* free-flowing emotion, ability to harmonize breathing with feeling; capacity to express a full range of human emotion, especially pain and sadness.
*Patterns of imbalance:* constricted feelings, particularly in the chest; internalized grief and melancholy, deeply repressed emotions.

**ZINNIA** *Zinnia elegans* (**red**)
*Positive qualities:* childlike humor and playfulness; experiencing the joyful inner child, lightheartedness, detached perspective on Self.
*Patterns of imbalance:* overseriousness, dullness, heaviness, lack of humor; overly somber sense of Self, repressed inner child.

# BACH FLOWER REMEDIES

This table, issued by The Bach Center and reprinted with their permission, lists the flower remedies and the negative states of mind that each can counter.

| Flower Remedy | State of Mind |
|---|---|
| Agimony | Those who hide worries behind a brave face. |
| Aspen | Apprehension for no known reason. |
| Beech | Critical and intolerant of others. |
| Centaury | Weak willed; exploited or imposed upon. |
| Cerato | Those who doubt their own judgment, seek confirmation of others. |
| Cherry plum | Uncontrolled, irrational thoughts. |
| Chestnut bud | Refuses to learn by experience—continually repeats same mistakes. |
| Chicory | Over-possessive—(self-centered)—clinging and over-protective especially of loved ones. |
| Clematis | Inattentive, dreamy, absent-minded, mental escapism. |
| Crab apple | The "cleanser." Self disgust/detestation. Ashamed of ailments. |
| Elm | Overwhelmed by inadequacy and responsibility. |
| Gentian | Despondency. |
| Gorse | Pessimism, defeatism, "what's the use!" |
| Heather | Talkative (obsessed with own troubles and experiences). |
| Holly | Hatred, envy, jealousy, suspicion. |
| Honeysuckle | Living in the past—nostalgic. Home-sickness. |
| Hornbeam | "Monday morning" feeling—procrastination. |
| Impatiens | Impatience, irritability. |
| Larch | Lack of self-confidence, feels inferior. Fears failure. |
| Mimulus | Fear of known things. Shyness, timidity. |
| Mustard | "Dark cloud" that descends, making one saddened and low for no known reason. |
| Oak | Normally strong/courageous, but no longer able to struggle bravely against illness and/or adversity. |
| Olive | Fatigued—drained of energy. |
| Pine | Guilt complex—blames self even for mistakes of others. Always apologising. |
| Red chestnut | Obsessed by care and concern for others. |
| Rock rose | Suddenly alarmed, scared, panicky. |
| Rock water | Rigid minded, self denying. |
| Scleranthus | Uncertainty/indecision/vacillation. Fluctuating moods. |
| Star of Bethlehem | For all the effects of serious news, or fright following an accident, etc. |
| Sweet chestnut | Utter dejection, bleak outlook. |
| Vervain | Over-enthusiasm—fanatical beliefs. |
| Vine | Dominating/inflexible/tyrannical/autocratic/arrogant. Usually good leaders. |
| Walnut | Assists in adjustment to transition or change, e.g. puberty, menopause, divorce, new surroundings. |
| Water violet | Proud, reserved, enjoys being alone. |
| White chestnut | Persistent unwanted thoughts. Preoccupation with some worry or episode. Mental arguments. |
| Wild oat | Helps determine one's intended path in life. |
| Wild rose | Resignation, apathy. |
| Willow | Resentment, embitterment, "poor old me!" |

**Rescue Remedy** A combination of cherry, plum, clematis, impatiens, rock rose, star of Bethlehem. All-purpose emergency composite for effects of anguish, examinations, going to the dentist, etc. Comforting, calming and reassuring to those distressed by startling experiences.

# HERBAL MEDICINE

## CHAPTER SIX

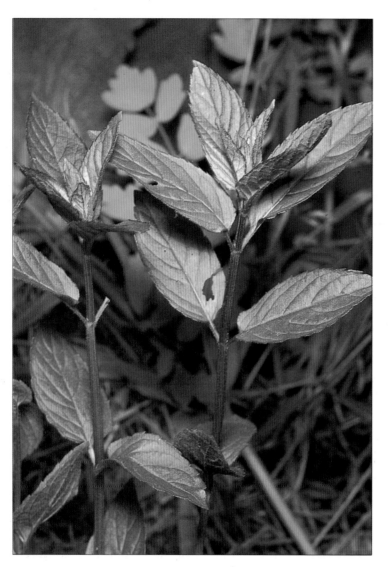

*H*erbal medicine is the use of whole plants, or parts thereof, for the treatment of disease and the maintenance of good health. It is the oldest form of medicine known and has been practiced for thousands of years. Although it is classed as being a "complementary" or "alternative" medicine in most Western developed countries, herbal medicine still remains the only form of medicine that is widely available to most of the world's population.

The history of herbalism is the history of medicine itself. There is even evidence that herbal medicine was practiced before written records began. For instance, in a Neanderthal grave which was excavated in what is now Iraq, pollen was found, indicating that the man who had been buried there was surrounded by flowers. This pollen was subsequently identified and was found to belong to plants which are closely related to the most common medicinal plants which are still widely in use by most Western herbalists today.

# HISTORY AND ORIGINS

The first written record of medicinal herbs comes from China, dating from 2800 B.C., and includes 366 plants. In other parts of the world, as soon as writing was adopted, information about herbs began to be recorded. The Greek physician Hippocrates left a list of 400 plants, many of which, including Elder, Garlic, Hawthorn, Henbane, Juniper and Thyme, are still in use today. Hippocrates is also notable for being what we would now describe as an "holistic" practitioner. He laid much emphasis on treating the whole patient, including physical, mental and emotional states. He saw the role of the physician as helping patients to help themselves, an idea to which we have only recently begun to return.

Holistic thinking received a setback under the system of Galen (A.D. 121-180), the personal physician to the emperor Marcus Aurelius. His system was a very rigid one. He

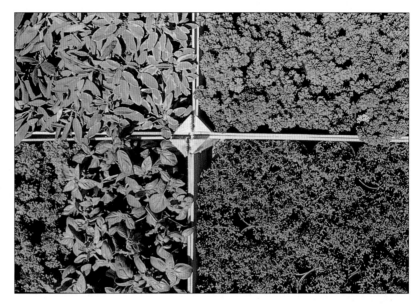

*Above: Parsley, Thyme, Basil and Sage are all culinary herbs. Thyme and Sage are rich in aromatic oils.*

classified plants according to their reaction with the patient's "humors" (choleric, phlegmatic, melancholic or sanguine), and designated a "temperament" for each herb with very strict rules about the conditions that indicated its use.

It was probably during Galen's time that the division began to appear in Western Europe between the "qualified" physician and the traditional healer. The former had

learned Galen's system and knew how the temperament of each plant reacted with the patient's humors; the latter simply knew that a specific plant was good for treating a particular condition. Galen also used inorganic compounds.

In ancient Britain, the native tradition of the Druids was enriched when Greek and Alexandrian knowledge was brought in by the Romans. In the sixth century A.D., the School of Physicians at Myddfai in Wales reflected the holistic approach of Hippocrates rather than the rigid system of Galen. Later on, medicinal herbs were used by monks to treat the sick, and medicinal plants were cultivated in monastery gardens.

There are several famous English herbals but the one with most historical significance was that written by Nicholas Culpeper and published in 1652. He was an apothecary who had achieved notoriety and incurred

## THE DOCTRINE OF SIGNATURES

This is another belief, which is widely held by many cultures. It states that a plant's appearance or characteristics holds a clue to its medicinal use. Thus plants that bear some resemblance to a part of the body might be used for treating disorders of that part. For example, liverworts resemble lobes of liver (albeit green ones) and were used to treat liver disorders. Lungwort (*Pulmonaria*), with its spotty leaves, is said to resemble a diseased lung and was used accordingly. There is no

scientific justification for this but it is interesting and, in some cases, it seems to work. Thus many plants that inhabit damp places, such as Meadowsweet, Birch and Willow, are used for treating rheumatism and arthritis, which are often brought on by damp conditions. Many yellow-flowered plants are useful for treating jaundice and other liver conditions, and an ancient long-lived tree, *Gingko biloba*, has been found recently to be of value in treating some of the problems of old age.

the wrath of the orthodox physicians when, in 1649, he translated their London Pharmacopeia from Latin into English. Thus it could be read and understood by other apothecaries who used it to treat poor people who could not afford a physician's fee.

Culpeper's herbal is significant in two respects:

■ It stressed the use of English herbs.

■ It reintroduced astrology into herbal medicine.

The use of herbs had always been associated with myth and magic to some extent, but Culpeper's timing was unfortunate, coming at a time when medicine was becoming "scientific." The use of inorganic poisons, such as mercury, lead, antimony and arsenic, had been introduced due to the influence of the Swiss-German doctor Paracelsus (1493-1591). Herbal medicine fell into disrepute because of its association with witchcraft and superstition. It was criticized by the Church of Rome and its practitioners were often burnt as witches. One of

## LATIN NAMES

Herbalists often use the Latin names of plants. This avoids the confusion that may arise from the use of common names, which vary between countries and between regions within countries. Thus the same name may be used to describe two unrelated species. The use of Latin names helps to ensure that the correct species is used.

the factors that particularly angered the Church was the knowledge held by "wise women" concerning fertility control and abortion.

Some of the so-called superstition associated with the gathering of herbs for medicine has now received scientific backing. Many plants were gathered at specific times: at sunrise, at dusk or during a particular phase of the moon. It ha been discovered that the alkaloid activity of many plants can fluctuate during the moon's cycle or even over a 24-hour period. For instance, the cardiac glycosides of the Foxglove decompose at night but are reconstituted in the leaves from morning onwards. Hence, it is better to gather them in the afternoon.

### A HERBAL MEDICINE REVIVAL

Throughout the seventeenth and eighteenth centuries, herbal medicine was still used in rural areas, but in the eighteenth century there came a revival in urban areas of Britain, brought by herbalists from America. They were descendants of the Pilgrim Fathers who had taken medicinal plants with them to the New World and, once settled, had learned from native Americans how to use the plants that grew in their adopted land. These were among the plants brought back to England and Europe.

Even today, North American herbs are prominent in the dispensary of a medical herbalist in the UK. For example, Capsicum (hot red pepper) is often used as a circulatory stimulant instead of the native British Horseradish. Nor would European herbalists wish to be without Echinacea for treating infections, or Wild Indigo, Black Cohosh, Golden Seal and many other American herbs.

Today, herbal medicine is a blend of tradition and modern science. Whereas many plants are still chosen on the basis of longstanding tradition passed down through the generations, others are finding new uses (or having their old uses justified) after detailed chemical analysis and clinical trials. Research is being carried out with the aim of increasing the efficacy and safety of herbal medicine while retaining the basic philosophy which stresses the healing properties of the whole plant.

## PHILOSOPHY AND OBJECTIVES

Herbalists aim to treat the person as a whole, using whole plant medicines to stimulate the body's own ability to heal itself. Herbs are chosen carefully to suit the patient as well as to treat the disease condition. Whereas an orthodox drug is a single compound, either isolated from a plant source or (increasingly) synthesized in a laboratory, a herbal medicine contains hundreds or thousands of different compounds. Sometimes it is possible for pharmacologists (who study the physiological activity of drugs) or pharmacognosists (who study plant medicines) to isolate and identify the active constituent(s).

However, herbalists believe that the activity and therapeutic effects of a plant medicine result from the combined action of the many constituents working together. In other words, "the whole is greater than the sum of the parts." There is evidence that this occurs, and a good example is found in Lily-of-the-Valley (*Convallaria majalis*). This plant is used by herbalists to treat heart

## CONDITIONS TREATED BY HERBAL MEDICINE

Herbal medicine can treat almost any condition that patients might take to their doctor. Common complaints seen by herbalists include:

■ Skin problems such as psoriasis, acne and eczema.

■ Digestive disorders such as peptic ulcers, colitis, irritable bowel syndrome and indigestion.

■ Heart and circulatory problems such as angina, high blood pressure, varicose veins and ulcers.

■ Gynecological disorders such as premenstrual syndrome and also menopausal problems.

Other conditions include: arthritis, insomnia, stress, migraine and headaches, tonsilitis, influenza and allergic responses, such as hay fever and asthma.

---

failure. It contains cardiac glycosides which are similar to those found in the Foxglove (*Digitalis spp*) but whereas the compounds in *Digitalis* can be isolated and shown to have pharmacological activity, those in *Convallaria* show very little activity as isolated compounds, but marked activity when combined in the whole plant. Both act to increase the power and force of the heartbeat without increasing the amount of oxygen needed by the heart muscle. *Digitalis* is also used extensively in orthodox medicine.

Another tenet of herbal medicine is that some constituents in the whole plant may "buffer" otherwise harmful side effects. There are plenty of examples of this occurring as detailed here.

■ Many orthodox diuretics (drugs that increase the flow of urine and often used to reduce body water content) have the unwanted side effect of depleting potassium in the body. The common Dandelion (*Taraxacum officinalis*), on the other hand, is an effective diuretic as well as a rich source of potassium.

■ Some orthodox anti-inflammatory drugs, including aspirin, have the unwanted side effect of causing stomach bleeding. Meadowsweet (*Filipendula ulmaria*) contains aspirin-related compounds which reduce inflammation. It is also a valuable antacid in the treatment of heartburn, gastritis and acid indigestion.

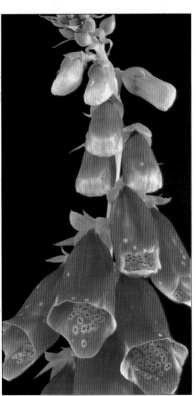

*Foxglove*

## CLASSIFICATION OF HERBAL MEDICINES

Because of their multiple constituents, most herbal medicines have quite a broad spectrum of uses. Nevertheless, they can be classified according to the body systems over which they have the most influence.

■ Nervines are used to treat disorders of the nervous system and include: Oats, St John's Wort, Valerian, Vervain and Skullcap.

■ Circulatory stimulants include: Hawthorn, Rosemary, Gingko, Capsicum, Ginger and Bog Myrtle.

The choice of remedies within each group will depend upon the individual case, since each remedy will have a slightly different emphasis in its action upon the system.

## VISITING A HERBALIST

At present there are various professional organizations of herbalists and many different training courses in different countries. For information on finding a herbalist, turn to the Useful Addresses section at the back of this book.

The first consultation will generally take at least one hour. The herbalist will take notes on your medical history and begin to build up a picture of you as a whole person. He may give you a physical examination or carry out some simple diagnostic tests, such as blood pressure measurement. Herbs may be prescribed in various forms: as teas, liquid tinctures or powdered in a capsule. Creams, ointments, rubbing oils and suppositories may be used in some cases. Treatment may include advice on diet and lifestyle as well as adminstering the herbal medicine itself.

A follow-up appointment will be arranged in two, three or four weeks, depending on the individual herbalist, the patient and the illness concerned. Thereafter any appointments are usually monthly until the problem is resolved. The herbs prescribed may be changed as the patient's condition changes. The duration of treatment is very variable but, as a general rule, chronic, longstanding problems will take longer to resolve than those that are more recent.

Where appropriate, a herbalist may sometimes suggest that a patient's condition should be seen by an orthodox medical physician or another therapist.

The safety record of herbal medicine is good, and side effects are rare. However, it cannot be assumed that because herbs are "natural" that they are always safe. They contain a complex mixture of chemicals and every patient is a unique individual with individual reactions. It is important to stick to the prescribed dose and report any problems to your practitioner.

## SELF HELP

Herbs can be used at home to treat minor ailments and to maintain good health. If you intend to do this a few common sense rules should be observed:

▓ Make sure that you have correctly identified the plant that you want to use. If in doubt seek advice.

▓ Consult a good herbal to make sure you are not exceeding a recommended dose.

▓ When taking plants from the wild, make sure they are plentiful in that area. Do not dig up wild plants. It is illegal in some countries to do so without the consent of the landowner and, anyway, they rarely survive.

### HERBAL TEAS

Herbal teas, infusions or tisanes can be made easily by adding boiling water to the herb in a cup or teapot. Use one or two teaspoonfuls of dried herb per cup (or 1oz to 1 pint), cover with boiling water, then leave for 10-15 minutes before straining and drinking. Teaball infusers are useful for making individual cups.

▓ Do not delay taking serious or persistent health problems to a doctor or qualified practitioner.

### HERBS FOR HOME USE
The following plants are all suitable for home use. They are either easy to grow yourself, common in the wild or readily available in drugstores and natural food stores.

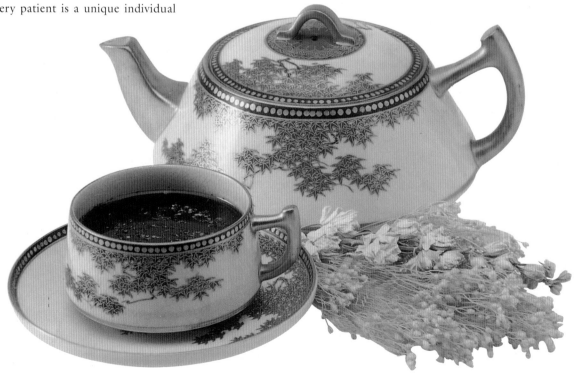

### Nettles

The common stinging nettle (*Urtica dioica*) is one of our most valuable remedies. It only grows in good, rich soil so is often found around compost heaps.

It is a rich source of nutrients including iron and vitamin C, making it ideal for anyone who is "run down" or anemic. It is also helpful in allergic complaints, particularly those affecting the skin, such as childhood eczema. Of course it is also a troublesome weed but worth leaving a corner of the garden for. Gather it wearing stout gloves, take it as a tea or cook it as a vegetable (the "sting" disappears on cooking or drying). Although common in the wild it may be contaminated by traffic fumes, pesticides or passing dogs!

### Marigold

The common Pot Marigold (*Calendula officinalis*) is antiseptic, anti-inflammatory and cleansing. The petals are used in many creams and ointments to sooth irritable skin conditions and insect bites. Make a hot infusion to add to your bath or take as a tea for lymphatic conditions or fungal infections.

### Cleavers, Clivers or Goosegrass

A common plant appearing in early spring. Pick the young leaves and shoots to eat in salads or make a tea. Take it as a spring tonic, particularly for swollen glands and lymphatic

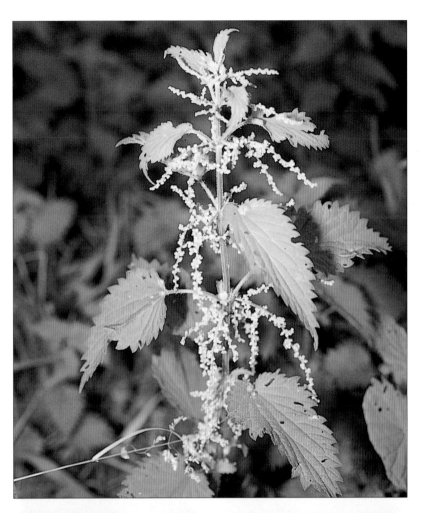

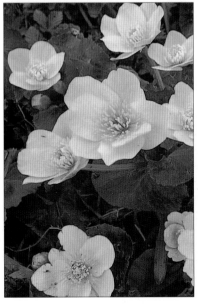

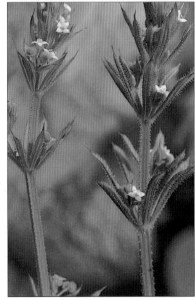

*Nettles (top), Marigold (right) and Goosegrass (far right) are all suitable herbs for home use and can be made into herbal infusions and teas. You can grow them yourself in the garden.*

disorders. It is rich in vitamin C. Later in the year the plant becomes tougher and less palatable. It produces the familiar stickseeds which cling to your clothing as you pass.

## Dandelion

Another plant best picked when young and tender and, like Cleavers, used in salads or tea. The leaves are good for stimulating kidney function, the root is good for the liver. Dried roots can be ground to make a pleasant (and healthy!) coffee substitute.

## Mediterranean herbs

Rosemary, Thyme and Sage are all Mediterranean herbs, rich in aromatic oils. The oils are antiseptic so infusions are good for bathing wounds, gargling when you have a sore throat or using as a mouthwash to treat gum infections.

Taken internally, as teas or in cooking, they have individual prop-

erties. Rosemary is a stimulant, particularly for the head. Try it for headaches, failing memory and falling hair. Thyme is a specific remedy for lung conditions. It also has antifungal properties. Sage reduces body secretions so try it for menopausal sweats or to reduce milkflow when it is time to stop breastfeeding.

## Yarrow

Yarrow is a common and attractive plant, flowering in grassy places during late summer. It has many medicinal uses: it may help in menstrual problems, in disorders of the blood vessels and it is a fever herb. It is rather bitter to take as a tea on its own. A traditional remedy for influenza and feverish colds is a tea made from equal parts of Yarrow, Elderflower and Peppermint. One ounce of the dried herb mixture should be infused in one pint of boiling water and drunk while still hot.

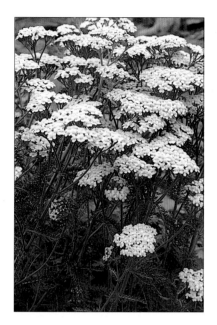

*Unlike Dandelion (below left), Yarrow (above) is rather bitter tasting and should be mixed with Elderflower and Peppermint in teas. Wild Thyme (below) has antifungal properties and is a remedy for lung conditions.*

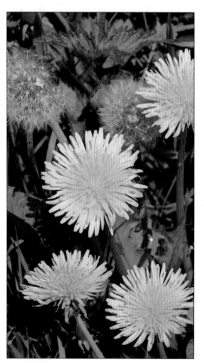

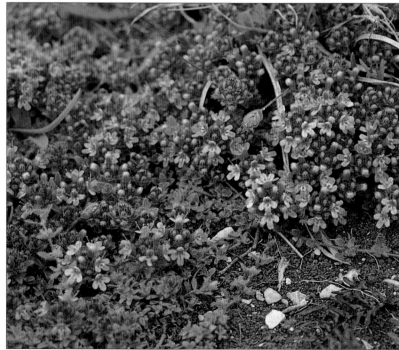

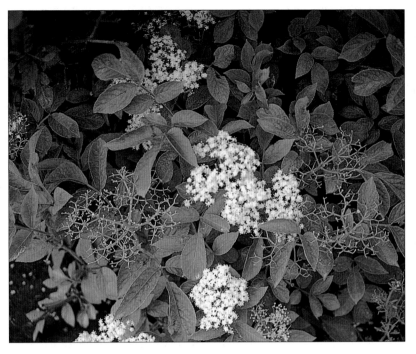

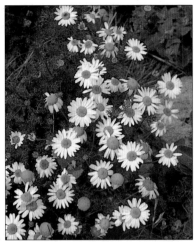

*Elderflower (left) and Chamomile (above) have valuable healing properties. Elderflower is good for treating colds and flu.*

## Elderflower

The Elderflowers in the mixture below make a pleasant, fragrant tea on their own, rich in Vitamin C and good for colds, influenza, sinusitis, asthma and catarrh. Gather them in May and use them fresh, or dry them or freeze them for later use.

### ELDERFLOWER CHAMPAGNE

1¼ pounds sugar
8 pints boiling water
2 tablespoons white wine vinegar
8 large elderflower heads
2 sliced lemons

Dissolve the sugar in the water. Cool and add the vinegar, elderflowers and lemons. Stir and stand for 24 hours. Strain and bottle, releasing the pressure daily if necessary. Store in the dark for three weeks.

## Peppermint

Peppermint contains volatile chemicals, including menthol, which help clear respiratory passages. It is also calming to the digestion.

## Lime flowers

These make another fragrant tea which calms anxiety and has a mild blood-pressure lowering effect.

## Chamomile flowers

These are anti-inflammatory and sedative. They calm stomach irritation and aid sleep.

## Echinacea

This is the Latin name for Purple Cone Flower, an attractive North American plant with several species, all used medicinally. Both the root and the green parts are used and Native American tradition assigns to them many properties. The one most valued by modern herbalists is Echinacea's ability to stimulate the immune system. Thus it is used in treating infections, particularly those of viral origin such as colds and influenza. It may also be taken as a preventative in those whose resistance to infection is impaired. While one must be cautious in making claims for the treatment of life-threatening conditions, there is reason to hope that it may be of value in the treatment of cases of HIV infection and in malignant disease. Echinacea is a bitter herb which may not be palatable as a tea. It can be obtained in the form of tablets and capsules.

### "TEA OF HAPPINESS"

Peppermint: 1 part
Chamomile: 1 part
Lavender: ½ part
Limeflowers: ½ part

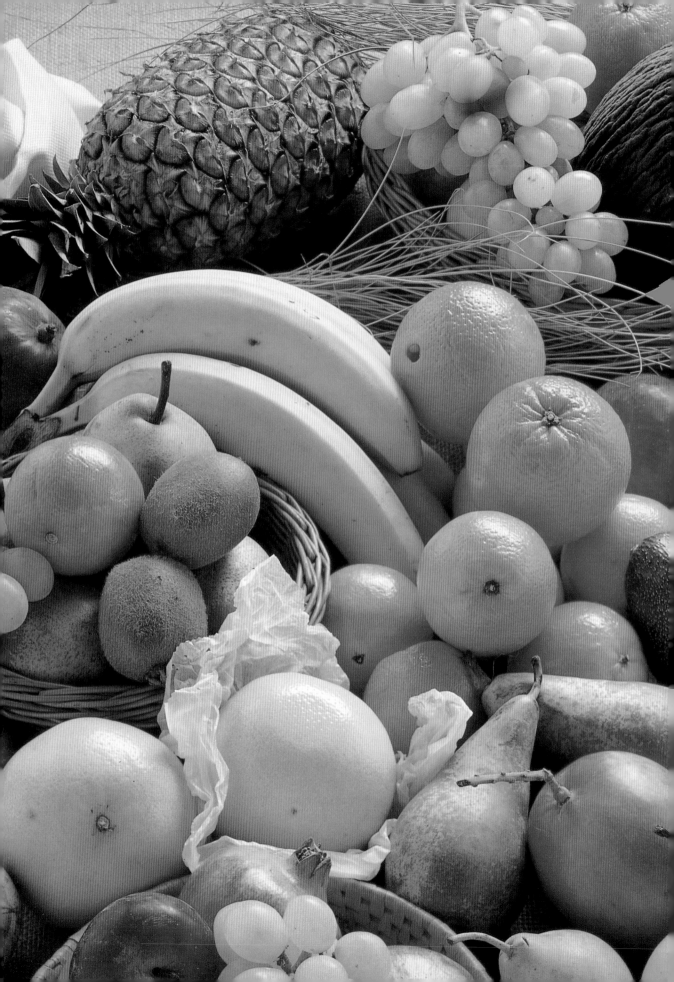

# NUTRITION AND DIET

## PART THREE

*Eating a healthy, nutritionally balanced diet is universally recognized as a way of promoting better health, physically, mentally and emotionally. The food we eat not only maintains health and prevents disease but it can also help us to regain our health. Hippocrates said, "Let food be your medicine and let medicine be your food" and 4,000 years later, this still holds true. Naturopathy is a system of healing which emulates the healing qualities of nature and stresses the importance of the body's natural vitality and capacity to heal itself.*

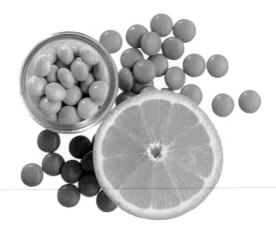

# DIET THERAPIES

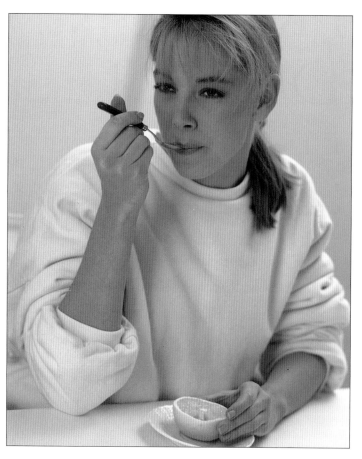

## CHAPTER SEVEN

Nutrition is a part of wholism. "You are what you eat" or "You are what you digest and absorb." These are common maxims in the world of nutrition. These simple adages refer to the belief that the human body is governed in almost every way by the food which it consumes and utilizes. This belief has expanded to such an extent that it has almost become a revolution. There are more positive relationships in scientific literature documenting nutrient deficiencies and nutrient restoration in the etiology and treatment of disease than there are for the drugs used by allopathic medicine to treat disease.

History tells us that changes in the beliefs and practices of medicine usually take a minimum of 40 years from their discovery until their general acceptance and use by practitioners. This is partially due to the difficulty in changing curriculums in medical schools and the reticence of practitioners to engage in an active review of new approaches when they are comfortable in their old methods. However, there is now a growing awareness among the general public as well as nutritionists, scientists and doctors that eating a "healthy" diet, which contains adequate amounts of all the essential nutrients our bodies need to function effectively, can help promote and maintain good health, both physically and mentally, and prevent disease.

## NUTRITION AND WHOLISM

Those who extol the benefits of nutritional awareness have an eager audience willing to participate. This is rooted in a revolution in information and thinking, one in which more and more people feel empowered to exert control over and take more responsibility for their own health. Nutrition is central to all of this, including food choice awareness, vitamins, minerals, amino acids, enzymes, phytochemicals and herbs. The public is discovering that through the manipulation of nutrition not only can we prevent disease but we can also treat many of the ailments known to man. This is diametrically opposed to our prior concept that whenever something

*Below: grains and pulses are a good source of protein, vitamins, minerals and fiber.*

## A BALANCED DIET

People often talk about eating a "balanced" diet, but what does this mean? Usually we choose to eat the food we like rather than the food that is nutritionally best for our health. Our diet is made up of a mixture of different foods, and this is how we obtain a supply of all the nutrients our bodies need. There is no precise prescription for the sort of food and the amounts we must eat in order to stay healthy, and individuals have differing requirements. We need to "balance" our food intake to meet our requirements for different nutrients. This means eating a range of foods from all the major food groups every day.

affects us or our wellbeing, we immediately go to the doctor who then dispenses drugs which only he has knowledge of.

## ALLOPATHIC AND ALTERNATIVE MEDICINE

We must define medicine as to its diverse applications. The use of drugs, and the use of surgery and radiation as treatment modalities have been referred to as "allopathic medicine." The western world has elevated these treatments into the primary healing category and has more or less defined the term "medicine" to mean allopathic medicine. The majority of the world does not employ allopathic medicine as their

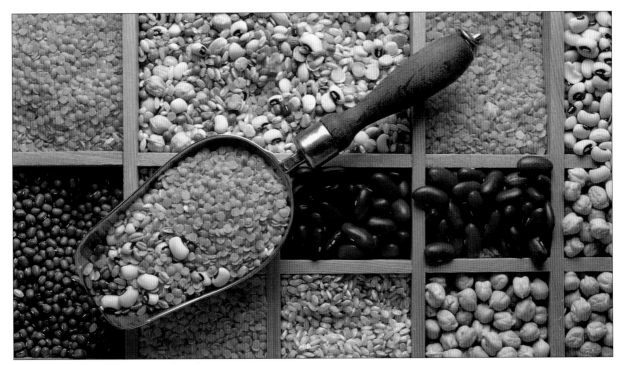

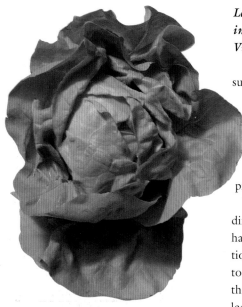

*Left: leafy green vegetables are rich in essential nutrients, especially Vitamins B and C, and minerals.*

surgery which allopathic medicine has specialized and honed to unbelievable heights. But they should bring us to the realization that the term "medicine" encompasses a whole realm of healing practices—and this includes nutrition.

In order to bring some kind of direction to nutrition, several groups have attempted to set up organizations to create ethical standards and to provide on-going education for the practicing nutritionist. This has led to guidelines and parameters which are followed quite widely by most nutritional consultants.

primary healing art; instead they engage in a variety of practices which range from acupuncture to shamanism. Careful examination of the results of such practices brings forth the astounding fact that these other healing practices may sometimes produce results comparable to and sometimes even better than allopathic medicine in chronic degenerative disease.

In no way should such facts deter us from the remarkable advances in

## A HEALTHY DIET

We need to eat a healthy diet and our requirements for specific nutrients will vary at different times in our lives—for example, in childhood, adolescence, pregnancy, menopause and old age. Eating too little or defective digestion or absorption of nutrients can cause deficiency diseases. Therefore it is

important to get the balance right, and we must ensure that we get sufficient but not excessive nutrients from the food we eat.

Most nutritionists would agree that a healthy diet would include adequate amounts of protein, carbohydrate, fat, vitamins, minerals and fiber. It is now widely accepted that it is prudent to reduce our fat intake—both visible and invisible. For instance, invisible fat is present in a wide range of foods, including cookies, cakes, ice cream, pastries and some processed convenience foods.

We should also ensure that we include some unrefined whole-grain cereals in our diet, as these are a valuable source of fiber which helps prevent constipation and may protect against common bowel problems.

It is also argued that a reduction in salt can be beneficial, and while it is acceptable to season our food with salt, we should take care not to eat too many processed and canned foods which often contain large amounts of it. Most people consume at least 50 percent more food than their bodies need, and high salt intakes have been linked in some cases with high

## VEGETARIAN DIETS

Many people are adopting a vegetarian diet and cutting out meat and fish and, in the case of vegans, dairy products, too. If care is taken to design a nutritionally balanced diet with adequate protein, it is possible to obtain a fully satisfactory diet and maintain good health. Lacto-vegetarians who consume dairy products and eggs have no nutritional problems. However, vegans who restrict their food intake to vegetable foods only must ensure that they eat a wide range of foods including whole-grain cereals,

beans and legumes, nuts, fruit, leafy vegetables etc.

Iron deficiency can be a problem as the iron in vegetable foods is not absorbed as well as the iron in meat, so there is a higher risk of becoming anemic. Vitamin B-12, which is found mainly in animal foods, may also be deficient, so vegetarians should take care that they obtain these essential nutrients. For more advice on vegetarianism, you should contact a nutritionist or one of the vegetarian societies and associations.

blood pressure. However, it should be remembered that a certain amount of sodium is essential for our health and wellbeing.

We all need to eat several servings of fresh fruit and vegetables daily (see the Pyramid Diet Table, right). They are good sources of vitamins and minerals and play an important role in health maintenance and disease prevention. As you can see from the pyramid, they should dominate the diet rather than being relegated to minor components.

## DIET SHOULD BE BASED ON THE DIET PYRAMID

### SUGGESTED DAILY FOOD GROUP INTAKE

This illustration offers a well-rounded balance of needed nutrients and can be easily varied to be more in line with individual tastes. Fortunately most nutritionists do not encourage or force radical dietary changes but instead concentrate on the elimina-

## THE PYRAMID DIET

**Fats, oils & sweets**
*use sparingly*

**Milk, yogurt & cheese**
*2-3 servings daily*

**Meat, poultry, fish, dry beans, eggs, nuts**
*2-3 servings daily*

**Bread, cereal, rice, pasta**
*3-5 servings daily*

**Fruit group**
*2-4 servings daily*

**Vegetable group**
*5 servings daily*

tion of refined sugar and flour from foods, and those containing partially or completely hydrogenated oils or margarine, and any foods that are so refined and contain so many additives that it's questionable whether they should be called foods. It's amazing how even small changes in the type of food consumed can increase your feeling of wellbeing.

**REDUCING FAT CONSUMPTION**
Reducing high fat consumption is another admonition which the nutritionist will give. Since fat increases the satiety value of foods, a high-fat diet will often reduce the amounts of cereal grains, vegetables and fruits you consume. Instead of being the mainstay of the diet, these three are relegated to minor intake resulting in a diet which must lead to health

*Left: bread is an excellent source of fiber, protein and B vitamins. It is best to eat wholemeal and whole-grain bread as it contains more fiber.*

## EXERCISE AND FITNESS

Most nutritionists also encourage the physical fitness aspects of health and will weave a lifestyle change into their recommendations. Walking on a regular basis (five times a week) is the most frequent suggestion, but for some the fellowship of group activity, such as dancing, playing tennis, bicycling or aerobic classes, is more acceptable. The more we learn about the effects of exercise, the less it seems we can truly say that one type of exercise is the best when one is only trying to increase motion and cardiovascular activity and not trying to create a marathon runner. In fact, jogging has many casualties among the older set because of the tremendous strain it places upon ligaments, tendons and cartilages which have been comparatively quiescent for many years.

problems. Fat should constitute approximately 20 to 25 percent of the diet with more being allowed in the cold climates and less in the temperate or tropical climates.

### VISITING A NUTRITIONAL CONSULTANT

There are trained nutritional consultants who have either attended classes on campus or received their education on a monitored home study program and have been certified as to their knowledge and are considered professionals in their field. There are also less qualified practitioners who have become enthusiastic about nutrition because of a personal experience and now want to share this with others. The non-professional often is not trained adequately to differentiate between nutritional problems and those problems that should be relegated to a more qualified practitioner of the healing arts. So the first piece of advice is to assure yourself that the person with whom you are going to consult has the background in nutritional training to be worthy of your trust.

### ■ Your first visit

In the first visit, the nutritionist will discuss your diet and general state of health with you, usually in an attempt to get a history of your food habits and your supplementation routine. In addition, you may have to fill out a form which is made up of known signs of nutrient deficiencies in order to determine whether you might have special needs for certain nutrients.

### ■ Deficiency signs

The various deficiency signs of two common nutrients—vitamin B-1 and potassium—are listed opposite. One would imagine that one was looking at clear-cut medical conditions and yet these signs are sometimes found in well-respected nursing and research publications and are classified as nutrient deficiencies and not diseases. One would not necessarily expect a doctor to prescribe vitamin B-1 or potassium to treat the deficiency symptoms listed, but the truth may be that doctors really should consider using such physiological "medicine."

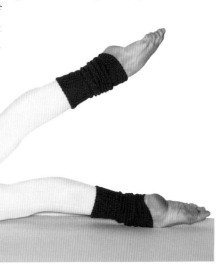

*Below: to achieve good health and a high level of fitness, it is a good idea to combine eating a healthy diet with taking regular exercise. You can choose from a wide range of options ranging from strenuous activities such as running to more gentle stretching and yoga.*

## SIGNS OF VITAMIN B-1 DEFICIENCY

- Heart palpitations
- Enlarged heart
- Diastolic blood pressure over 90
- Hurt all over, but can't pinpoint area
- Lack of elbow and/or knee reflex
- Muscular weakness
- Vague fears, feeling of persecution
- Excessively fatigued
- Loss of appetite
- Forgetfulness

## SIGNS OF POTASSIUM DEFICIENCY

- Swelling of the ankles
- Muscular weakness
- Rapid heartbeat
- Irregular heartbeat
- Nervous
- Dry skin
- Insomnia
- Elevated blood pressure

## DEFICIENT DIETS

The concept of deficiencies in the diet was recently put into perspective by an article published in the United States which was entitled: *Diet Falls Short*. In a survey of diets it was found that:

- 50 percent of people get less than RDA of calcium.
- 80-90 percent get less than RDA of vitamin E.
- 25 percent get less than RDA of vitamin C.
- 25 percent get less than RDA of folic acid.
- 25-50 percent get less than RDA of vitamin A, etc.

This was the result of a massive survey of random citizens of the United States. Considered to be the wealthiest nation in the world with possibly the best supply of a variety of food stuffs, these results act as a warning to all who have subscribed to the myth that food can supply all our needs.

Unfortunately, the appearance of some foodstuffs is sometimes ranked higher than their nutritional content, which may not even be considered. Thus it becomes apparent that food supplementation is very important for people on poor diets, which are deficient in specific nutrients.

To compound this problem it appears that we are not only eating nutrient-deficient diets but we are also in serious need of reconsidering the "recommended daily allowances" of many nutrients. Many research scientists now question the recommended daily requirements and state, for example, that vitamin E may help to prevent heart attacks but never at the present suggested daily amounts. This leads us to believe that the recommended intake of nutrients may be guided by the amount necessary to avoid frank deficiency signs rather than what is needed to promote optimum nutrition.

What is clear is that in order to enjoy good health, you should eat a healthy, nutritionally balanced diet which contains adequate amounts of protein, carbohydrate, fat and all the essential vitamins and minerals. Reducing your consumption of convenience foods, sugar, salt and fat, and increasing your intake of wholegrain cereals, fruit and vegetables will help promote a more healthy eating regime.

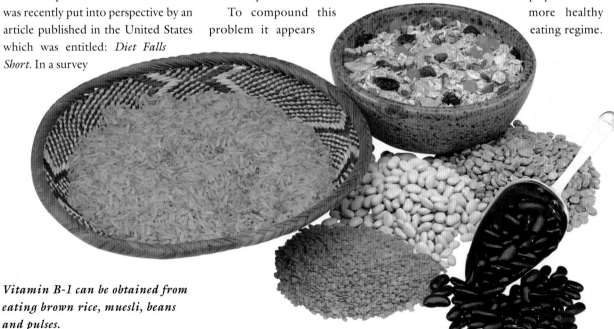

*Vitamin B-1 can be obtained from eating brown rice, muesli, beans and pulses.*

# IS FOOD SUPPLEMENTATION DANGEROUS?

Nowadays many people have concerns, often unwarranted, about the use of food supplements. In general, food supplements have been proven safe by repetitive testing all over the world although it is generally acknowledged that it is difficult to set a "recommended daily allowance," and for all nutritionists to agree on a recommended daily intake of any specific nutrient which is considered to be "safe."

Of all the nutrients, there are only a very few that really need some restriction knowledge. These include the fat-soluble vitamins (A and D) which dissolve in fat and can be stored in the body, as opposed to water-soluble vitamins (e.g. the B group and Vitamin C) which dissolve in water and cannot be stored by the body. Thus excessive intakes of these vitamins are excreted harmlessly from the body.

### ▪ VITAMIN A
This should not be taken in high doses, especially during the first trimester of pregnancy as it has anti-angiogenic properties which might lead to birth defects. On the other hand, a deficiency of Vitamin A during pregnancy might, in some circumstances, lead to birth defects and other problems.

### ▪ VITAMIN D
Excessive intakes of Vitamin D (10,000 IU daily) can cause hyper-calcemia of soft tissues leading to arteriosclerosis. Vitamin D is toxic if taken in excess. However, we need an

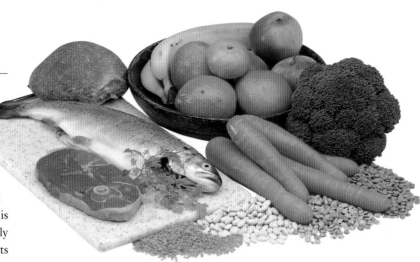

adequate supply for the maintenance of healthy bones. Some research studies have concluded that Vitamin D can help in the prevention of several forms of cancer.

### MODERATION IS BEST
It should be obvious that moderation is a good practice in all things in life, including supplementation. Occasional use of high dosages have not been shown to be harmful and may have an almost miraculous benefit for some people under the proper guid-

*Above: fish, red meat, beans and pulses, carrots and broccoli are good sources of the mineral potassium.*

ance of a nutritionist who can be on the look-out for any untoward effect.

Vitamins and minerals are classed as micro-nutrients because we only need small amounts of them in our daily diet, as opposed to macro-nutrients such as protein and carbohydrate. Vitamins and minerals are measured in units known as micrograms and milligrams.

## SUMMARY

As the interest in self-responsibility for personal health expands, nutrition becomes an obvious avenue to explore for people who care about their health. Science and research support nutritional concepts and the role of nutrition in preventing disease and maintaining good health. The major trend is to learn about nutrition for personal use and evaluate which supplement is best for the individual's needs. More doctors and scientists are recognizing the important role of a nutritionally balanced, healthy diet in promoting and maintaining good health. The probability is that in the near future, diet and food supplementation will be a much larger part of "medicine" than they are today.

# VITAMIN DEFICIENCY SIGNS

## VITAMIN A
▦ Do you catch cold easily?
▦ Do you have a predisposition to infections of the throat and lungs?
▦ Do you have frequent infections of the bladder or urinary tract?
▦ Do you suffer from sinusitis?
▦ Do you often have absesses in the ears?
▦ Do you see poorly in dim light?
▦ Do you have rough, dry, scaly skin?
▦ Do your eyelids become swollen and pus laden?
▦ **Female:** Difficulty in getting pregnant?
▦ **Female:** Have you had a spontaneous abortion?

## VITAMIN D
▦ Do you have poor bone development?
▦ Have you had rickets?
▦ Do you have osteomalacia (soft bones)?
▦ Do you have arthritis?
▦ Do you have an abnormal number of tooth cavities?

## VITAMIN E
**Female:** Have you ever had any spontaneous abortions, uterine degeneration or sterility?
**Male:** Do you have a low sex drive?
▦ Do you have muscular-type problems?
▦ Do you suffer from angina pains?
▦ Have you had a heart attack?

## VITAMIN C
▦ Do you have little pink spots on your skin?
▦ Do you have ruptured blood vessels in either eye?
▦ Do you have inflamed gums?
▦ Is your hair falling out abnormally?
▦ Do your gums bleed when you brush your teeth?
▦ Do you have cartilage problems?
▦ Do you have cataracts?
▦ Do you have excess oil on the skin near the fold of the nose?

▦ In children, restlessness and irritability?
▦ Do you have joint pains?

## VITAMIN B-1
▦ Do you have heart palpitations?
▦ Do you have an enlarged heart?
▦ Do you have a diastolic blood pressure over 90?
▦ Do you hurt all over, but can't pinpoint an area?
▦ Have you lost your elbow and/or knee reflex?
▦ Do you have muscular weakness?
▦ Do you have vague fears or feelings of persecution?
▦ Are you excessively fatigued?
▦ Have you lost your appetite?
▦ Do you suffer from forgetfulness?

## VITAMIN B-2
▦ Do you have cracks and sores in the corners of the mouth?
▦ Do you have a red-purple shiny tongue?
▦ Do you have a sensation of sand on the inside of the eyelids?
▦ Are the whites of your eyes bloodshot?
▦ Are your eyes sensitive to bright light?
▦ Do your eyes get easily tired, do they burn and itch?
▦ Do you have an abnormal number of cavities?

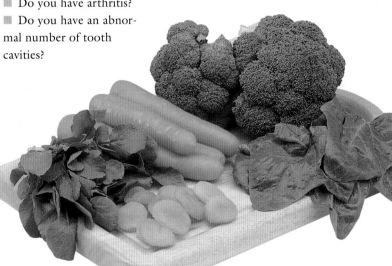

*Green leafy vegetables, carrots and apricots are sources of Vitamin A.*

# VITAMIN DEFICIENCY SIGNS

## NIACIN (NIACINAMIDE)
Do you suffer from chronic inflammation of the skin?
- Have you lost your appetite?
- Do you have canker sores in the mouth?
- Do your hands and/or feet often feel like they are hot?
- Have you ever been diagnosed as a schizophrenic?
- Do you feel like your hands and/or feet go numb quite often?

## VITAMIN B-6
- Are you dizzy often?
- Do you have more than two colds per year?
- Do you suffer from nausea?
- Are you a smoker?
- Do you feel confused?
- Female: Do you suffer from PMS?
- Do you have kidney stones?
- Do you have edema?
- Ever observed a greenish tint to your urine?
- Do you have numbness of hands and/or feet?

## VITAMIN B-12
- Is your tongue often sore?
- Do you have frequent skin inflammations?
- Do you suffer from insomnia?
- Do you have tingling of the extremities?
- Do you have pernicious anemia (diminished reflexes, diminished sensory perception, ataxia, stammering, jerking of limbs)?

## PANTOTHENIC ACID
- Do you have chronic headaches?
- Do you suddenly feel dizzy?
- Do you feel lightheaded when getting up out of a lying or sitting position?
- Does your heart beat fast upon exertion?
- Have you been diagnosed as an arthritic?
- Have you been diagnosed as a hypoglycemic?
- Do you occasionally have a burning sensation of your hands and/or feet?

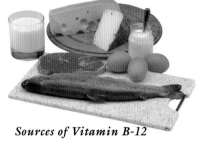

*Sources of Vitamin B-12*

- Do you have periods of deep depression?
- Do you have numbness and any tingling of the hands and feet?

## BIOTIN
- Do you have a sore tongue and dermatitis?
- Do you have loss of appetite and nausea?
- Do you have sleeplessness?
- Do you have muscle pain?
- Do you have low-grade anemia?

## FOLIC ACID
- Do you have macrocytic anemia?
- Did you have a cleft palate?
- Do you have a smooth, very red tongue?

## PARA-AMINO-BENZOIC ACID
- Do you suffer from chronic gastrointestinal disorders?
- Do you have patchy, pigment loss in skin (vitiligo)?
- Are you chronically irritable with periods of depression?
- Do you have Lupu Erythematosis?
- Do you have scleroderma (hardening of skin)?

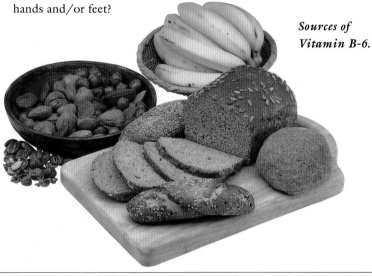

*Sources of Vitamin B-6.*

# MINERAL DEFICIENCY SIGNS

## CALCIUM
- Did you have stunted growth?
- Do you have frequent leg cramps?
- **Female:** Do you have excessive menstruation?
- Are you nervous and irritable?
- Are your teeth crowded, with poor placement in the mouth?

## PHOSPHORUS
- Do you have poor bone and tooth structure?
- Do you have arthritis, pyorrhea or rickets?
- Are you mentally and/or physically fatigued?
- Do you have irregular breathing?

## POTASSIUM
- Do you have swelling of the ankles?
- Do you have muscular weakness?
- Do you have rapid heartbeat?
- Do you have an irregular heartbeat?
- Do you consider yourself nervous?
- Do you have dry skin?
- Do you suffer from insomnia?

## SODIUM
- Do you have a dry mouth and dry skin?
- Do you have chronic indigestion?

## MAGNESIUM
- Do you think you have irritable nerves?
- Do you think you have irritable muscles?
- Do you have muscle cramps?
- Do you have nervous tics and twitches?
- Do you have an irregular heartbeat?
- Do you have convulsions and/or seizure?

## IRON
- Do you suffer from anemia?
- Do you have unusual shortness of breath?
- Are you a vegan?
- Have you lost your appetite?

## ZINC
- Are you readily fatigued?
- Are you very susceptible to infections?
- Do skin wounds heal slowly?
- Do you have a poor appetite?
- **Male:** Do you have a swollen prostate?

## IODINE
- Do you have cold hands and feet?
- Do you have dry hair?
- Are you a slow starter in the morning?
- Do you tend to gain weight easily?
- Do you have a goiter?

## MANGANESE
- Do you have weak ligaments and tendons?
- Do you have a neuromuscular disease?

## SELENIUM
- Do you have cancer?
- Do you have atherosclerosis (heart disease)?
- Are you prematurely aged?

## VANADIUM
- Do you have diabetes or a tendency to it?

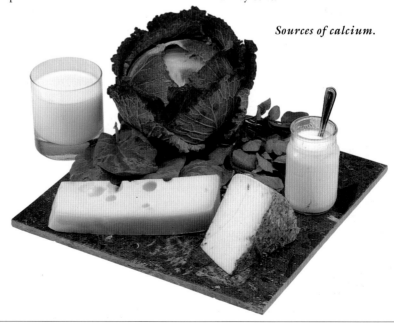

*Sources of calcium.*

# SPECIAL DIETS

Most modern nutritionists would recommend that a person should eat a varied "healthy" diet, which provides all the essential nutrients we need for the proper functioning of our bodies. They advocate that foods from all the major food groups should be eaten every day.

Special emphasis is put on eating fruit, vegetables and whole-grain cereals. This message was reinforced by the World Health Organization's report on diet, nutrition and the prevention of chronic disease. What is most important is that our diets should provide an adequate and constant supply of all the essential nutrients.

However, there are still nutrient deficiencies in certain groups of people due to their:

▓ Failure to consume adequate food, e.g. the elderly and some people on slimming diets.

▓ Tendency to eat the wrong foods, e.g. teenagers and people who consume a large amount of highly refined, processed foods which are high in sugar and fats.

Below are outlined three examples of the many diet therapies which have been conceived. We do not recommend that you follow these—they are given only as examples of the wide range of alternative diet therapies to the "healthy' one that is outlined in this chapter.

## THE ATKINS DIET

The Atkins Diet is the result of Robert C. Atkins, M.D., then specializing in bariatrics or the treatment of overweight problems, seeking the ideal diet. The basis of this diet is the induction of "ketosis" which is the burning of stored fat for energy. His clinical observations led him to publish that such a diet also worked for a variety of other problems and particularly cardiovascular, arthritis and a host of chronic degenerative diseases. The diet was referred to as the "Atkins Low Carbohydrate Diet." The following is an outline of food regulations on this diet:

▓ **Animal foods (meat, fish, fowl, shellfish)**

All are allowed, unless sugar, MSG, corn syrup, cornstarch, flour, pickling, nitrites or other preservatives are use in the preparation.

▓ **Fats and oils**

Despite the furor over "high-fat diets," many fats, especially certain oils, are essential to good nutrition. We must include a source of gamma-linolenic acid and omega-3 oils (salmon oil, flaxseed oil). Olive oil is valuable. The best vegetable oils are walnut, soybean, sesame, sunflower and safflower oils, especially if they are labeled "cold pressed." Butter is always superior to margarine. Mayonnaise is permitted. The fat that is part of the meat or fowl you eat is permitted. For salad dressings, use the desired oil plus vinegar or lemon juice and spices. Grated cheese, chopped eggs or bacon may be added.

▓ **Cheese (hard, semisoft, aged, yellow)**

Examples are Swiss, American, Cheddar, Brie, Camembert, Blue, Mozzarella, Gruyère, etc. Goat's cheeses are fine. Fresh cheeses: Cottage, Farmer, Pot, Ricotta and Soybean cheese (Tofu). Avoid "diet" cheeses, cheese spreads or cheese foods. From three to sixteen ounces per day is allowed according to your doctor's recommendation.

▓ **Eggs**

Permitted without restriction.

▓ **Salad vegetables**

Leafy greens (lettuce, romaine, parsley, collards, endive, spinach), mushrooms, cucumbers, celery, radishes, peppers, bean sprouts. From two to six cupfuls per day according to your doctor's recommendation.

▓ **Other permissible vegetables**

Asparagus, broccoli, string or wax beans, cabbage, beet greens, cauliflower, chard, eggplant, kale, kohlrabi, mushrooms, tomatoes, onions, spinach, peppers, summer squash, zucchini, okra, pumpkin, turnips, avocado, bamboo shoots, bean sprouts, water chestnuts, snow pea pods, sauerkraut. This use is defined as part of the "Salad vegetables" and use is governed by those restrictions.

▓ **Sweeteners**

Sorbitol, honey, fructose, lactose, sucrose, maltose, dextrose are not allowed.

▓ **Liquids**

The best liquids are water and herbal teas. Spring and mineral waters are preferred to tap water or club soda but all are allowed. Herbal teas should be free or caffeine, sugar or barley.

▓ **Alcohol**

Not permitted.

**Note:** Although Dr. Atkins was criticized by many, he has stood firm because of his thousands of clinical success stories. Recent findings document that his moderately high protein and fat diet is not bad advice and his severe curtailment of sugars is beneficial to many.

## THE MACROBIOTIC DIET

The macrobiotic diet, also known as the Zen macrobiotic diet, consists mainly of cereal products with the major one being rice. Individuals following the diet must not eat any sugar, meat, or animal products and must restrict their intake of fluids. There are many variations of the macrobiotic diet which range from very strict to somewhat moderate.

The principle of the macrobiotic diet that some doctors and nutritionists object to is the restriction of fluids in whatever form. The body desperately requires almost three-and-a-half pints of fluid per day to properly carry on metabolism. Restriction of fluid can create serious problems over a period of time.

The concept of not consuming sugars, fatty meats or anything artificial certainly can apply to all those seeking a better eating style. However, the more rigid macrobiotic regimes are seriously deficient in many vitamins, minerals and amino acids.

It probably would hurt no one who is moderately healthy to follow the diet for two weeks or less, provided they consumed at least three-and-a-half pints of fluid every day. This could have certain detoxifying benefits and give the digestive tract a complete new menu to break down. Long-term adherence could create major deficiencies even in the healthy person.

## THE GERSON DIET

The Gerson Diet is a therapeutic diet for the treatment of cancer and was the brainchild of Max Gerson, M.D., a German physician who fled the ethnic and political unrest in his native country and established a practice in the United States. Dr. Gerson was one of the few of his era who made any correlation between diet and illness, particularly cancer. His original and probably most valid concept was that the level of potassium must be increased in the body and the level of sodium decreased. He also advocated the use of natural foods, saying "it's safer to use foods in the most natural form, combined and mixed by nature and raised, if possible, by an organic gardening process, thus obeying the laws of nature."

### Structure of the diet

Dr. Gerson felt that 75 percent of a person's diet should include the following:

▦ **All kinds of fruits,** mostly fresh and some prepared in different ways: fruit salads, cold fruit soups, mashed bananas, raw grated apples, applesauce, etc. Using nothing from cans, the recommended fruits are apples, grapes, cherries, mangoes, peaches, oranges, apricots, grapefruit, bananas, tangerines, pears, plums, melons, papayas and persimmons. Pears and plums are more easily digested when stewed. Dried fruit may be eaten if unsulfured, such as apricots, peaches, raisins, prunes or mixed fruit. Forbidden are all berries, pineapple, nuts, avocados and cucumbers.

▦ **All vegetables** are recommended to be freshly prepared, some stewed in their own juices and others either raw or finely grated, such as organically grown carrots, cauliflower or celery, vegetable salads and soups. Some dried vegetables were permitted, but not frozen ones. Potatoes should be baked in their own skin, never fried but can be boiled. Salads of green leafy vegetables are desirable. Recommended vegetables are: carrots, peas, tomatoes, Swiss chard, spinach, string beans, Brussels sprouts, artichokes, beets cooked with apples, cauliflower and red cabbage, all prepared without salt and in their own juices, not cooked in water.

▦ **Unsalted bread** from whole rye four or whole wheat flour or a combination of both is allowed. Oatmeal should be used freely. Buckwheat is acceptable.

▦ **Brown sugar,** honey, maple sugar and maple syrup are optional.

▦ **Dairy products** such as pot cheese and other cheeses which are not salted are acceptable as are buttermilk and yogurt.

▦ **Preserved or salted meats** are not to be used.

# NATUROPATHIC MEDICINE

## CHAPTER EIGHT

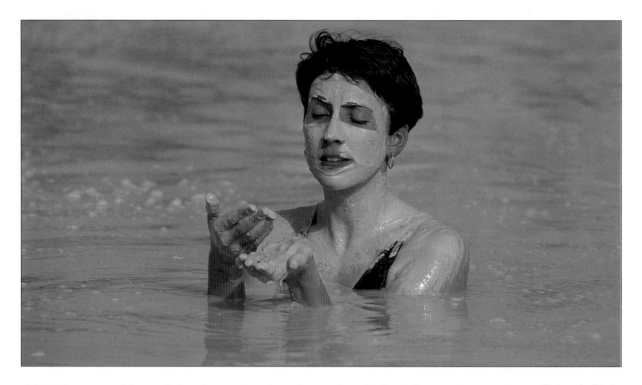

*N*aturopathic medicine is an American invention derived from a European tradition, which
came together at the turn of the twentieth century. Its antecedents emerge from prehistoric
times. In fact, several of the methods commonly in use in naturopathic medicine today are employed
by animals, and are instinctive to the pursuit of healing after injury or disease. These include
fasting, hydrotherapy, botanical medicine and other techniques.

    The immediate precursors to modern naturopathic medicine include European and native
American herbalism, the Physical Culture and health food movement of the late nineteenth
century, the hydrotherapy tradition popularized by Preisnitz and Kneipp of Europe, the emerging
homeopathic medicine of Europe and America, the natural hygiene movement, the public health
movement, and the mechanotherapy and physiotherapy developments of the nineteenth and early
twentieth centuries. Elements of these traditions literally came together in convention about 100
years ago, invented a new medicine, and called it "naturopathy."

## DEVELOPMENT AND GROWTH

This new system of healing thrived. It rapidly became popular in America and Germany, and by the 1920s had 22 colleges in the United States. First licensed in California in 1906, by 1950 it was a licensed medical practice in 26 states. But by 1955 those were reduced to eight states, primarily as a result of a major "anti-quackery" campaign by the AMA, and no school was offering the ND degree any longer. The profession was considered obsolete.

To prevent it dying out, several of the practitioners in the Northwest chartered a new college through the Oregon legislature, the National College of Naturopathic Medicine, in 1956. In the late 1960s, interest in "alternative" medicine began to increase, and the school began to grow. A decade later there was enough interest to found a second school in Seattle, followed by a

third in Toronto in the early 1980s, and a fourth opened in Arizona in the fall of 1993. Currently, there are a number in planning around the country, and legislative efforts toward licensure are proceeding in at least 18 states.

Naturopathic medicine is now re-emerging. It is in a state of dramatic resurgence, invigorated by a society hungry for relief from the ills common to modernity, especially the chronic and degenerative problems, and seeking solutions which are health generating rather than drug based. In this climate, the naturopathic medical profession has found a renewal.

*Below: naturopaths believe that it is important to eat a balanced healthy diet that contains all the essential nutrients we need for maintaining good health.*

## PARADIGMS OF MEDICAL THOUGHT

### THE CONVENTIONAL PARADIGM

The practice of what the popular press is increasingly referring to as allopathic medicine, the medicine of the AMA, is based upon a simple and elegant paradigm: "the diagnosis and treatment of disease." This describes in a succinct way what the doctor is expected to do. He or she determines the specific nature and name of the disease process that ails the patient (diagnosis) and then brings to bear the various tools or weapons that science and experience have provided to eliminate the disease from the body (treatment).

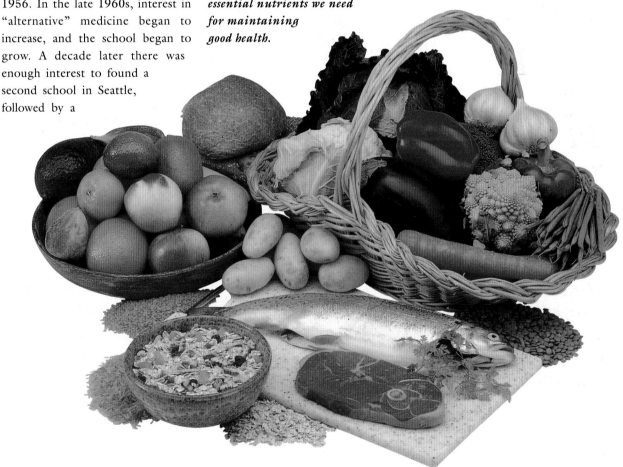

This is taken as self-evident and unquestioned. Upon analysis, however, it contains at least three assumptions:

1 That there are distinct disease entities which exist separately from the individuality of the patient.

2 That these disease entities can be identified.

3 That these disease entities can be removed from the patient through treatment.

In this system, the doctor identifies the disease, and then "does battle" with it, almost as if the patient were a neutral field upon which this battle takes place. The "weapons" that the doctor uses include drugs, surgery, chemotherapy, radiation, and a few other techniques.

This system of approaching illness works well in certain circumstances, less well in others, and not at all in some. For instance, acute bacterial infection has demonstrated the excellence of conventional medicine, in eliminating some of the major disease killers of the nineteenth century, such as pneumonia and tuberculosis. Through the meticulous pursuit of microbiological science, these maladies were identified to be due to specific microorganisms.

Further research, and a bit of luck and providential intervention, provided new tools in the form of antibiotics which could kill these microorganisms, yet not harm the body, at least not in a significant way. A shot of penicillin in the bottom, and the pneumonia clears up as the pneumococcus bacilli die from the effects of the antibiotic. Tuberculosis is a bit more difficult, but a long-term regimen of Rifampin, Streptomycin and Isoniazid, and the scourge of the 1800s clears up, and the patient is left disease free.

*Left: meditation and yoga are sometimes recommended by naturopaths to aid good health and general wellbeing.*

There are increasingly, however, problems that do not respond to this approach. The most obvious, perhaps, is CFIDS, more commonly known as chronic fatigue immune deficiency syndrome. In this increasingly widespread phenomenon, a person, often functioning at a high level of productivity, suddenly loses all energy, is often unable to get out of bed, succumbs to flus and colds much more than ever before, and develops a pattern of illness involving painful lymphatic swelling, frequent sore throats, headache, chronic debilitating fatigue, and immune deficiency, which may last for years.

In this problem, which not all physicians recognize (in part because it does not fit the model

## THE ELEGANT PARADIGM

Arthritis, multiple sclerosis, and similar "auto-immune" diseases present a similar problem for the paradigm. Although diagnosis is much more certain, treatment is not. There is usually nothing to kill, so the goal becomes suppression of symptoms. In the case of arthritis, all of the drugs used to suppress the symptoms carry consequences. The most potent drug, prednisone, causes osteoporosis, immune deficiency, poor wound healing, mild psychosis, and other problems with long-term use, and such use does not cure the disease. It may decrease the severity of symptoms, but even that only temporarily. Again, the elegant paradigm breaks down.

described above), there is sometimes a recognizable chronic viral infection, such as Epsteint-Barr or Cytomegalyovirus, but often not. And no treatment is consistently helpful. There is nothing to kill. In this problem, the disease is vague and diagnosis is uncertain. There is no recognized or effective treatment. So how is the doctor supposed to function? He or she is not able to "diagnose and treat the disease."

## THE NATUROPATHIC PARADIGM

Naturopathic medicine has a different paradigm, and operates upon different assumptions. In naturopathic medicine the emphasis is upon health restoration rather than the disease treatment.

The naturopathic physician does not do battle with a disease entity. Instead, he relies upon the healing wisdom, vital energy and intelligence of the organism to restore normal and healthy function. The work of the naturopathic physician is to invoke healing by helping patients to create or recreate conditions for health to exist within them. Health will occur where the conditions for health exist, and disease is the product of conditions which allow it to exist. To accomplish healing, naturopathic physicians study health and its determinants, evaluate the patient relative to that which determines health, and advise upon the changes which would create more healthy conditions for the organism. As necessary, they stimulate the process of restoration through a system of therapeutic interventions, which are rationally applied, and have the capacity to do this while inducing

no further harm to the body.

It begins with an observation of the organism in nature, that it constantly seeks to nourish and restore itself, and to protect and heal itself. Paracelsus, the great iconoclastic physician of the sixteenth century, taught this in response to the formalized and dogmatic medicine of his time. He would say that the snake is a better physician than any doctor, for no doctor can heal even a cut, while any snake will heal itself if left alone to do so. Discussed in a different way, a wound heals by "first" or by "second intention." The wound will heal if the edges are reoppposed, with stitches, or if left open. The first way it will heal more rapidly, with less scarring. The second way, it will heal from the bottom up, with quite a bit more scarring. Either way, the healing occurs. It is the nature of the body to heal; the physician, at best, can assist the process.

## A MODEL OF HEALING

The healing process can be modelled very generally through a simple diagram (above right). As the person moves down this diagram recognizable pathology appears, as if these pathological events were entities rather than an organism in the process of challenge, reaction, and degeneration.

In this model, consider a person demonstrating normal health. There may be an optimal health which sits above the normal, but attainment of that is unusual, and most people begin with a normal degree of health. Something, usually a multiplicity of things, disturbs this normal state.

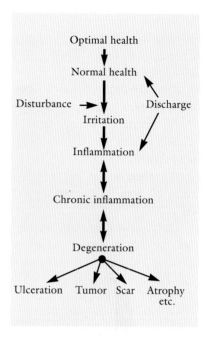

This can be any number of things, such as dietary factors, trauma, exposure of various types, stresses, emotional disturbances, etc. If the disturbance is severe enough, tissue will become irritated. When tissue is irritated, it will generate an inflammatory process.

Inflammation is caused by the release of several chemicals from injured or irritated tissues, such as kinins, leukotrienes, prostaglandins, etc. These chemicals cause several events to occur. Among these are vasodilation, increased vascular permeability, chemotaxis, diapedesis, nerve stimulation, and so forth. These are generally experienced by the patient as the cardinal signs of inflammation: heat, redness, swelling, and pain.

Upon simple analysis, these can be seen to be intelligent and healing phenomena. The increased blood flow from vasodilation, the increased vascular permeability, the increased availability of white blood cells, etc.,

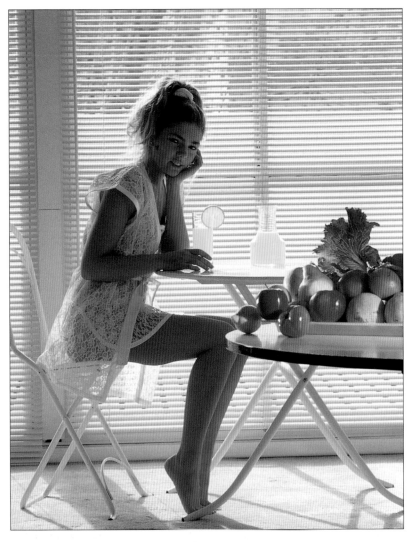

result in the symptoms of inflammation. The increased blood flow brings increased oxygen, increased numbers of white blood cells, and other healing elements into the disturbed area. These are the front-line healing processes which the body employs. They are obviously intelligent and wise things for the body to do to heal itself. This is an example of what is meant by *vis medicatrix* nature.

If the disturbance is single, or short lived, these processes will bring the body, or the involved tissues, back to a normal state. The inflammation

*Above: naturopaths recommend a healthy diet and may even advocate a detoxifying 24-hour "juice-only" fast initially.*

will be followed by a discharge and then by resolution. This can most easily be seen with the common cold.

Most of us have experienced this phenomenon. It begins with a degree of fatigue and malaise, followed by a sore throat, perhaps a fever, and proceeds through a cough, runny nose, and the whole process resolves in a week or two: disturbance, inflam-

mation, discharge, resolution. These are variations which may involve facial sinuses, headache, various degrees of respiratory system involvement, etc.

### Causes and healing processes

At the root there are causes. The common cold is not a disease entity; it is a healing process. Most commonly, the causes are a multiplicity of factors involving the various aspects of life habits. The person is living in such a way that he is accumulating physical and/or emotional disturbances. Diet and digestion are central, as the basic causes of "toxemia," combined with stress, which also impairs digestion. The person hurries around, worries about finances, or relationships, eats inappropriately, doesn't digest well, accumulates a level of metabolic toxins and irritants from poor digestion that begins to interfere with function, and then is subjected to another stress, like a change in the weather.

A cold ensues, which requires the organism to rest and clean out some of the toxemia. Stress levels are reduced, digestive capacity is increased, discharge takes place in some form, and restoration occurs. The worst thing one could do would be to suppress the process with drugs, which interfere with the process of inflammation, discharge and recovery.

## THE ORIGIN OF CHRONIC DISEASE

If any process of acute, restorative inflammation is suppressed, usually by drugs, the disturbing factors persist. The level of toxemia grows. Function is increasingly disturbed, and inflammation becomes more persistent or recurrent. This is the origin of chronic disease. As disturbing factors persist and as the natural inflammatory response is suppressed, the disturbing factors penetrate more deeply into the organism, and thus chronic inflammation is the obvious response. Which tissues become involved will depend upon inherited weaknesses, acquired weaknesses and mechanical stresses, the nature of the specific toxins, etc.

Consider arthritis as an example. Arthritis in general is an inflammatory disease characterized by pain and degeneration. Cause is not conventionally understood, and conventional treatment is directed at reducing the pain and inflammation, which is partially successful, but the various treatments (drugs) generally create their own pathology, which may become devastating, including immune suppression, osteoporosis, ulceration of the gut, etc.

Following the naturopathic model presented above, the physician works with the patient to identify and remove or ameliorate the causes of toxemia, primarily found in diet and life-stresses. The patient is advised and helped to establish more healthful habits, improve digestion, and, if necessary, stimulate the self-healing potential, or act to overcome the obstacles to it through the therapeutic modalities of hydrotherapy, homeopathy, acupuncture, manipulation, botanical medicine, specific nutrition, etc. What one can expect to see is the rapid improvement of the chronic inflammation and the decrease of pain. In fact, this is what is usually seen. And it occurs rapidly and almost inevitably.

## TOXEMIA

Toxemia, of course, is the inappropriately high level of metabolic waste products and exogenous toxins in the blood. Most of it is due to the bacterial production of such toxins generated by their metabolism of poorly digested dietary elements in the large intestine. One simple example of this is the inappropriate bacterial degradation of phenlyalinine in the large intestine in which phenol is generated. Hundreds of these reactions occur generating hundreds of different toxins. These products are absorbed into the blood, become a cause of tissue irritation and thereby the physical basis of most chronic inflammation, and increase one's susceptibility to acute disease. This is the most common "disturbance" in the model described above.

Maldigestion is caused by eating foods which are inherently not well digested by a particular body, by

## CASE STUDY

Consider the case of a woman suffering with a recalcitrant dermatitis, who sought cure rather than more cortisone. First, a diet designed to improve digestion to decrease the toxemia was recommended. Any chronic skin condition is simply a vicarious elimination of toxins through the skin, which are irritating the skin and causing inflammation.

Second, constitutional hydrotherapy was then applied to improve digestion and drive the healing process forward. Third, a simple herbal digestive tonic as an adjunct to improve stomach and intestinal function. After several days of treatment she began to feel better in some ways. She reported more energy, feeling lighter, sleeping better, though her skin got a bit worse. This is typical. She was improving from the center, outward, with an increased discharge through the skin. She was given a homeopathic remedy to help with some discomfort. After about three weeks, much to her surprise, she began to see better. She was also suffering from retinitis pigmentosa.

When she began with the naturopathic physician, both she and the doctor knew that the retinitis was incurable. That is not why she came to see him. She wanted help with her skin. She was originally led up to the doctor's office by a friend; she could not see well enough to come alone. But now she was starting to see better. After several weeks, she was able to see the features of the doctor's face, which previously had been obscure, and to read large print books. She could come to the office alone.

What happened? The treatment was not directed at her eye disease. They were not treating her diseases, her skin condition or her eye problem, *per se*. They were treating her, to improve function and restore health. Her body was able to improve the retinitis condition and to reverse some of the blindness. What had been done was to remove causes of disturbed function and stimulate the self healing potential. The result was that the patient's health improved, following the lines earlier described in the diagram, including an increased discharge through the skin, followed by a resolution.

inappropriate food selection or preparation, by overeating or other inappropriate eating patterns, and by stress. Excess stress or unmanaged stress causes increased adrenal activity, which decreases circulation to the digestive system through the mediation of cortisol and adrenalin. The digestive processes are heavily dependent upon free and appropriate circulation of blood to function properly during the active phases. Adrenalin and cortisol, intrinsic or extrinsic, will reduce this circulation and thereby reduce the effective functioning of digestion. As poorly digested food passes through the digestive tract, it is subject to the bacterial action, i.e. fermentation and putrefaction, described above.

**The process of disease**

Stress and dietary choices determine toxemia. Toxemia disturbs cellular function and results in inflammation. Other factors may disturb normal function: exogenous toxins, climactic or other exposure including pathologic bacteria or virus, physical injury, negative family history, etc. Cellular irritation results in inflammation. If the disturbance is singular and short-lived, the inflammation will return the body to a normal state. If the disturbance persists, the inflammation becomes persistent, and over time may cause degenerative changes. Suppression of inflammation will result in a deepening of the effect of the disturbing factors, resulting in the development of disease deeper in the organism, i.e. affecting more centrally important systems or organs.

To reverse this process, one removes the disturbing factors, or ameliorates them, and the process will reverse. If some suppression has occurred, or if the disease has deeply penetrated or damaged the organism, there will likely be a return of acute inflammation as the organism moves back toward health. This is the "healing reaction" or "healing crises." This process of healing is the reverse of the process of disease. It is the inherent nature of the organism to do this, and this has been observed and reported upon over many centuries, beginning with Hippocrates, and then proceeding through Galen, Paracelsus, Ibn Senna, Sydenham, Preissnitz, etc. This process is the theoretical basis of naturopathic medicine.

## THE HIERARCHY OF THERAPEUTICS

In facilitating the process of healing, the naturopathic physician seeks to use those therapies which are most efficient and which have the least potential to harm the patient. The concept of harm includes suppression of natural healing processes, including inflammation and fever. These precepts, which are coupled to an understanding of the process of healing, result in a therapeutic hierarchy. This hierarchy is a natural consequent of how the organism heals. Therapeutic modalities are applied in a rational order, determined by the nature of the healing process.

### THE HEALING PROCESS

If one examines the healing process, one can come to an understanding of appropriate therapeutic

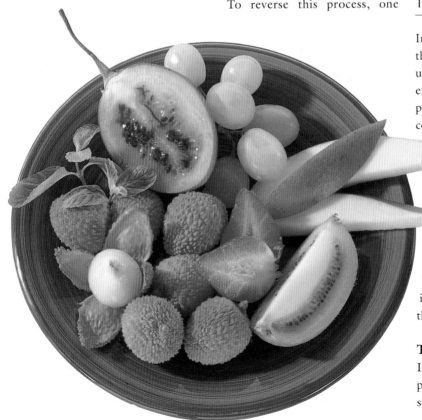

intervention and its natural order. This process is defined by four principles as follows:

1 Re-establishing the basis for health.
2 Stimulation of the vital force.
3 Tonification and nutrition of weakened systems.
4 Correction of structural integrity.

First, the physician must identify the nature and causes of whatever is disturbing the organism, resulting in the symptoms presented. The physician will then advise or otherwise work with the patient to remove or ameliorate the disturbing factors. The first intervention will include at least three therapeutic elements:

1 Talking with the patient (counseling).
2 Dietary and nutritional assessment and modification.
3 Stress assessment and modification.

These three elements generally manifest as dietary changes and other lifestyle modification, including exercise prescription. They may also require specific attention to psycho-spiritual dysfunction.

The second part of therapeutic intervention is that which seeks to move the process "upward," therapies designed to stimulate the healing process. This would begin with those therapies which most generally, most gently and most effectively stimulate the healing process, and, if needed, proceed toward those which are more

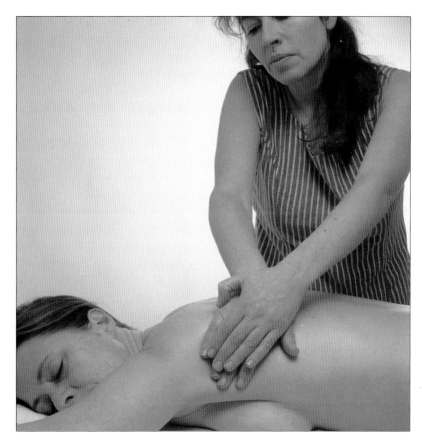

*Above: naturopathy can be used successfully in conjunction with many other forms of alternative medicine including therapeutic massage.*

## CASE STUDY

A first year student from a National College in the U.S. consulted with one of her teachers because a sprained ankle would not heal. She was in a state of chronic fatigue and subject to frequent headaches. She could not think or study well. She was frequently ill. She had taken "tons" of immune-enhancing herbs, such as echinacea, which, she said, only made her worse. And nothing seemed to help her ankle.

A diet was prescribed for her based upon improving digestion and removing food intolerance. She began a series of hydrotherapy treatments. She began to feel better and think more clearly. Then she got "the flu." Her body temperature, which was "normally low" began to rise. As she continued with the hydrotherapy treatments, she developed a fever. She went through three days of nausea, vomiting and diarrhea. At the end of this period of discharge, her body temperature was 98.6 degrees, and she reported feeling better than she could remember. Although this intense discharge is unusual, this is a classic example of the model that is presented above: chronic disease → acute inflammation → discharge → normalization.

specific, more invasive, more potentially harmful, more potentially suppressive, etc. A natural hierarchy results from an examination of potential therapies *vis-à-vis* the above parameters. In my experience, such a hierarchy presents as follows:

## 1 Re-establishing the basis for health

This is most efficiently accomplished through constitutional hydrotherapy: a method designed to stimulate circulation to the digestive and eliminative organs, stimulate the nervous system, the function of the digestive organs, and the "vital force." This treatment is applied similarly to everyone, i.e. it is not specific, and constitutes the most pure form of general stimulation of the VMN.

## 2 Specific stimulation of the vital force

■ Homeopathy: a patient specific system of stimulation of the "vital force."

■ Acupuncture: this is also a patient specific system of stimulation and balancing, but more invasive than homeopathy.

## 3 Tonification and nutrition of weakened systems

■ Glandular and protomorphogen supplementation: a system of providing specific nutrition and stimulation to the various organs and tissues of the body.

■ Botanical medicine: this is an organ specific system of stimulating or normalizing function, with a potential for suppression or toxic reaction.

■ Therapeutic exercise: specific exercise prescriptions which are designed to strengthen weaknesses or enhance circulation and mobility.

■ Physiotherapy: this is an organ specific system of stimulating function which applies electro-

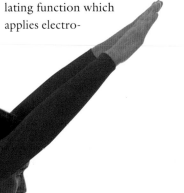

magnetic or mechanical forces to the organism.

■ Specific nutrition through vitamin and mineral supplementation, principally used as a form of pharmacology.

■ Pharmacology: the use of drugs, natural or synthetic, to control function, which generally carry toxic manifestations and the greatest suppressive potential.

## 4 Correction of structural integrity

■ Manipulation: a specific system of force applied to reintegrate structure, primarily to spinal vertebrae.

■ Surgery: the most invasive therapy, with the highest potential for irreversible harm, reserved for repair, emergency, and as a last resort.

The specific placement of therapies in this "hierarchy" may be debatable, but it is based upon an increasing potential for harm, the level at which they work in the organism (e.g. more general toward more specific), and their potential for stimulation of the *vis medicatrix*.

This is a refinement of the philosophy presented earlier. One reason why people will experience failure with an alternative medical approach concerns the order of therapeutic intervention. Naturopathic medicine is not simply the substitution of "natural" medicaments for the conventional drugs and surgery. One can take "tons" of echinacea, or other appropriate therapies or remedies, and leave out that which must come first: dietary correction. If the cause of the disturbance continues to be fed into the system, therapeutic intervention at a lower level in the therapeutic hierarchy will rarely be curative, and may exacerbate the body's inflammatory response.

In general, one should use those therapies highest on the above lists most often, or at least with the understanding that one is affecting the organism with different potential for ultimate return to normal by utilizing different therapeutics. Those highest in the hierarchy have the greatest potential to return the organism to normal unsupported healthful function, and toward optimal function. Those lower in placement have lower potential to truly bring about permanent cure.

Further, to send one's patient out the door with a box full of supplements, without first having plumbed the causative elements of dietetics, digestion and stress, and acted to correct them, will generally not result in permanent nor efficient cure.

condition, family and other relationships, exercise pattern, rest and recreation. This will be followed by a physical examination pertinent to the nature of the problem.

Having gathered the appropriate information, the physician will analyze it and then discuss with the patient the findings and conclusions to which the physician has come. This will be followed by the development of a treatment plan, usually following the outline discussed above, with modifications based upon the individuality of the patient.

Most often, the patient will be sent home with a new understanding of their maladies, and a plan to correct them, a few medicinal agents and a new diet. They will visit the physician on a regular basis for office treatments and reevaluation

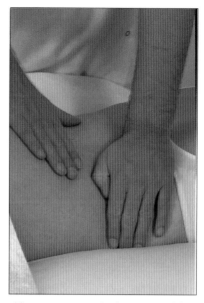

*Above: naturopathy interacts with other therapies and many naturopaths are also practicing osteopaths.*

until the problem is cleared and the health is restored.

## A TYPICAL VISIT

Most naturopathic physicians spend about one hour with a new patient, and about 30 minutes with a returning patient. A new patient visit usually will consist of information gathering. In some manner the patient will be encouraged to tell his story. This is usually facilitated by a patient information form which has been filled in prior to the visit. Either through a form, or directly from the patient, the physician will develop an understanding of the patient's past medical history and current status. This will include a review of all of the systems of the body, and a symptom picture from head to toe. The physician will inquire about the patient's dietary habits, and other aspects of lifestyle: occupation and working

## CONCLUSION

Naturopathic medicine is defined by a philosophy of healing which is focused upon restoring health rather than upon destroying disease. This is accomplished by a system of therapeutics which is the natural result of the philosophy. The therapeutics function best, and fulfil the philosophy, when they are applied in a rational order which is defined by the natural healing process of the organism. This hierarchy of therapeutics is a further refinement of the definition and philosophy of naturopathic medicine. A two stage process is defined which is based first upon creating the conditions within the organism which allow health to occur and which remove from the

organism those elements which disturb function, and secondly upon the application of appropriate therapies in a natural order which stimulates the healing process.

Naturopathic medicine is thus based upon a rational theory which can be applied consistently in a healthcare situation, the positive outcome of which can be anticipated and relied upon. This being true, the outcome of naturopathic medical application should be predictable, observable and repeatable. The repeatability and predictability of this system is therefore testable in clinical situations, and thus presents a scientific basis for evaluation, as well as for practice.

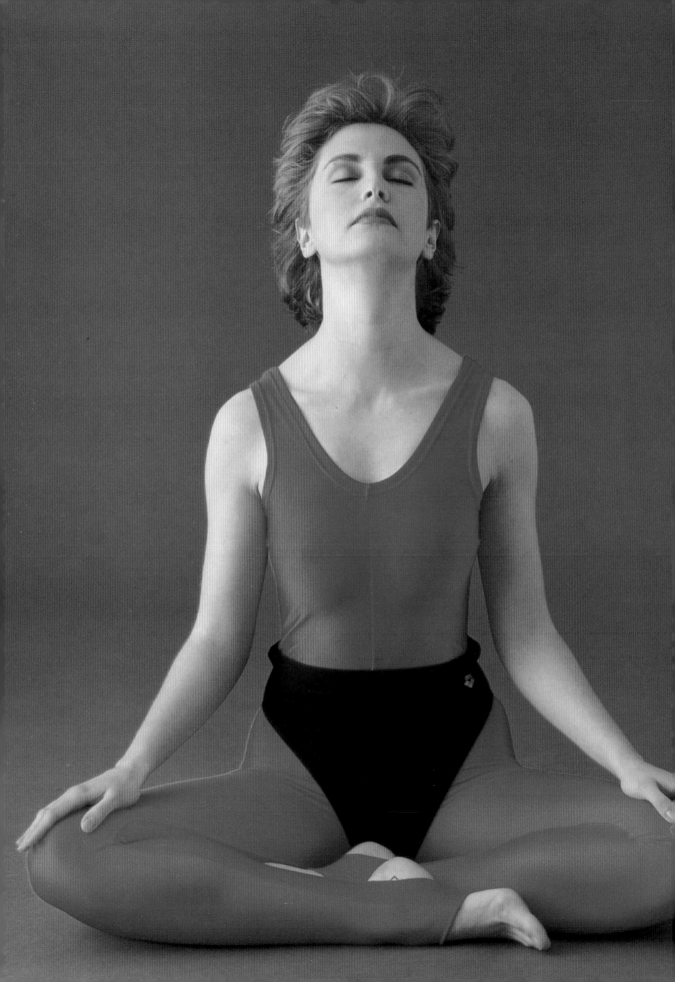

# MOBILITY AND POSTURE

## PART FOUR

*The therapies featured here include therapuetic methods and systems of healing, such as osteopathy, chiropractic and yoga. The Alexander Technique can help you to increase your conscious awareness and understanding of your body, improving posture and mobility. Chiriopractic, osteopathy and cranial osteopathy are all forms of manipulation therapy, correcting misalignment and increasing mobility. Rolfing is a form of structural integration, while dance therapy uses bodily movement to promote health. Yoga seeks to achieve a balance between body, spirit and mind.*

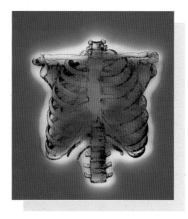

# ALEXANDER TECHNIQUE

CHAPTER NINE

*The F. M. Alexander Technique is a century-old process of awakening self-awareness of movement and its relationship to health and performance. The process is educational, rather than therapeutic, in orientation. The student learns to identify and exercise control over physical habits of excess tension, internal stress, posture, breathing and movement, as well as habits of thinking that interfere with natural ease and flow in everyday activity and skilled performance. As this interference is diminished and more natural functioning restored, specific symptoms and overall health frequently improve.*

*Today there are over 3,000 Alexander Technique teachers throughout the world, with training centers and national professional societies. As the medical community and the general population are finding increasing benefits in low-tech, personal, preventive and educative approaches to healthcare, the Alexander Technique offers a great variety of potential help to individuals in private, institutional and corporate settings.*

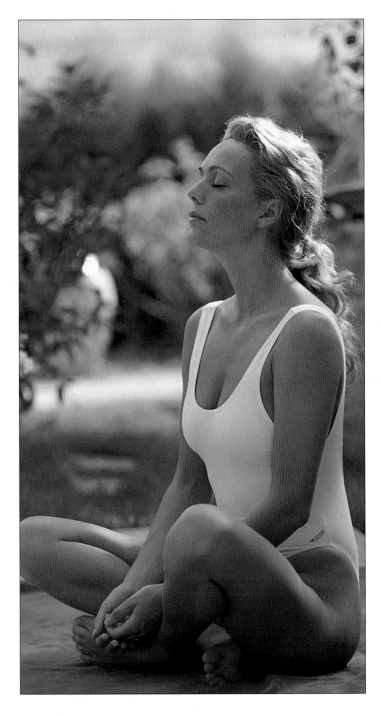

# ORIGINS

F. M. Alexander (Australia, 1869-1956) was an orator and also a Shakespearean actor who, at a critical time in his career, developed a chronic loss of voice in performance. Palliative recommendations from physicians and voice specialists, including extended vocal rest, were to result in a brief recovery between performances, but upon returning to the stage Alexander's vocal loss recurred.

Persistence and a decade-long process of self-observation with the aid of mirrors led to him developing what today is known as the Alexander Technique. Alexander succeeded in identifying previously unconscious, habitual patterns of head movement, neck tension, back compression and forceful breathing, which together had the effect of causing a lack of sufficient breath support for his voice, and destructive pressure on his vocal apparatus.

More important to his own learning and eventual teaching, he operationalized a means of breaking the habitual cycle of destructive response patterns set in motion by the stimulus to speak and perform. In doing so, Alexander was able not only to regain the use of his voice in performance, but also his vocal quality was much improved.

The improvement in his voice corresponded with a dramatic, evident change in his physical stature and respiratory function; in less tension and more balance throughout his body; and an unanticipated improvement in his general physical health. Over a period of years, Alexander developed his teaching and

## PHILOSOPHY AND OBJECTIVES

Following a simple, and somewhat mechanistic formula that "use affects function," the technique explores the relationship between how we "use," or coordinate ourselves—our thinking, consciousness, perception and physical structure—and how we function. Regardless of our unique anatomical differences and limitations, a teacher's job is to help the student maximize that potential for movement, breathing, and functioning in any context, by restoring balance to that function. The results are often improved health, wellbeing and enhanced performance.

he performed less, as first performing artists, and later medical patients, with various respiratory and physical ailments found their way to him for vocal, breathing and physical or movement re-education.

## BALANCE AND POSTURE

Successful integration of movement function demands balance. As vertebrate animals, we are designed to move in such a way that the head leads our movement along the spine, and the body follows. This move-

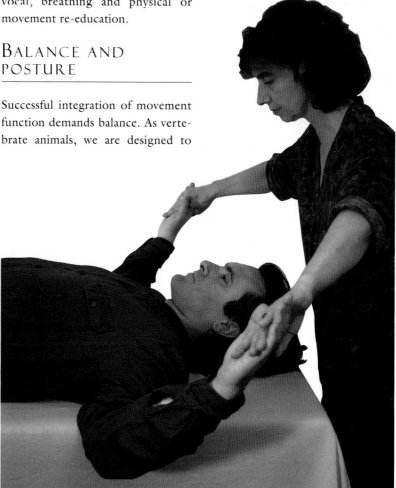

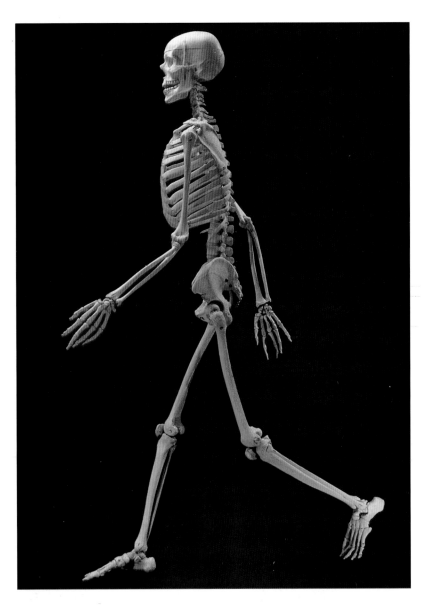

In most instances, the balance of our head to our spine is innate. Most healthy newborns explore and maintain this balance developmentally as they grow. Over time, under constant stress and maladaptive accommodation to our environment, we tend to lose this delicate balance.

## BALANCED, DYNAMIC POSTURE

The Alexander Technique focuses on restoring a balanced, dynamic posture, or coordination of the head and the spine. While posture is frequently thought of as a position in which to sit or stand, a dynamic posture is one that maintains a balanced relationship between the head, neck, and torso in movement, continually changing in response to the demands of activity, yet maintaining an underlying integrity or principle. This is characterized by:

▥ A perceptible and altered relationship of the head to the neck and back.

▥ A corresponding activation of deep postural antigravity musculature specifically.

▥ A re-balancing of the generalized tonus of the external musculature.

▥ An increased length along the spine.

▥ Freedom and mobility of the joints.

▥ Ease and increased flexibility of movement.

This organization creates a pattern of efficient muscular distribution of effort and a natural upright buoyancy that is characteristic of children and animals. As animals, we too are designed to move with freedom, vitality and balance. Distortion of this dynamic postural coordination leads to stress, wear and tear.

ment is an upward, vital direction in response to gravity, distinct from our movement in space, which is often horizontal (for example, walking or running along the horizontal surface of the ground).

In animals, the head leading horizontal movement is clearly evident. Any animal searching out its prey, for example, can clearly be seen to orient its movement by the head, where the primary organs of sight, smell and sound are located. Watch the intensity of a cheetah in motion and you can see clearly that the head is leading, the spine is following, and it almost seems as if the legs are merely catching up. Conversely, to restrict movement, to stop a horse for example, we pull back on the reins. This pulls the head back, directing forces in the animal's body into the opposite direction from the one in which the horse is moving.

## WHAT IT IS AND HOW IT WORKS

The Alexander Technique is a process of learning, or re-learning balance. The process of re-education is neuro-muscular, referring to the central nervous system which includes the brain. This system serves to transmit signals through the spinal cord and nerves to the musculature for balance and movement. It also serves trans-mission in the opposite direction, sending sensory-motor information from muscles and joints back to the brain in an ongoing feedback loop.

These signals are a form of thought, although we do not usually think of them that way. Virtually every action we take as human beings, if the thought is in any way expressed, is expressed through movement. To simplify, some examples would be movement of the respiratory and vocal apparatus, lips, tongue and jaw for singing or speech, movement of the arms and hand to conduct, write, etc.

While any potential students may initially come to the Alexander Technique for relief of physical (or psychological) symptoms or problems, the teacher's job is to teach, not to treat or diagnose. These are beyond the scope of an Alexander teacher's practice and his training. Observation and assessment of patterns of malcoordination and, in particular, postural response are what are addressed. Students learn to stop doing things that get them into physical trouble and excessive stress. Learning occurs in several stages:

### ▮ Insight

Initially students gain greater and greater conscious insight into habits of unnecessary tension, poor posture, ineffective thinking, shallow breathing, stress and fear patterns that get in their way and can lead to physical (or psychological) distress, pressure, pain and malfunction—"dis-ease," or under-performance.

### ▮ Control

With insight comes control. A critical component of the lessons is experiencing the immediacy and results of clear, directed thought and intention. We can have clear intention to do something, as well as not

---

## SUCCESSFUL INTERVENTION

In many instances of potential injury or strain, early detection is a key to successful intervention. Greater kinesthetic sensitivity provides earlier perception of discomfort. This offers the opportunity to modify behavior before conditions become more aggravated. A mindset of consciousness, and the ability to take greater responsibility (as opposed to blame) for effective functioning, lead to greater confidence and a sense of control when things go wrong. This can give even those in chronic pain a sense of psychological wellbeing and hope.

---

## POSTURE

*Developing good posture and control is very important to prevent putting pressure and strain on the spine, joints and musculature. You should not compress your spine or slump when sitting or standing.*

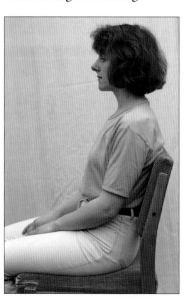

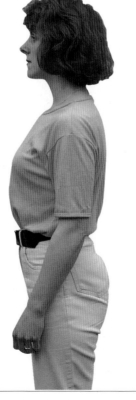

to do something. For example, a student may recognize a tendency to tighten her neck, collapse her torso and compress her spine when she stands up or sits down (slumps). This can exert enormous pressure and strain on the spine, joints, and musculature. She can equally make a decision not to do that.

This sounds easier than it is when dealing with internal movement patterns in the musculature (or deeply held emotional patterns), and often may require confronting perception and belief systems. This is why an Alexander Technique teacher is so crucial. The teacher is there to assist in the process, through the means of sophisticated sensory guidance with the hands, as well as providing verbal or demonstrative instructional guidance and feedback.

The student must resist the temptation to do what is very familiar. When successful, the student will do something else, and that "something else" is almost always easier and freer, less stressful and more mechanically efficient.

## CHANGING HABIT PATTERNS

Through movement repetition, over time, new neuromotor patterns replace less useful ones, and gradually the student's general sense of self and overall standard of functioning improves. While experience of relief and freedom may come early under a teacher's guidance, it is in a later stage of learning that symptoms of "dis-ease" tend to either disappear or diminish dramatically, as fundamental habit patterns have changed.

Most likely, the aggravating, contributing behavior has been eliminated—or is no longer a dominant response. The student's whole system has changed its internal environment by means of improved respiration and circulation, reduced spinal and joint pressure, improved neuromuscular control and postural tone, more even distribution of

effort, all of which may allow healing to occur and prevent recurrence of functionally-related health problems.

The technique is taught against a backdrop of our own internal sense of feeling and motion—our kinesthetic sense. How accurate our sense perception is (which Alexander maintained was not very well developed)—how "in touch" we are with our bodies, and how "present," or aware we are—will, to a great extent, influence the course of lessons and speed of learning.

## THE LESSON

The purpose of a lesson is to facilitate the student's learning about the coordination of the head, neck and back as a basis for all movement, and of the inseparability of the human being into parts, whether they be a "mind" and a "body," a "leg" and an "arm," a "psychological," "emotional," "intellectual" or "physical."

The Technique recognizes the body/mind as one. Every activity engages the entire system. There may be greater or lesser emphasis on a specific dimension of the person, on specific muscle groups, perhaps, but the whole person is engaged. It is a tenet of the Technique that every part of the self affects the whole. Almost a century ahead of his time, Alexander was insistent that the distinction between body and mind was a false one, and that the scientific tendency towards reductionism was not only false, but dangerous to the well being of the individual.

To the initial observer or student, a typical lesson of 30 to 45 minutes is likely to appear as a form of sophisticated postural adjustment, and a process of learning how to sit, stand and walk correctly under the teacher's guidance. Movement guidance includes touch—a sophisticated use of the teacher's hands and verbal instruction. Some work is also usually done lying down, giving the student the opportunity to undo tension patterns associated with supporting the structure upright, while the teacher may be moving limbs and encouraging lengthening of the spine.

## THE ALEXANDER TECHNIQUE IN PRACTICE

A performer might be interested in dealing directly with speaking, singing, conducting or playing a musical instrument; an athlete with swinging a tennis racket; a computer operator with sitting, supporting the arm, dealing with a mouse and keyboard.

For example, a student may learn that while waiting to return a tennis serve, there is an unconscious, habitual pattern of contracting the neck,

*Right: a good teacher will work with the student during a course of lessons.*

over-tightening leg muscles and the hip joints, tightly clutching the racket and collapsing the torso. These may be manifestations of a desire to concentrate hard on returning the serve. Unwittingly, these may actually contribute to ongoing physical and respiratory problems, as well as performance deficits. The teacher may then guide the student into a preparation that is different in its fundamental organization (the position may be the same, while the quality is different), representing a new neuromuscular pattern that is biomechanically more efficient and less stressful to the body, that elevates alertness. This is both motor learning and attentional instruction on a fine and fundamental level. Continual repetition serves to:
- Give a reinforcing experience to the student.
- Lay a new neuromuscular movement pattern and attentional process.
- Bring an awareness to the process of achieving the movement on a regular basis. Thus, not only does the new pattern become learned but, perhaps most important, the awareness brought to the process of employing the new pattern itself becomes habitual.

## EXPLORING OURSELVES

As students advance, lessons represent a paradigm for observing habits of response in general, an opportunity to bring consciousness or mindfulness to our generalized reactions, and a greater connection between ourselves and the environment. This model is then transferable, through conscious choice, to

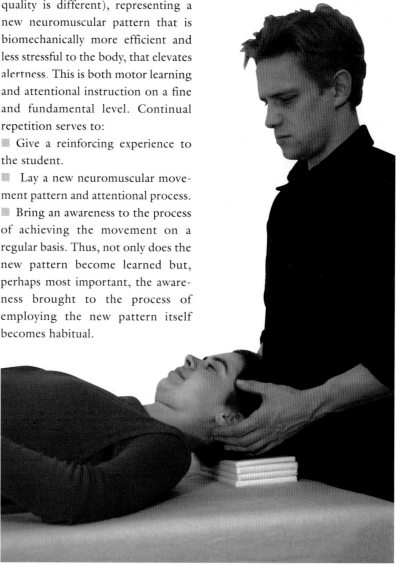

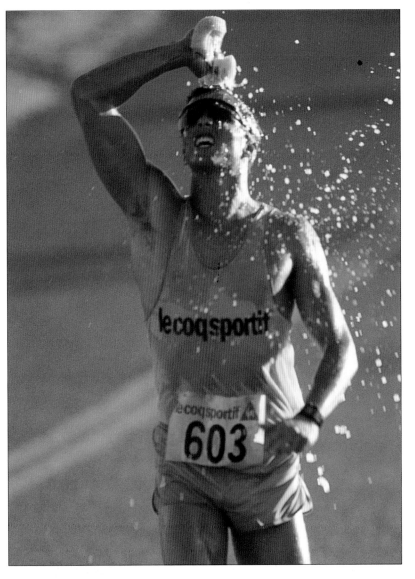

*Left: athletes who are pursuing peak performance can benefit from the Alexander Technique.*

increased, energy and vitality are increased, wellbeing is enhanced, and perception and attention are clearer. It is as if you were walking around in heavy shoes all day long and were not aware of their weight until you removed them at the end of the day. Skilled performers reduce stress, fear and risk of injury, as they increase expressiveness, and gain a sense of inner connectedness and wholeness.

## APPLICATIONS

The Alexander Technique has a wide array of applications because it deals with various key elements of human functioning within our control including: consciousness, attention, habit structure, learning, coordination, flexibility, neuromuscular processing, posture, breathing, vocal production, and physical and emotional expressiveness. For this reason, students of the Technique range from actors and musicians, to airforce

any arena. On this level, the lesson bears the same relation to sitting and standing as a Japanese Tea Ceremony does to drinking tea—very little. Study becomes about exploring ourselves. The activity fades into the background, as our awareness is drawn more and more into our internal process of functioning, being, in any situation, faced with any activity, including emotional response. As study continues, a generalized sense of wellbeing, calmness, health, control and confidence tend to increase as constant stress, injury, discomfort, and feelings of "being at the effect of..." tend to subside.

## BENEFITS

The effect of balance is to frequently leave the student with an absence of habitual sensation. Simple everyday movements, such as walking or sitting and standing, become light and seemingly effortless, flexibility is

## ENDORSEMENTS

Two of the century's leading Nobel Prize winning physiologists, Sir Charles Sherrington and Nicholas Tinburgen, have endorsed the Technique, the latter devoting half of his 1973 Nobel Prize winning acceptance speech to the subject. Private orthopedists and other physicians refer patients, as well as others from medical institutions including in the Unites States: Mount Sinai School of Medicine; Westchester Medical Center, Section of Spinal Surgery; The Miller Institute for Performing Artists; St. Luke's/Roosevelt Hospital; and Columbia-Presbyterian Medical Center. A selection of artistic institutions that represent the Technique in their theatre and/or music curricula in the United States and England includes the Juilliard School, the University of California, Los Angeles, the Aspen Music Festival, the American Conservatory Theatre, the Royal College of Music, and the Royal Academy of Dramatic Arts. The Israeli Airforce uses the technique for stress reduction and rehabilitation of injured pilots.

pilots, to athletes in pursuit of peak performance, to self-seekers, to those suffering from poor posture and low self-esteem, stress, headaches, muscle tension, repetitive strain injury, spinal injury, neck pain, back pain, arthritis, or various other forms of joint dysfunction. The common denominator is an active student interested in learning about habit patterns within their control that impede performance and function.

## INTERACTION WITH OTHER DISCIPLINES

The nature of the Alexander Technique is interdisciplinary. It is most widely known in the performing arts. In addition, the Technique provides a natural alliance with physicians, orthopedists, chiropractors, psychologists, physical therapists, occupational therapists, ergonomists, human resource directors, athletic trainers, and other holistic healthcare professionals.

## FINDING A TEACHER

It is generally not advisable to attempt learning the Alexander Technique without the aid of a teacher, unless you intend to duplicate Alexander's ten-year process! Outside feedback and the hands-on experience are essential to the learning process.

Most teachers of the Alexander Technique teach privately but many also teach small groups and in institutional or University settings. Generally it is recommended to study on a weekly basis, and sometimes more frequently. A student who is seriously interested in lasting change in habit pattern and

function should consider studying for a minimum of six months, or approximately 30 to 40 lessons. However, there are no fixed rules or prescriptions, and many have found benefit in five lessons and others have studied for years.

All certified teachers of the Alexander Technique undergo a minimum of 1600 hours of specialized training over a period of approximately three years. To locate a certified teacher of the Alexander Technique, turn to the useful addresses section at the back of this book.

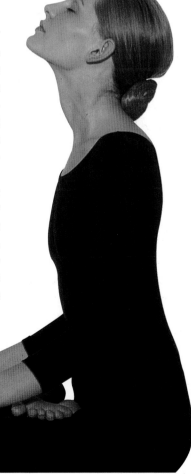

# CHIROPRACTIC

## CHAPTER TEN

*T*he word "Chiropractic" came from the Greek words cheir and praktikos, which mean "done by hands." Chiropractic treatments began thousands of years before the birth of Christ. Early missionaries who visited China found an ancient manuscript called the Cong Fou Document, which was written around 2700B.C. This ancient Chinese paper shows definite details of practitioners using soft tissue manipulation to treat a variety of problems.

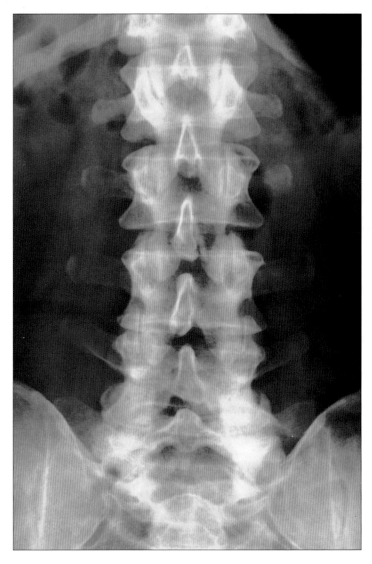

*The Greeks were also known to use manipulation, as far back as 1500B.C. Recovered writings of that period have been preserved on the original ancient papyrus. These manuscripts from antiquity give instructions on how to manipulate the spine. Other early civilizations also treated conditions of the spine with crude manipulation. Among the many peoples around the world who have used this simple but effective treatment were the early Babylonians, the Egyptians, the Japanese, the Indians of Asia, and many more ancient civilizations.*

# HISTORY OF CHIROPRACTIC

Most people today think of Hippocrates as the father of modern medicine. He was, however, a practitioner of spinal manipulation as well as a learned man, scribe and physician. He wrote a number of remarkable and informative books on methods of realigning the spine, to correct illnesses, and mechanical problems of the neck and back. Born in 640B.C., he lived to be 73 years old, writing a book for almost every year that he lived. Two great works of medical significance, which are as valid today as when they were first written, are: On Setting Joints by Leverage, and Manipulation: An Importance to Good Health. A quote directly attributed to Hippocrates is "Get knowledge of the spine, for this is the requisite for many diseases."

Approximately 500 years after Hippocrates popularized and legitimized manipulation, another Greek physician, Galen, became famous after he cured a paralysis of the right hand of a well-known Roman scholar, Eudemus. History records that he worked on the patient's neck, causing what we would term today a Chiropractic manipulation. He was thereafter given the title "Prince of Physicians." Galen continued to validate and expand Hippocrates' theory of Chiropractic, when he said: "Look to the nervous system as the key to maximum health."

Chiropractic never became a valid, written science until the latter part of the nineteenth century. Manipulative therapy, however, continued in various forms throughout the many centuries in between. In Europe, the art of manipulation was practiced by people who were called "bonesetters." Bonesetting was an art that was handed down through families. Eventually these bonesetters became famous as healers, and were accorded great respect and considered gifted in the healing arts. In 1867, the British Medical Journal featured an article by the famous surgeon Sir James Pagget, who wrote a paper entitled, "Cases that bonesetters cure." Although Chiropractic in various forms of crude manipulation and bonesetting was practiced in Britain, Europe, and throughout Asia, it was never truly researched or formulated into a specific healing science. The education and practice was haphazard; no one person ever came forth to define this healing art, and put it on a legitimate level with the accepted medical treatments and theories of the day.

## DANIEL DAVID PALMER

D.D.Palmer is considered to be the father of modern Chiropractic. A former grocer and teacher, his interest in healing the sick led him to an apprenticeship with Paul Caister, a practitioner of magnetic healing. His first documented case of the effects of Chiropractic manipulation occurred with his successful treatment of a man, Harvey Lillet, who had been deaf for 17 years. It came to D. D. Palmer's attention that Lillet's deafness appeared to have been caused by a spinal injury, and he treated him by adjusting his spine in the neck region, where the original injury occurred. After Lillet's neck was realigned, his hearing was restored, and modern Chiropractic began.

## PHILOSOPHY AND OBJECTIVES

Medicine is a very broad term, and deals with various forms of therapies that are used to treat the human condition. The local family medical doctor is really only one of many types of physician. He is a student of a branch of medicine called Allopathy. This holds that most illnesses that affect mankind are due to

## EARLY CHIROPRACTIC

In Tahiti, gentle movement of the spine has been used for hundreds of years as a treatment. On examination of these old records, their diagrams and treatment manuals; it would appear that the initial types of manipulation practiced were very simple and over-forceful compared with today's gentle scientific approach. The one thing that holds true, and which still is at the heart of Chiropractic is the concept of moving the bones of the spine as a physical way of treating a variety of mechanical problems of the neck and back.

One of the cruder methods of manipulation was used by the North American Indians. They would walk on the back of the person being treated, thus forcing a type of harsh spinal realignment to take place. Winnebago, Sioux and Creek Indians were some of the more notable tribes who participated in this activity of rough adjustment. In Central and South America, the Mayan and Inca Indians were also practitioners of this ancient art of manipulation.

## MODERN CHIROPRACTIC

In order to be at the birth of what we consider to be modern Chiropractic, we must look to the United States, in the year 1895. At that time there were no real doctors who treated the sick in the sense that we have them today. There was no standardization of education to arrive at a degree of Doctor of the healing arts. In many cases, a person who would treat the sick or injured, was considered a physician or healer, simply by the acquisition of some very basic skills and knowledge of what was available at the time, either via an apprenticeship or through a process of self-training.

This usually consisted of a mix of many different healing aspects, ranging from blood letting, purging, bonesetting and herbal medicine, to religious and magnetic healing, all of which were acceptable and popular therapies at that time. As there was no standardized formal education or knowledge available, the patient could not be sure of the safety or efficacy of any practice or practitioner.

Therefore, it is no wonder that the average person's lifespan at that particular time was limited to what we now consider to be middle age. It should also be noted that in that era, surgery was performed without any anesthesia or regard to cleanliness, and possibly in some areas by the local barber.

Disease was the greatest killer of the time, causing a very high mortality amongst children in particular. Sanitation was almost unheard of. Into this arena came a grocer and former teacher turned healer called Daniel David Palmer (see page 111) who is considered to be the father of modern Chiropractic.

the intrusion of some invading agent. The Allopathic Doctor treats his patients with manufactured drugs and biological products, or with surgery. This type of treatment could be deemed crisis therapy, in that the patient is treated chemically, once the symptoms begin and have been identified into a specific pathology. Drug therapy is either continued until the symptoms disappear, or continued indefinitely, if needed, from the allopathic viewpoint.

In order to treat any condition, a very specific diagnosis must be made to pinpoint a specific cause. This involves the grouping together of certain symptoms and then the classification of a highly specific diagnosis. This then demands a very specific chemical agent to combat the problem. At times many conditions can cause similar symptoms or, indeed, there may be no symptoms at all, until the condition is well advanced, and in some cases irreversible. The similarity of symptoms can at times create a situation where a drug that is used is ineffective or indeed dangerous.

### MEDICATION AND SIDE EFFECTS

It is a well-known fact that almost all medication has side effects. Sometimes a patient who is treated with drugs may develop another condition because of the toxicity of the very medication that was prescribed for him in the first place. This often leads to another medication to undo the damage from the first medication. Although prescription drugs have to be tested and given a government license, they usually have a list of possible adverse reactions. The colossal human experiment here is that the medication you take was not tested on you specifically, and you may have your own individual biological adverse reaction to the medication. Finally, these medications may not have ever been tested together, and certainly their combined chemical compounds have never been tested on you.

This is not meant to be a condemnation of allopathic medicine for there are many circumstances that would be fatal to mankind were it not for the great discoveries of life-saving, enhancing and prolonging medications. Advances in surgical techniques over the last century have also helped to save many lives. However, with all its advances and benefits, allopathic medicine lacks the preventative and curative effects of manipulation that are used in Chiropractic health care.

### RESTORING SPINAL BIO-MECHANICAL BALANCE

Whereas medicine gathers its forces of treatment to eliminate symptoms, Chiropractors are more concerned with the restoration of the spinal bio-mechanical balance, as these directly affect the musculoskeletal, neurological and vascular health systems of the human body. Chiropractic philosophy is to take a physical approach, to allow the body's nervous system to function at its maximum, and to restore the patient to a healthy state. The main avenue of treatment is by manipulation of the spine, to remove mechanical stress that can be affecting the discs, joints, nerves, supportive and connective structures, and even the spinal cord itself.

## CHIROPRACTIC TREATMENT

This is soundly based upon certain accepted, scientific and biological principles. The Central Nervous System is composed of the brain and the spinal cord; this is the body's "master system," under which all body functions are controlled and monitored.

### ▇ DISEASE PROCESSES

These may be affected by disturbances of the nervous system, such as lack of exercise, poor nutrition, obesity, dangerous chemicals in our food chain, contaminated food, air and water, stress, injury, germs, and musculoskeletal imbalance. It is the Chiropractic philosophy that a healthy, strong, flexible and aligned spine is necessary for an uninterrupted communication between the various body parts and systems, and the brain itself.

### ▇ MALFUNCTION OF THE NERVOUS SYSTEM.

This may be caused by the vertebrae of the spine being displaced, resulting

*Right: the chiropractor works to restore the spinal bio-mechanical balance by using a process of manipulation.*

in what is known as a classical subluxation. There are also conditions that affect the spine that could be termed muscular compression syndromes where the vertebrae may not be misaligned, but rather compressed due to injured or over-used muscles that have gone into spasm, and thus hold the vertebrae in a painful vice-like grip. This condition may cause one or several discs to be irritated, painful, and ever so slightly swollen. There are nerve fibers in the disks

which are called sensory, and will send a pain signal to the brain.

A swollen disk could also cause pressure on the nerve as it exits from the spinal canal—a trapped nerve. These muscle spasms can also jam and irritate the joints at the back of the spine. In these two cases there may be no perceptible misalignment of the spine, but there may be pain and dysfunction, due to this neuromusculoskeletal compression syndrome. This could affect all

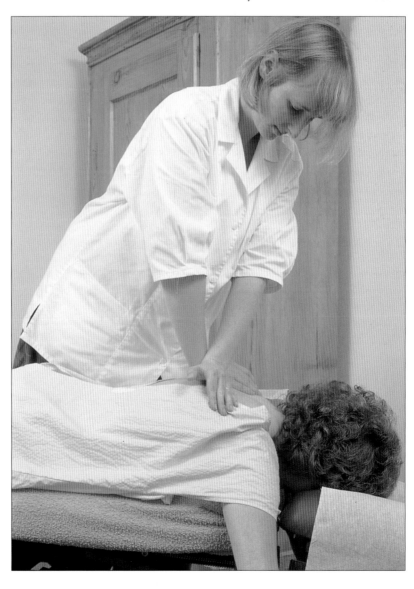

the supportive structures of the spine, including the spinal column itself. Pressure and irritation to these parts could build up tremendous pain that could cause the local muscles to go into spasms or sustained contractions. If these defects were allowed to continue for an extended length of time, they could cause irreversible degenerative changes to all structures involved.

This neurological chaos, is a destructive electrical charge that could also affect internal organs and other body systems. This could then create a vicious circle where a trapped nerve causes a muscle spasm which compresses a vertebrae, thus squeezing the disk, which then further traps the nerve, and then the nerve causes the muscle to go into spasm. It is an anatomical and neurological fact that when a main nerve trunk exits the spine, it will send some nerves to muscles and other connective tissue, whilst also sending some of its fibers to the internal organs.

It is important to understand that a so-called back problem could indeed eventually cause a major problem to the internal organs. Dysfunction of the spine may disturb and create imbalances in different parts of the body causing the system to malfunction, and thus be more susceptible to disease. This can affect body parts and body systems. Most elderly people will tell you that a severe lower back pain affects their bladder. Imagine what your state of health would be if you were unable to empty your bladder and rid your body of the toxins and waste products that your kidneys have filtered. Without an unencumbered nerve supply, the kidneys would not work at all.

# HOW DOES CHIROPRACTIC WORK?

Chiropractic is a physical approach to mechanical problems of the spine and its supportive and related structures, which could also be the cause of other pathological problems. The Doctor of Chiropractic treats his patient by adjusting or manipulating the spine. When this structure is in its proper and normal position, the nervous system can send out signals from in between the vertebrae, via the spinal nerves, to every part of the body. These signals will go to the top of the head, and to the tip of the toes. They will tell the heart to beat over 100,000 times a day. They will control the movement of over 600 muscles.

Generally, when a patient visits a Chiropractor, they present three problems.

## 1 PAIN
They have got pain, and this is the main reason for their visit.

## 2 TIGHTNESS
There is a tightness that is part of the pain portrait; this can be localized to the muscles of the neck, mid-back, or low-back. It may also run into the shoulders or down the legs and arms. These muscle spasms are caused by the pain itself, and can become a problem in themselves, which aggravates and perpetuates the original pain at the spine.

## 3 WEAKNESS
This is usually the condition that allowed the problem to occur in the first place. The weakened state of

## CHIROPRACTIC TECHNIQUES

Chiropractic works in a very natural way, because there are no drugs or surgery. The Doctor of Chiropractic uses his hands to gently move the spine, and unlock jammed vertebrae. There are many different techniques that Chiropractors use. Some will work on the muscles first, and then the spine. Some Chiropractors may use different physiotherapies to release muscle tension and spasm, reduce swelling, or increase the circulation to the areas that are being worked on. These therapies may precede or follow the adjustment.

The Chiropractor will treat the spine and the person as an integrated system, trying to free up abnormal spinal positions, and letting the body get back to its normal healthy condition. He will also consider other predisposing factors that may have brought the patient to him. If someone is clearly overweight, this creates a burden on the spine, which has been built specifically to the individual's own unique normal, healthy weight.

In many cases a Chiropractor will recommend a weight loss program to his patient to be followed in conjunction with the treatment to help eliminate one of the probable causes of the person's spinal problem. An overworked spine becomes a weak spine, which, in turn, becomes an unhealthy spine.

the muscles in the back is one of the factors that causes them to lock up, in order to support the person. It is a vicious cycle: trapped nerves, compressed disks, and jammed posterior facet joints can send pain signals to cause weak muscles to lock up, which can further irritate and compress the spine, thus trapping nerves whose irritation signals the muscles to lock up more.

## THE OBJECTIVE OF THE CHIROPRACTOR

This should be to get the patient out of pain, rehabilitate the injured/dysfunctional area, and to provide a proper exercise programme, which will keep the patient healthy and help prevent the problem reoccurring.

In most circumstances where there is pin-point pain, either in the spine, the hips, or down the legs and arms, it is usually caused by some sort of inflammation. This is the body's response to injury, or pathological process; it consists of pain, swelling, heat, at times redness, and loss of function. Through manipulation, the Chiropractor can gently, over a period of time, unlock and unjam those areas of the spine and pelvis that have seized up.

It is most important at this time for the Chiropractor to instruct the patient not to aggravate the condition further; many times, bed rest is one of the doctor's best tools. When a person has a severe back condition they either rest it, and allow it to heal, or they aggravate it and make it worse. The Chiropractor will often recommend the use of ice packs on areas of pin-point pain. This helps to reduce the swelling that the inflam-

mation may be causing to the disk, joint or nerve. A hot soak bath may sometimes be recommended, as the general heat of the water that surrounds the larger muscles of the back would aid the circulation, thus relaxing the muscles and giving further pain relief.

There are certain treatment tables that some Chiropractors use that help in the treatment of neck and back problems. One such table, called the Anatomotor, has two rollers. As the patient lays on their back, the rollers gently go up and down the spine, causing an intermittent, intersegmental traction. This action moves the spine from top to bottom many times, in a gentle, soothing, massage-like action, encouraging the spine to loosen up and gently realign itself. At this point, the Chiropractor can adjust the patient with a minimum of force, and still achieve maximum movement.

### FREQUENCY OF VISITS
The Chiropractor may only see a person a few times for a minor problem but in circumstances where the problem and pain are severe, treatment may be required three or more times a week, over an extended period of time. For example, a stiff neck and shoulder that resulted from gardening yesterday might be resolved in two or three visits. However, migraine headaches, whose symptoms may have accumulated over months and years, due to emotional or occupational stress, or even an automobile accident years previously, may require months of treatment to normalize the neuromusculoskeletal conditions that are causing the problems.

## THE HUMAN SPINE

A person's spine, when viewed from the back, is supposed to be straight. All 24 vertebrae, and the disks in between, should be properly aligned with one another. This bony structure, unlike a solid pipe, should be capable of some gentle movement, whilst the disks provide a cushioning effect. The muscles of the back, as they are attached to the spine, should supply support, mobility, and locomotion to the individual. If the spine is observed from a side view, four distinct curves are noticeable. This arrangement is again for mobility and support, and allows for a greater range of motion. It is also important for a creature that stands erect on two feet, to have this shock-absorbing and spring-like structure. The Chiropractor's job is to keep the spine mobile, aligned, flexible and uncompromised.

When a patient notices a reduction of pain, the Chiropractor can then begin to prescribe some gentle stretching exercises to increase flexibility, and thus gently coax the tight muscles to loosen up. This increase in the range of motion and movement also increases the circulation to the spine and muscles. A good analogy here for the patient to use might be to think of the muscles of the back as a sponge. If a sponge isn't used, it will dry out, shrivel and shrink. If you take that sponge and immerse it in water, and gently squeeze and release, you will get the water engorging the sponge, increasing its size, and restoring it to a useful state. It is like this with the muscles and lig-

## QUESTIONS PATIENTS ASK

Here are some of the most common questions that many patients ask a Chiropractor. They are as follows:

- How many visits?
- How many treatments?
- How often?
- How long?

Although there are no magic formulas to answer these questions, there are certain guidelines that can be used to gauge the person's progress, and therefore decrease the frequency of their visits.

There are five helpful criteria that can be used by the doctor in helping him determine when the patient can be treated less frequently. These are related to the patient's perception of their own pain. They are:

- Intensity
- Duration
- Frequency
- Location
- Nature of the pain

aments that support the spine—use it or lose it.

As the patient continues to benefit from the treatment and the stretching exercises, the treatment might be decreased in chronic, severe cases, down to twice a week, while increasing the amount of stretching exercises. When the pain intensity, frequency, duration and location reduce further, the doctor can introduce strengthening exercises to further stabilize the spine, increasing the circulation and using the body's self-healing natural ability.

Eventually, and in most cases, the patient who has had this intensive treatment and has been given a self-help exercise program, becomes pain free.

The heart and spirit of the Chiropractic treatment is not only just to get the patient out of pain, but to rehabilitate him, correcting the mechanical problem if possible, and setting up a home exercise program to try and prevent the problem from returning. It is also the practice in the United States to see patients on a monthly basis, once they have completed their initial treatment program. It is a system that some 60 million Americans a year continue to benefit from.

### PREVENTIVE MEDICINE

Since Chiropractic teaches us that total health depends upon a healthy, functional spine and central nervous system, it makes sense to keep the spine, and its supportive structures as strong and flexible and as properly aligned as possible. The Chiropractic philosophy is to add years to your life, and life to your years. The monthly maintenance programs have shown a proven advantage over crisis therapy.

## VISITING A CHIROPRACTOR

There are a number of different Chiropractic approaches to treatment, and these vary depending on the patient's condition. There is one approach which is highly technical and orthopedic in its examination and evaluation, whereby the Chiropractor, along with taking an extensive and complete history of

the individual, will also utilize an extensive series of orthopedic and neurological tests, possibly with X-rays, to arrive at a diagnosis.

The other school of thought is more concerned with the presenting pain and problem, and the Chiropractor might simply ask the patient to point to where it hurts, ask how it happened, and when.

### X-RAYS

The purpose of X-rays is to find breaks, fractures, and gross misalignments, but the average person coming in with a back or neck problem may have a misalignment or compression of their spine that can't be detected by X-ray. In most of the cases, there are no breaks or fractures anyway. Obviously, if the patient had suffered a recent traumatic injury, such as a fall or an automobile accident, then X-rays would be indicated, but most problems of the neck and back usually involve a muscle in spasm, compressing the spine and causing pain in the disk and joint, whilst trapping the nerve. An experienced Chiropractor should be able to diskern the problem simply by talking to the patient, and having him show where the pain is.

### THERAPIES AND ADJUSTING TECHNIQUES

Some Chiropractors will use therapies prior to adjusting the spine, while others simply adjust. Some will use very gentle adjusting techniques, while others will be more forceful. The Chiropractor should loosen up the spinal muscles, and physically move the spine to relieve the pressure. However, this treatment should not be painful in the extreme but how does one define what is too painful and what's not enough?

A good answer to this question might be the following analogy. If a person who was in relatively good shape worked out with a personal trainer, he would probably be a little sore and stiff afterwards. He would have performed a healthy, beneficial activity, but there would be some slight diskomfort, due to the use of muscles and joints that had not really been physically used in a while. The manipulation, like the exercise, may move parts that have been jammed or locked up. This sometimes creates a little diskomfort, but not always, and never extremely. In most cases the patient will notice a slight reduction in the pain of their condition, and an increase of their range of motion.

## A HEALTHCARE SYSTEM

Whilst Chiropractic is the healthcare newcomer in some countries, in the United States where it originated, and has been perfected, it is consid-ered part of the mainstream health-care system. The US Public Health Service classifies Doctors of Chiropractic among "medical specialists and practitioners." The United States court system has officially recognized the Doctor of Chiropractic as a qualified specialist in neuromusculoskeletal injuries; and has designated them as expert witnesses in litigation cases. In the USA, Chiropractors are licensed by the Government in each State, and have to graduate from a Government Accredited University. There are currently some 50,000 Chiropractors in the United States.

In the United Kingdom, the Medical Research Council has carried out a number of projects, testing the efficacy of chiropractic healthcare, comparing it with standard British hospital care, for the treatment of neuromusculoskeletal problems. The results demonstrated that not only did the patients respond to Chiropractic care, but that their responses were better than those treated with standard medical care. They also stated that the beneficial

## CLOTHING

One minor difference between the examination technique of the British and American Chiropractor is that some British Chiropractors will require their patients to strip and wear a gown. Their American colleagues are taught to examine the patient fully clothed for the most part, and do not find it necessary to use a gown.

results from the Chiropractic treatments lasted longer.

Major private healthcare companies in the United Kingdom are now covering Chiropractic care for their clients as it becomes more generally accepted in orthodox medical circles. The Institute for Complementary Medicine in London, has created a register of those qualified chiropractors who are acceptable for their standards.

## SLIPPED DISK

At times, some disk injuries are wrongly described and diagnosed as being a "slipped disk." However, the disk cannot actually "slip" as it is held in place by fibers that run from it to the vertebrae above and below. But this flexible pad can bulge, tear, rupture, herniate, prolapse or even disintegrate.

It is important to understand that because the disk is not just slightly out of place, the injury will take time to heal, if it does at all. Therefore a patient should never expect a Chiropractor just to "slip" a disk back into place.

## TREATABLE CONDITIONS

The following list highlights some common treatable conditions which any qualified American, British or European Chiropractor would be expected to treat. The most commonly seen conditions include the following:
- Arthritis
- Numbness
- Pins and needles
- Back, arm or leg pain
- Sports injuries
- Whiplash
- Migraine
- Strains
- Sprains
- Neck and shoulder pain
- Insomnia
- Trapped nerves
- Muscular cramps
- Stiffness
- Work injuries
- Disk degeneration

# OSTEOPATHY

## CHAPTER ELEVEN

*O*steopathic medicine arose in the heartland of the United States as an alternative to many of the ineffective and dangerous medical practices of the late nineteenth century. In the United States, osteopathy has subsequently gained full legal and professional recognition as a parallel and distinctive healing profession. The osteopathic approach has maintained its distinctive patient-oriented philosophy while combining it with the ever-expanding medical sciences. This high-tech, high-touch approach to patient care has made it the fastest growing arm of the health delivery system in the United States.

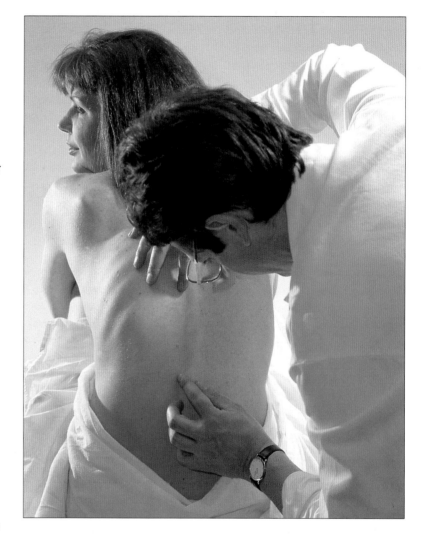

Today, doctors of osteopathy (D.O.) constitute five percent of American physicians with full, unrestricted licenses, but they are the healthcare provider choice of nearly 10 percent of the population. Providing health care to over 20 million individuals annually, over 39,000 American D.O.s continue to offer the general public an alternative to the conventional allopathic medical approach.

# ORIGINS OF OSTEOPATHY

The founder of osteopathic medicine was an American frontier physician named Andrew Taylor Still, M.D. He had practiced "regular" medicine in the mid-western United States and served as a surgeon during the Civil War, but he concluded that disease-oriented medicine was ineffective.

In 1874, he began practicing a system emphasizing health rather than disease and developed an approach to improve the body's own self-healing mechanisms. His system of palpation of the musculoskeletal dysfunction and manipulation to return optimal function was the most obvious difference in his therapeutic approach. Still selected the descriptor, "Osteopathy"— meaning, literally, "bone suffering"— to describe his distinctive new approach.

In 1892, at the age of sixty-four, Still founded a college in Kirksville, Missouri, to "improve our present system of surgery, obstetrics and treatment of disease generally, and place the same on a more rational and scientific basis, and to impart information to the medical profession." Although he could have granted the allopathic M.D. degree, he chose instead to call his graduates "D.O.s" to set them apart from those doctors practicing traditional medicine. When Still died in 1917, there were more than 5,000 D.O.s in the United States and abroad.

## MODERN TRAINING

Today, distinctive osteopathic principles and practices (OPP) and osteopathic manipulative treatment (OMT) are integrated into the training of every D.O. A parallel

## PHILOSOPHY AND OBJECTIVES OF OSTEOPATHIC MEDICINE

The 100 million patient visits to osteopathic physicians are provided by practitioners in every specialty field, all of whom share the common unifying philosophy developed by A.T. Still. Osteopathic education emphasizes four basic osteopathic tenets, which are as follows:

### 1 The body is an integrated unit

The physical body is made up of a number of interrelated organs and systems, all working in unison towards maintaining health. Likewise, the mind, body and spiritual being of each person are inseparable and interdependent. This belief in wholism is built into the osteopathic educational system to such an extent that all D.O. specialists are first trained to be generalists. The position of the American Osteopathic Association is, "Proper balance among the parts means health while improper balance can mean susceptibility to disease and illness."

### 2 Structure and function are inter-related

Dysfunction in the musculoskeletal system frequently contributes to pain, poor blood flow, and even changes in the way in which organ systems work, leading to constipation, headaches, fatigue and increased susceptibility to disease. Conversely, problems in different body functions will typically present neuromusculoskeletal system clues which the osteopathic physician has been trained to find. This additional knowledge leads to early diagnosis, often with fewer expensive tests. Understanding the inter-relationship between structure and function provides the D.O. with additional diagnostic and therapeutic options. D.O.s will frequently use OMT (see above) as part of a treatment plan to improve structure-function relationships.

### 3 The body has self-healing, self-regulating mechanisms

D.O.s respect the wisdom and experience of the body which is continuously treating and healing itself: fighting invading bacteria, forming clots and eventually new skin over cuts, even seeking out and destroying cancer cells. A D.O. strives to protect and assist these natural processes. Thus, osteopathic treatment emphasizes preventative practises, such as nutrition and exercise, but it also includes careful decision-making about when and how to prescribe medication. Because the root word for "doctor" means "teacher," doctors of osteopathy also recognize the responsibility to teach the patient to make their own wise decisions to enhance self-healing.

### 4 Rational osteopathic treatment is based on applying the first three tenets

This is the most defining of the four osteopathic tenets. While the other three tenets are individually considered to be true statements by almost all healing professions, only the osteopathic profession has elected to, and has the means of, applying all three to the core of its educational and practise philosophy and therefore to the care of its patients.

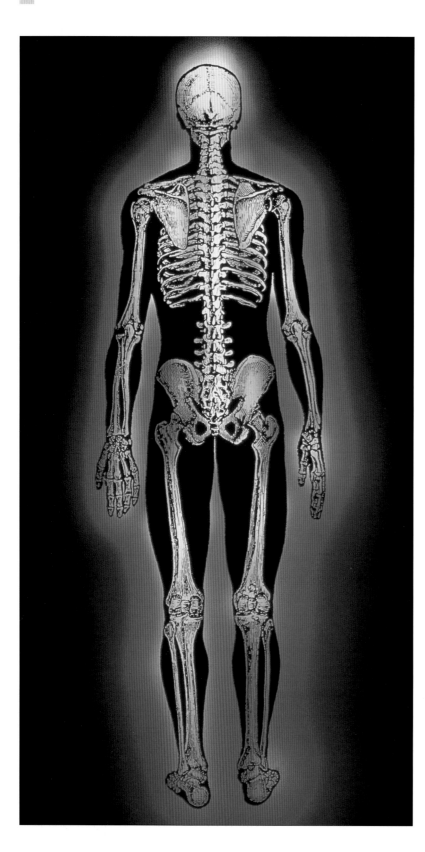

educational, postdoctoral training and specialty licencing system ensures that the distinctive osteopathic education in 16 U.S. colleges of osteopathic medicine (1996) is fully accredited as are its state, national, and specialty testing boards.

## PATIENT-CENTERED TREATMENT

Applying the osteopathic philosophy provides patient-centered rather than disease-centered treatment. Otherwise traditional treatment modalities, including medication, surgery, injections, braces and psychotherapy, are all used by U.S. osteopathic physicians, but the component parts of each treatment are tailored to each individual patient. Osteopathic manipulative treatment (OMT) may or may not be a part of a given patient's treatment. When it is employed, it too is selected for its role in applying the osteopathic tenets. Physiologist I.M. Korr, Ph.D., summarized the integration of OMT in applying the philosophy:

"Osteopathic manipulation is a whole system of diagnosis, appraisal and therapy designed to preserve health and prevent the spread of disease. Even when being applied primarily for the relief of symptoms, such as backache and headache, or for the treatment of diseases, manipulative therapy places the individual as a whole on a more nearly healthy, functioning path. That path, unique for each individual, leads the well person towards greater wellbeing and a lowered susceptibility to illness in general, and the ill person toward recovery and toward the cure, which, if it comes, must come from within."

## HOW OSTEOPATHIC MEDICINE WORKS AND ITS PRACTICAL APPLICATION

The neurologic and physiologic bases of the osteopathic tenets have been well documented.

### 1 THE BODY UNITY CONCEPT

Now known to have a neuroendocrine mechanism, the body unity concept has long been demonstrated by the relationship between chronic pain and depression. Current research in psychoneuroimmunology demonstrates the clinical impact of stress and emotional status on the ability of the body to resist infection and to fight cancer. Applying this tenet is illustrated by the following case reported by an osteopathic internal medicine specialist:

"When I went into the practice of internal medicine, most internists were in the cardiac field, which takes about 70 to 80 percent of an internist's attention. Once my practise was established, 1 was greatly surprised to find that a high percentage of my referrals were coming to me from M.D. internists. Their patients would be suffering from all the signs and symptoms of coronary heart disease, acute coronary attacks, or anginal attacks, but electrocardiography (ECG) and all the other tests had disproved it was a coronary.

"Yet the patients were still suffering from chest pains. Sometimes it was persistent; sometimes it was intermittent; sometimes with exertion, or without. They were referred

to me because they were termed cardiac cripples. They were afraid psychologically.

"One man had suffered an attack of chest pains and was too frightened to go to work. He was afraid to mow his lawn or do anything that required physical exertion. Even though he'd been assured by the M.D.s that he had no evidence of coronary heart disease, he was convinced psychologically that he did have."

The osteopathic spinal examination in these cases frequently reveals somatic dysfunction of the upper thoracic vertebrae and ribs. Treatment in ECG and enzyme-negative cases consists of OMT to correct the dysfunction, and patient reassurance. Said the osteopathic internist of this approach, "Their pain left and they no longer suffered from this syndrome."

### ■ Assessing the whole person

In approaching each patient, the D.O. assesses the total person. For some, the hands-on approach is as reassuring to the patient as it is diagnostic; for others, the palpation uncovers specific physical clues needed to begin treatment. Regardless of the treatment selected—medication, manipulation, surgery or psychotherapy—the D.O. will educate and reassure the patient about the suggested approach and will further involve the patient in the healing process.

### 2 STRUCTURAL DYSFUNCTION

This is consistently found in a number of disorders associated with neurologic reflexes, including referred pain. These somatic (body framework) clues also provide reflex evidence of visceral problems. Treatment of somatic dysfunction

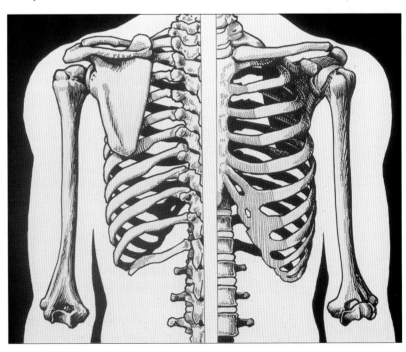

*Right: this image shows the front and back views of the spine and rib cage, the framework for the upper body.*

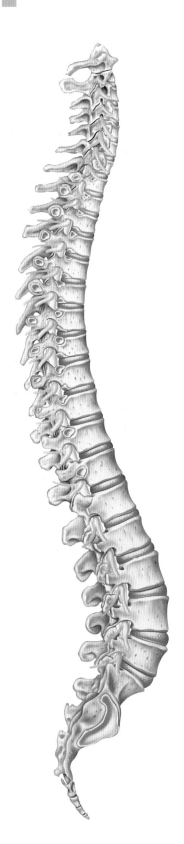

*Left: the spine is made up of 26 separate bones with cushioning disks in between the vertebrae. The back muscles provide support, mobility and locomotion.*

with manipulation is advocated and effective in acute low back pain and a number of myofascial pain syndromes. Additionally, treatment modifies a variety of physiologic parameters important in the care of patients in and out of the hospital. Somatic dysfunction has been studied extensively. Furthermore, the osteopathic profession has hosted a number of international conferences in which research and understanding of this phenomenon has been objectively studied.

The expanded physiologic effect of somatic dysfunction might be better understood if the dysfunction is thought of as a "neurologic lens." In essence, painful stimuli from various problems report to the spinal cord where they sensitize (or facilitate) the cord to any other stimulus. These facilitated segments neurologically focus physical and emotional stressors to other structures innervated by that segment, disturbing the physiology and blood supply to those tissues. Knowing these neurologic connections improves diagnosis. Managing these connections with OMT permits the patient to better handle stressors by removing the neurologic lens.

## 3 HOMEOSTASIS (SELF-HEALING)

Nutritional and other preventative strategies have a checkered scientific basis, but most health professionals support the rational basis for such approaches in supporting homeosta-

### VISITING A D.O. – WHAT TO EXPECT

The focus of an osteopathic examination is the patient. The D.O. will take a thorough history that includes questions on the patient's response to stress and effects of prior trauma to the body framework. All appropriate traditional physical examinations are likely to be used. These may range from the pelvic examination to a neurologic examination; from examining the eye grounds to the patient's arches on the soles of the feet. The D.O. will also incorporate a special examination, referred to as the osteopathic structural examination.

sis (self-healing and self-regulating). Patchy research also underlies the use of OMT in homeostasis. Several studies show reduced hospital length of stay when OMT was added to total osteopathic care. There is also a decreased mortality and morbidity when OMT is applied in the cardiac care unit to patients who have had heart attacks.

In all of these cases, OMT was added to recognized medical and surgical interventions as a means of addressing the self-healing mechanisms and reducing pain. Other studies measure physiologic effects of OMT on blood pressure and respiratory function, on urinary output and bowel contractions. One hundred years of use has convinced the osteopathic profession that OMT is safe and probably widely applicable in patient care.

A past president of the American College of Osteopathic Family Physicians, Dr. Korr, discussed his approach

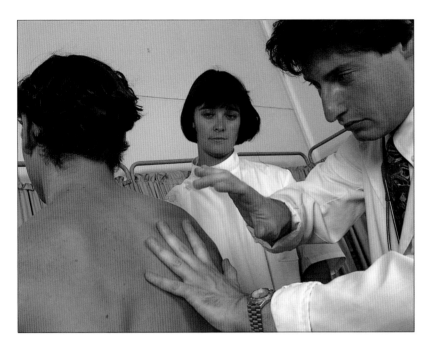

*Above: the osteopath will carry out a thorough physical examination as well as exploring the patient's medical history.*

to a patient with pneumonia:

"My first step is to utilize osteopathic manipulative treatment (OMT) as a way of establishing an adequate blood and nerve supply as well as lymphatic drainage. This is an additional aid to any drug therapy that might be available, such as appropriate injections of penicillin. Many times OMT is remarkably successful in speeding up the recovery process."

### 4 HEALTH MAINTENANCE

Dr. Korr summarizes the practical application of the osteopathic approach in today's health care arena as follows:

"It is becoming more and more widely appreciated that the prevailing healthcare delivery system is a monstrous anachronism. Technologically advanced as medicine is, its prac-

tice—with its social, political, and economic aspects—is geared to an era that has long passed. The acute infectious diseases and the quick killers (especially of the young) that prevailed a half-century and longer ago have largely been replaced by long-term illnesses of the adult, the aging, and the aged. These diseases cripple and kill gradually. A system which continues to be based on episodic treatment is absurdly and tragically

inappropriate at a time when the need is for a shift from periodic individual visits to extended continuous care, from sick care to well care, from emergency, finger-in-the-dike care to preventive 'flood control,' from the palliation of disease to the maintenance of health."

## THE OSTEOPATHIC STRUCTURAL EXAMINATION

■ The D.O. will gently palpate the head, neck, back, sacrum and extremities.

■ He will look for areas that are different from the surrounding regions.

■ Individual spinal and extremity joints will be checked for motion restriction, pain on motion, and malalignment.

■ Muscle spasm and chronic muscle shortening will be noted.

■ In areas of somatic dysfunction, neurologic reflex changes will produce tissue texture changes.

Years of training allow the D.O. to sense relatively small yet clinically important changes indicative of somatic dysfunction.

## SOMATIC DYSFUNCTION

This is a codable diagnosis. Officially the criteria for diagnosing somatic dysfunction can be remembered by the mnemonic "TART"—tenderness, asymmetry, restricted motion and tissue texture change. Once a diagnosis of somatic dysfunction is made, the D.O. will then attempt to interpret whether it is primarily a musculoskeletal clue or whether it is related to an

underlying visceral or systemic process.

A complete history is important for proper interpretation of the palpatory findings and for applying the osteopathic tenets. The historical and physical examinations also provide an insight into the most efficient, effective and safe manipulative techniques which should be selected in order to accomplish clinical goals.

# CONDITIONS WHICH OSTEOPATHIC MEDICINE ADDRESSES

Philosophic emphasis on the whole patient parallels the osteopathic profession's emphasis on primary care. Approximately 60 percent of D.O.s become primary care physicians who apply the osteopathic approach to all conditions. This means that regardless of whether a patient is suffering from a cold, pneumonia, diabetes or congestive heart failure; regardless of symptoms of headache, constipation, or low back pain; regardless of an impending birth or an impending surgery, the D.O. will apply the four tenets in caring for the person who is their patient. Osteopathic specialists, who have the same initial training as osteopathic general practitioners, may limit their practices to pediatrics or to patients with a specific group of problems, but most find ways to demonstrate their osteopathic heritage.

OMT is only one treatment tool available to osteopathic physicians but it is an active means of supporting body homeostasis. Occasionally it is the only specific treatment a patient will receive, whereas in other situations the physician may decide that its use in a particular situation is not needed.

When OMT is used, it may play a role in helping to thin sinus secretions, relieve headache and dizziness, diminish facial pain, and manage ear infections. It may assist in stabilizing heart rhythms, improving breathing mechanisms and regulating bowel and bladder functions. It provides patient comfort, enhances immune function and may prevent the need for more invasive procedures. It is the individual osteopathic physician who can decide when and how to integrate OMT with all of the other diagnostic and treatment methods at his disposal.

Not only is patient satisfaction high, but studies show that for a number of conditions, the osteopathic approach is extremely cost effective.

*Below: osteopathic treatment may consist of palpating the patient's head, neck, back, sacrum or extremities. The osteopath will look for areas that are different from the surrounding regions.*

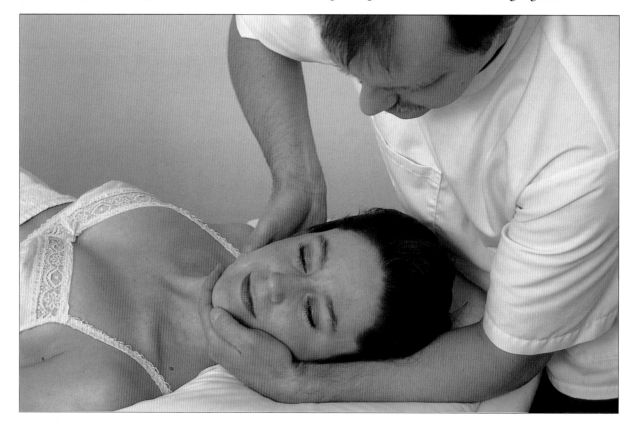

# INTERACTION WITH OTHER THERAPIES

The osteopathic approach integrates a wide range of therapeutic modalities in designing an individualized program to fight disease and/or to promote health in each patient. Osteopathic physicians interact side-by-side with allopathic physicians in hospitals, teaching institutions, health bureaus, and outpatient clinics throughout the United States. They make up a parallel but distinctive profession—parallel in scope of practice, but distinctive in their education, philosophy and patient care.

D.O.s and M.D.s make up the only two professions in the U.S. with unlimited license to incorporate any recognized health care practice—alternative or mainstream—which might benefit their patients.

■ Both D.O.s and M.D.s weigh the health benefits to the risks when they are determining a therapeutic approach.

■ Both are held to the same high standard accepted and required of all American physicians.

Osteopathic medicine, however, is possibly the only health profession whose colleges accord a central position to the importance of the patient and his/her neuromusculoskeletal system in the maintenance of health, the diagnosis of disease, and the relief of illness, while also teaching the use of all proven diagnostic and therapeutic modalities available to modern medicine. Thus the D.O. is likely to modify a given treatment regimen specific to the individual needs of the patient, while consistently practicing the physician's principle: "first do no harm."

# FITTING OSTEOPATHY INTO YOUR LIFESTYLE

**MAKING IT WORK FOR YOU**
Because health care works best when both the physician and the patient work together with common goals, the first step in fitting osteopathy into your lifestyle is to decide what your goals are.

■ Are you wanting to maximize your level of health or seeking relief from a particular symptom?

■ Are you hoping for assistance in modifying your diet or willing to accept the advice resulting from a general physical examination?

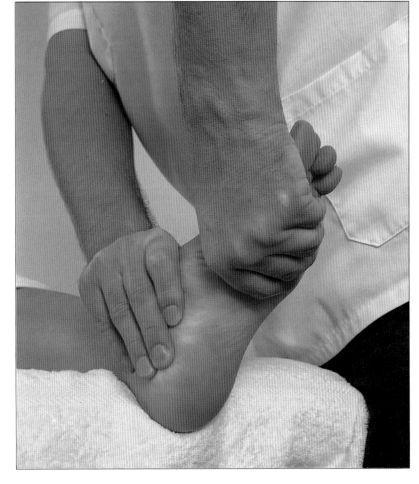

*Right: osteopathy is a "high-touch" system of practice, which emphasizes the patient's health, physically, mentally and spiritually. Your osteopath may suggest a broad program for you to implement, including exercise and diet.*

## FIND AN OSTEOPATHIC PHYSICIAN

Seek out an osteopathic physician who meets your needs and goals. Often friends who enjoy osteopathic care can provide you with recommendations. The Useful Addresses at the end of this book can help you to locate an osteopathic physician close to you. A few questions over the phone to the receptionist will determine whether the osteopathic physician you are considering is a general practitioner, an obstetrician-gynecologist, or a cardiovascular surgeon. Select the appropriate type of practitioner you need and schedule an appointment. At your initial appointment, discuss both your problems and expectations. You are looking for a "doctor" who can help to "teach" you how best to reach your health goals, so look for an osteopathic physician with whom you are comfortable. Remember that physicians are people too and have as wide a range of personalities. Provide the physician you ultimately select with a full and honest history. Some points that you consider unimportant may be valuable in providing insight into your care.

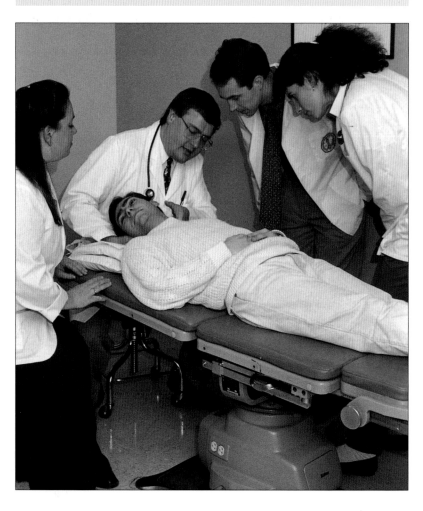

## SELF-HELP

**PRACTICAL MEASURES THAT YOU CAN DO YOURSELF TO COMPLEMENT THE TREATMENT YOU RECEIVE**

Your osteopathic physician will encourage you to play an active role in your treatment protocol. D.O.s often emphasize diet and exercise while stressing preventive health practices. They will teach or provide educational materials to help you make wise health decisions. Being as compliant with the treatment protocol as possible is, of course, the best way of maximizing the osteopathic prescription. If you don't understand why you are asked to do something, let your physician know this. Knowledge helps you to comply and empowers you to play an active role in maximizing your health.

## UNDERSTANDING THE OSTEOPATHIC APPROACH

As you come to appreciate that the body is a unit, you might set aside some time for activities designed to improve not only your physical health, but also your mind and spirit. Take some time for introspection, meditation and/or prayer. Build positive relationships with your friends and family. If you have a chronic condition, inquire about positive support groups. Laughter, peace of mind and

*Left: osteopaths receive a very comprehensive training before they qualify. In the United States, there are 16 colleges of osteopathic medicine.*

supportive relationships have all been shown to maximize health. Your osteopathic physician can suggest these things but only you can accomplish them.

Knowing that your own body is responsible for healing and grasping the relationship between structure and function, will encourage you to exercise, eat properly, and avoid extrinsic substances harmful to your body. Your "doctor" can teach and suggest but, for the most part, implementation of the program that you mutually agree upon is left up to you.

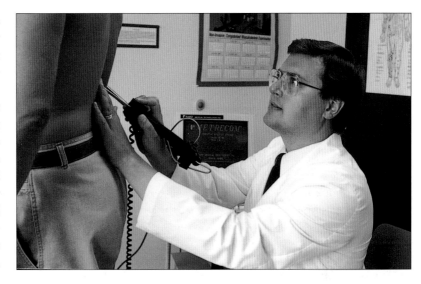

## SUMMARY

Osteopathic medicine provides an alternative to allopathic medicine practiced by M.D.s. It is a complete system of practice which emphasizes health and the patient while possessing all diagnostic and treatment modalities needed to control illness and disease. Its distinctive mission is primary care, its distinctive philosophy recognizes the primacy of the neuromusculoskeletal system, and its distinctive approach remains holistic. It is simultaneously "high-tech and high-touch." Attractive for these reasons, it is the choice of many families for their complete health care needs.

*Above: It is important to examine the patient thoroughly and to assess the problem before deciding on a course of treatment. The experienced DO is able to sense relatively small yet clinically important changes indicative of somatic dysfunction.*

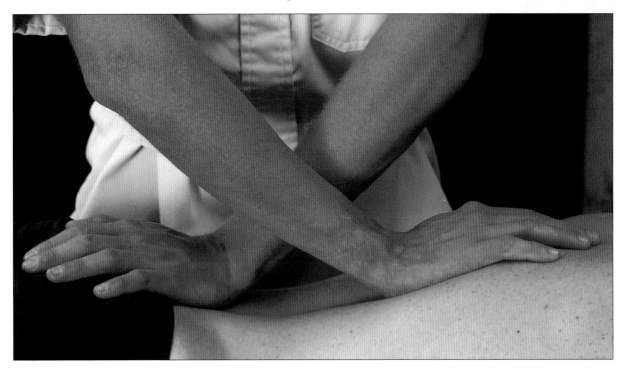

# CRANIAL OSTEOPATHY

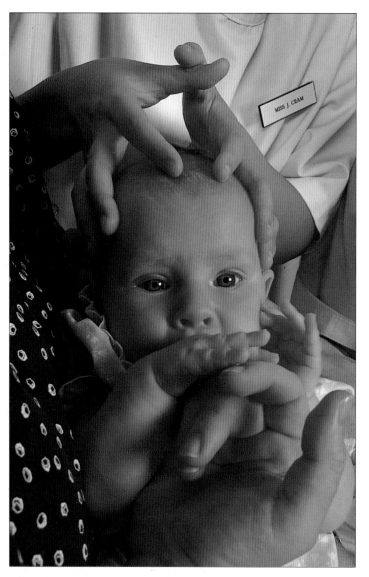

## CHAPTER TWELVE

*C*ranial osteopathy is an extremely subtle and profound form of osteopathic manipulative treatment, focusing as it does on a subtle and profound fluctuation of fluid within the body. This treatment may benefit a wide range of common health problems and medical disorders, ranging from conditions such as colic in the newborn, recurring ear infections in children, back pain in pregnancy, and migraine headaches, to difficulty in breathing and dizziness in the elderly. It may reduce the cost of orthodox allopathic medicine and may even help to establish a firm diagnosis, even in cases in which conventional medicine can find no cause or cure for the affected individual's symptoms. As we shall see, cranial osteopathy accomplishes the release of the restrictions on motion and helps to promote the body's natural self-healing mechanism.

# HISTORY AND ORIGINS

Cranial osteopathy originated with William Garner Sutherland, D.O. (1873-1954). While he was a student at The American School of Osteopathy in Kirksville, Missouri, in 1899, he pondered a specially prepared skull, which was put on display by his teacher, the founder of osteopathic medicine, Andrew Taylor Still, M.D. This "disarticulated" skull revealed all the fine details of the cranial bones as they come together in joints, called "sutures."

Dr. Still taught his students the osteopathic principle that each of the body's functions determines a particular structure, and that each structure has a function. Sutherland wondered what the function of these complex sutures could be. A flash of inspiration struck him that a design for a respiratory motion is evident in the sutures. All of the textbooks of anatomy stated that the sutures are fused and are unable to move in adulthood. Sutherland resisted the idea that the skull moves, but he could not let it rest, and soon it became the motivation for his singular, detailed and prolonged study of inanimate skulls and his experimentation upon his own head.

As a result of Sutherland's insight and detailed research, he discovered a previously unrecognized phenomenon, i.e the "primary respiratory mechanism." In time, his discovery may be regarded as one of the most important in physiology. He found that:

**1** The central nervous system inherently moves in an organized cycle of swelling and receding.
**2** The fluid it manufactures (the cerebrospinal fluid) fluctuates in rhythm with it.
**3** The skull, spine and sacrum and the tough membranes (*dura mater*) encasing the brain and spinal cord accommodate for this motion.

This swelling and receding can be felt by the trained individual in all areas of the body, including the cranium and sacrum.

# MAINTENANCE AND SELF-HEALING

In essence, Sutherland maintained that this motion is the mechanical manifestation of the body's dynamic system of maintenance and self-healing. The fluctuation brings nutrients, peptides, hormones and other essential substances to all the cells of the body, and washes away the waste products. This fluctuation of fluid is associated with an electromagnetic energy which also cycles from positive to negative. It works within the extracellular fluid which contains the connective tissue, the final common area of all.

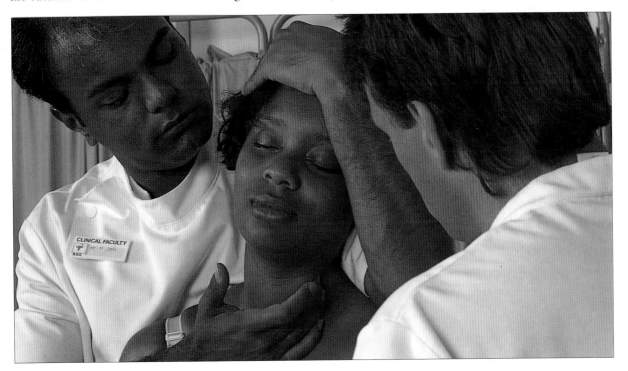

## BENEFITS OF CRANIAL OSTEOPATHY

Besides relieving symptoms of biomechanical imbalance and nerve dysfunction, such as pain, numbness, weakness, and tingling, cranial osteopathy is thought to reduce swelling, improve vision, sharpen cognition, improve functioning of organs, enhance breathing, increase energy levels, allow restful sleep and relaxation, and provide a sense of wellbeing, confidence and self-awareness. This treatment provides healing, as distinguished from the goal of conventional medicine: to fight disease. Cranial Osteopathy stimulates the body's own resources to generate its own healing.

■ Fluids (blood, lymph, cerebrospinal and cellular).
■ Physiologically active substances (peptides, hormones, immune regulators and more).
■ Nerve endings, as they all influence the cells.

The connective tissue touches every cell, and sheets of it (fascia) surround every organ, muscle, nerve and vessel. These sheets conduct this fluctuation of fluid and energy.

## RELIEVING RESTRICTIONS OF MOVEMENT

Areas of mechanical restriction are thought to serve as focal points for the origin of disease processes, as Dr. Still taught, since they impair the normal function of joints, nerves, and the flow of blood and lymph. A goal of the osteopathic physician is to relieve the patient's body of these restrictions of motion. With this goal in mind, many forms of osteopathic manipulation are employed.

Cranial Osteopathy accomplishes a release when the physician identifies by palpation, the exact conformation and location of the restriction, and accordingly recreates the position of injury. The connective tissue holds the force of trauma via the shape and charge (piezoelectric quality) of its collagen fibers. The treating physician must achieve a balanced tension of all the injured parts in order to release:

1 The distorted shape and charge ("tissue memory").
2 The restricted motion.
3 The diminished healing potential there.

Often, the positioning of these tissues requires very little gross motion on the part of the physician, but, sometimes, great amounts of force are specifically applied to achieve a release. This is why the physician's knowledge of the details of anatomy are vital. This practice represents the art and the science of medicine coming together in a practice of healing.

## TREATMENT

In a typical session, the clothed patient usually lies face up on a comfortable table as the physician gently places his hands lightly upon various areas of the body to identify where the fluctuation of fluid is diminished or distorted, and assists in its normalization, thereby promoting healing. The physician pays particular attention to the cranium, sacrum, spine, pelvis and diaphragm, but treats any part of the body where there is such a restriction of motion. When the fluctuation is normalized in a particular region, he moves on to the next area. A treatment usually lasts between 20 and 60 minutes.

## EFFECTS AND RESULTS OF TREATMENT

■ The effects of this treatment may be immediate and/or accumulative, at times avoiding the need for surgery and drugs. The treatment is usually very relaxing, and sometimes induces a trance-like state or sleep. There may be some physical discomfort as an area of major trauma is addressed but this is only short-term. Emotional discomfort, such as fear or grief, may arise. This usually happens as the physician recreates the position the body was in at the time of the original trauma. It is in this manner that healing of the whole person occurs.
■ Results of treatment vary according to the severity and acuteness of the problem, and the general health of the individual. Younger patients generally respond more quickly and completely. In acute conditions, these patients will require one to three treatments, one week apart. Difficult, chronic conditions might be treated weekly, perhaps for several months.

## TREATING BABIES, CHILDREN AND ADOLESCENTS

In the newborn, this treatment is applied at its best. As opposed to adults, a baby may be permanently changed by treatment, preventing the possibility of illness in later years.

Indicators of the need for treatment in infancy include such factors as difficult, prolonged or precipitous birth (including Caesarean section in the case of a difficult labor), excessive crying, poor sleep, poor ability to suckle, spitting up and a distorted face, neck, shoulders etc.

In the childhood and teenage years, scoliosis can often be managed very well, frequently eliminating any sign of a lateral spinal curvature. With cranial osteopathy, children with learning disabilities, in many cases, will be better able to focus their attention. Childhood allergies respond to treatment of the cranium, sternum, diaphragm and related structures. When treated early in life, asthma may resolve. Likewise, recurring ear infections may improve, if mechanical blockage is the issue.

## CONDITIONS IT CAN BE USED TO TREAT

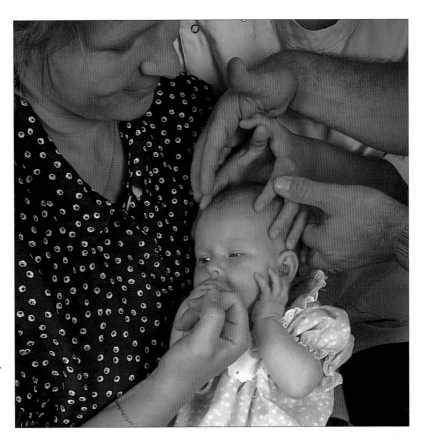

At any age, some causes of ringing in the ears and dizziness may respond well to cranial osteopathy. Colitis, urinary incontinence and painful menstrual periods may be helped. It can be successful in relieving many painful conditions, including low back pain, neck pain and headache, even migraines. It helps in many cases of facial pain, such as trigeminal neuralgia and temporomandibular joint dysfunction. It also helps restore the facial weakness of Bell's Palsy. Chest pain, abdominal pain and pelvic pain may respond very favorably, especially if there is some history of trauma to the spine, ribs, pelvis or extremities. Difficulties with pain, tingling or weakness in the extremities may often be successfully treated, including such problems as carpal tunnel syndrome, sciatica and thoracic outlet syndrome.

There are instances when Cranial Osteopathy is successful in treating ruptured intervertebral discs and injuries resulting in fractures and sprains. Any time there is involvement of the soft tissues, Cranial Osteopathy can be helpful, even when a fracture of a bone exists, or if surgery is necessary. It may be important to integrate physical therapy or a specific exercise program to optimize the healing process, in conjunction with the manipulative treatment.

## CHOOSING AN OSTEOPATHIC PHYSICIAN

Paramedical practitioners learn a simplified version of Cranial Osteopathy called "Craniosacral Therapy." Osteopathic physicians are trained to diagnose and treat patients by receiving a comprehensive medical education that provides them with a thorough understanding of the function and dysfunction of the human body. To be assured of the best possible care, choose a qualified osteopathic physician, medical doctor or dentist who has a Certificate of Competency in Cranial Osteopathy. For further information, turn to Useful Addresses section at the back of the book.

# ROLFING

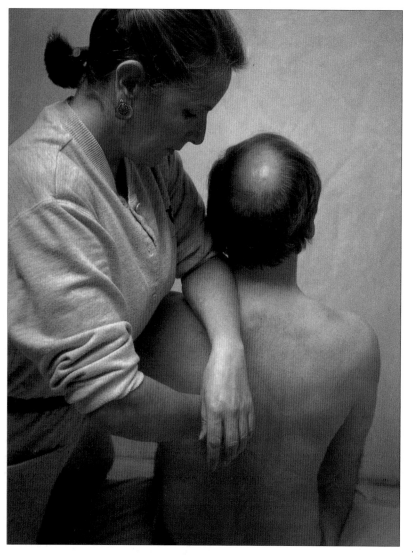

## CHAPTER THIRTEEN

*R*olfing is the holistic philosophy, science and art of releasing, enhancing and integrating the structural, functional and energetic organization of the human body in gravity. Developed by Dr. Ida P. Rolf (1896-1979), Rolfing was originally called Structural Integration but the public preferred the eponymous title and the nickname remained. The official non-generic, service-marked name of this work is Rolfing Structural Integration. It is a unique somatic practice designed to proactively explore, improve and balance a person's structural/somatic "pattern" within gravity.

If you can imagine how it feels to live in a fluid, light, balanced body, free of pain, stiffness and chronic stress, at ease with itself and the gravitational field, then you will understand the purpose of Rolfing. World-class athletes, musicians, artists, actors, business people and people from all walks of life and of all ages have sought the benefits of Rolfing. Not only do people seek Rolfing as a way to ease pain and chronic stress, but also as a way to improve performance in their professions and daily activities.

## PHILOSOPHY OF ROLFING

"Before" and "after" photographs of once-slouching clients who appear to have grown an inch or two are evidence that, at the very least, Rolfing improves posture and elongates the body. But the more profound results of this approach are located within the "subjective" experience of the client. It is the "experience" of being supported in gravity and the individual's perception of imminent change that Rolfers are working toward. Rolfing is not a form of massage, deep tissue or otherwise, nor is it simply a type of myofascial or osseous release therapy, although all of these respective approaches rest upon Dr. Rolf's pioneering work. Instead, it is an entirely holistic form of education and manipulation that deals with the whole person in relation to gravity.

Rolfing is as much a philosophical stance as it is a concrete, hands-on therapy. For example, if someone came up with a way to structurally organize a person within gravity by merely waving a hand over a body without ever touching the person, that could be considered Rolfing because the holistic intent was balancing the whole person in gravity. Merely facilitating relaxation, fluid flow, and/or symptomatic relief through superficial or deep tissue techniques is wonderful—however, it's not Rolfing. The view of gravity's impact on human structure is the hallmark of Rolfing and distinguishes it from all other types of somatic approaches.

## DR. IDA P. ROLF

The founder of Rolfing, Dr. Ida P. Rolf, was born in New York and graduated from Barnard College in 1916 with a bachelor of science degree. In 1920 she received her doctorate in biochemistry from Columbia University's College of Physicians and Surgeons. During the 1950s, after 25 years of developing her revolutionary work, Dr. Rolf presented Structural Integration in the United States, Canada and Great Britain, primarily to osteopaths and chiropractors. Most "deep-tissue" therapies and many other types of soft tissue manipulation developed in this country have been influenced by Dr. Rolf's work, along with that of some of the early osteopaths including Drs. Still, Sutherland and Ward. In the 1960s, she was invited by Fritz Perls, founder of Gestalt Therapy, to teach at Esalen Institute in Big Sur, California. During this time, Rolfing rose to unprecedented popularity and, possibly, because many in the Gestalt/Human potential movement flocked to Rolfing and promulgated numerous accounts of profound transformation, Rolfing developed a reputation as a desirably cathartic form of emotional processing and release. To this day, many university psychology texts include descriptions of Rolfing.

## ROLFING AND SCIENCE

Beginning with the insight that the human body is a unified structural and functional whole that stands in a unique relation to the uncompromising presence of gravity, Dr. Rolf asked this fundamental question: "What conditions must be fulfilled in order for the human body to be organized and integrated in gravity so that it can function in the most economical way?"

Science has known for years that proper physiological function and anatomical structure are related. Dr. Rolf agreed, along with her peers in Osteopathy and Chiropractic, that the body as a whole functioned better when local areas of dysfunction were resolved, when bony segments were in proper alignment, and when joints exhibited proper mobility. But she realized that a long-lasting and profound transformation in our bodily being, alignment, and overall sense of wellbeing and freedom, required a more far-reaching understanding of the impact of gravity on our bodies. Dr. Rolf was not only concerned with creating a system of manipulation that could ease the pain and stresses of human life by properly aligning the body, but she was also profoundly interested in creating a system that could transform the whole person at every level.

## ROLFING AND FASCIA

Rolfing achieves its remarkable results by manipulating the myofascial system. The medium that is so radically influenced by gravity is fascia. Fascia is a continuous web of thin, elastic (connective) tissue throughout the entire body. It binds muscle fibers together, and attaches muscles to bones and to each other, covers organs and blood vessels and provides the individual shape of the human form. Eighty percent of the body's protein is utilized to create and maintain this intricate system. Fascia can be distorted due to injury, emotional trauma and poor postural habits. It adapts to these insults by contracting and bonding, thereby shortening and thickening. Basic physical movements become complicated and too much energy is then required for a simple task. Rolfing attempts to reverse this process by systematically and sensitively freeing fascial adhesions and, then, introducing more efficient movement options which reinforce the structural change. The proactive nature of the work is another characteristic that distinguishes the process from other deep-tissue techniques.

## ROLFING AND PAIN

Our bodies must deal with gravity like other material structures. When we are out of alignment, gravity drags us down, just as it drags down a building that has lost its architectural integrity. Whether from poor posture, injury, illness or emotional distress, a misaligned or "random" body is at war with gravity. We experience this war as pain, stress, and depleted energy.

Rolfers are similar to archeologists while working with the body in that they are involved in the process of "uncovering." Does the archeologist, upon discovering something old and significant, pull out a jackhammer and desecrate the site? Instead, precise tools and brushes are used to patiently extricate the underlying material. In the same manner, Rolfers are trained to sensitively uncover patterns of holding and shortening in the body that may or may not be tolerably painful. If there was no accumulated trauma in bodies, there would be no pain whatsoever.

The most common misconception about Rolfing is that the technique consists of gratuitously painful pressure that is applied to the client, but that is not the case. In fact, the Rolfer's eyes, more than his hands, are the primary tools used to "see" the structural patterns that have emerged over the course of a person's life. To the Rolfer's trained eyes, the all too prevalent examples of bodily disorder, such as slouched postures with head and neck too far forward, hyper-erect structures that bow backward, knock knees or bowed

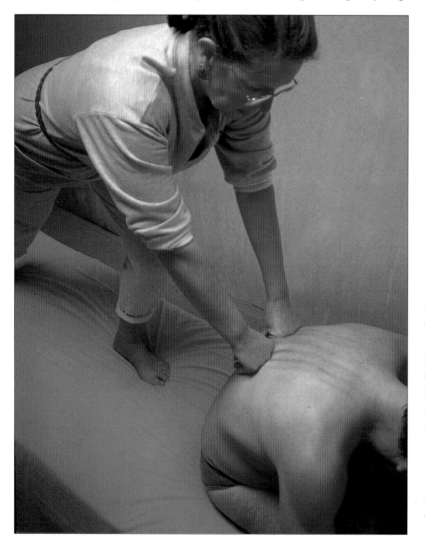

*Left: the Rolfer uses educated hands to improve and balance a person's structural/somatic "pattern" within gravity.*

legs, flat feet or high arches or excessive spinal curvature, all display complicated patterns of strain, tightness and thickening of the connective tissue.

But, rather than merely doing something to the body, especially something that does not honor or moves beyond the client's boundaries, Rolfers approach their objective to introduce options for change with finesse. Metaphorically, as a type of "dialogue" with the body, Rolfing is more about listening and suggesting, rather than shouting or demanding.

Through refined and intelligent pressure applied by the educated hands of the Rolfer, layer by layer of fascia is softened and lengthened, allowing the body to effortlessly right itself in gravity. From the Rolfing perspective, if the whole body is not properly prepared to receive the effects of local manipulations, either the change will not be maintained or strain will show up in other areas. Photographs may be taken before and after the work to show changes in the body. Rolfing is an on-going process of change that may continue after an initial series. Advanced sessions are available after a period of integration.

Rolfing Movement Integration is a system of movement education that continues the process of change by promoting more harmonious and efficient movement within gravity, thereby continuing the process of embodiment.

*Right: Rolfing achieves its results by manipulating the patient's myofascial system.*

# RECENT RESEARCH

Research conducted at UCLA by Dr. Valerie Hunt, showed that Rolfing:
■ Creates a more efficient use of the muscles.
■ Allows the body to conserve energy.
■ Creates more economical and refined patterns of movement.

More recent research conducted at the University of Maryland demonstrated that Rolfing:

■ Significantly reduces chronic stress and changes body structure for the better.
■ Significantly reduces the spinal curvature of subjects with lordosis (sway back).
■ Enhances neurological functioning in general.

Surprizingly, these changes in structure and function are long lasting and rarely require maintenance sessions.

## FINDING A ROLFER
Rolfing practitioners and movement teachers are trained and certified at the International Rolf Institute in Boulder, Colorado, which continues to be the leader, pioneer, and the source of the most advanced forms of myofascial manipulation and body integration anywhere in the world today.

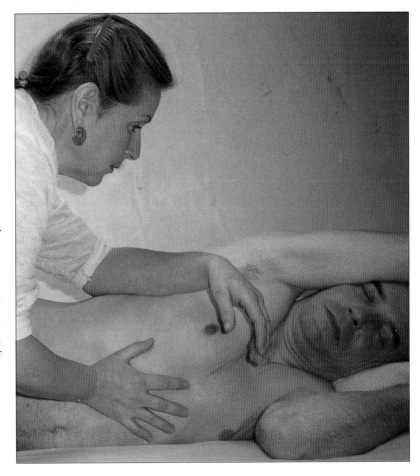

# DANCE THERAPY

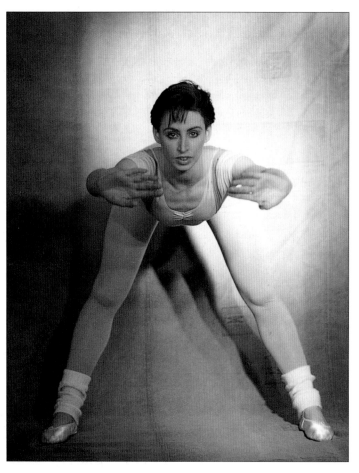

## CHAPTER FOURTEEN

*D*ance movement therapy is a healing art, using movement of the body to promote growth and health. Since the personality and emotions are thought to be rooted in the body, changes made on the body level can affect a person's total functioning. The dance movement therapist creates dance actions to relate and respond to each patient's needs.

In 1942, Marian Chace, a former member of the Denishawn dance company, was working in Washington, D.C. Psychiatrists in the area became aware that their patients were deriving therapeutic benefits from studying dance with Chace and asked her if she would "teach" psychotic patients at St. Elizabeth's Hospital. The mental health field was in flux; psychiatrists and administrators of mental health facilities were looking for new ways to treat the large numbers of returning servicemen, many of whom were unable to communicate, to express their feelings or to participate in group activities. Chace, who was accustomed to inspiring dance students to extend themselves physically and emotionally, used her skills to transform disabled and traumatized patients into social human beings.

At the same time, Trudi Schoop, a dancer and a mime artist, was volunteering her services at Camarillo State Hospital in California. She used her skills with schizophrenic patients and labeled her work "ego body" technique. The time was ripe for a body-movement therapy that could reach large numbers of dysfunctional people. The modern dance movement combined with the insights of psychology provided the impetus for a new profession—dance movement therapy.

## THE DEVELOPMENT OF DANCE THERAPY

There are three major areas from which dance movement therapy has developed: dance, psychology and movement observation techniques.

### DANCE

Throughout the ages, dance has been used to commemorate significant events. People have always expressed themselves by moving together to a common rhythm. They danced to honor significant events in their lives, to share strong feelings, to heal the sick and the disaffected, and also to maintain a communal bond. The sense of community that comes from people dancing together to a common beat is an important feature of dance movement therapy. The improvizational and creative component of dance is a direct outgrowth of modern dance which departed from the set structure of ballet.

Modern dancers portrayed their personal feelings as well as their reactions to contemporary issues and events. Expressing, modifying and controlling feelings through dance actions are basic foundations of dance movement.

### PSYCHOLOGY

The second influence in the development of dance movement therapy was the growing interest in psychology. Dance movement therapy pioneers, such as Liljan Espenak, Blanche Evan and Mary Whitehouse, applied psychological theories to their work with neurotic and psychotic people. For example, Marian Chace was influenced by the interaction theory of Harry Stack Sullivan; Evan by the psychodynamic theory of Sigmund Freud; Whitehouse by Jung's concept of creative imagination; and Espenak by Alfred Adler's views on inferiority and the importance of aggression.

The work of Wilhem Reich also made a major impact in the field of dance movement therapy. He was the first psychoanalyst to explore the relationship of muscular rigidity (character armor) to psychic disturbance. This allowed him to analyze the somatic manifestation of the unconscious.

## MOVEMENT OBSERVATION TECHNIQUES

These techniques, particularly those of Rudolf Laban, have enabled dance movement therapists to understand the meaning of movement behavior. Labananalysis, a system to observe, record and analyze the behavior of individuals, allows for devising movement profiles, researching movement behavior and monitoring change on the movement level.

## BODY AND MIND

Dance movement therapists espouse a unitary relationship between body and mind. They believe that the body manifests the subtleties of the mind. Bodily feelings affect mental states and, conversely, our thoughts and feelings are expressed in muscle tension and movement patterns. Emotions, accidents, abuse and injury are locked into the body. Personality style, coping skills, feeling states and ego functioning can be

## AIMS OF DANCE

The overall objective in dance movement therapy is to enable clients to understand how and why they function as they do and to help them explore and choose new ways of behaving. A significant aspect of dance movement therapy is that it develops the strengths of people by reinforcing what they are able to do physically, psychologically, intellectually and socially.

■ On the physical level, the dance movement therapist aims at decreasing bodily tension, reducing chronic pain and enhancing circulation and respiration.

■ On the psychological level, the aim is to ameliorate depression, fear, anxiety, and suicidal feelings, to express anger, experience joy and learn self-control.

■ On the intellectual level, the goal is to increase attention span, verbalization and the use of imagery.

■ On the social level, the dance movement therapist helps to decrease isolation, foster solidarity and increase communication skills among patients.

Working simultaneously on all these levels allows for integration of body and mind and the connection of self to others.

seen as a person moves. Unexpressed feelings are seen in chronic muscle tension and restricted movement patterns. The dance movement therapist deals with these physical manifestations of the psychic process. Intervening with dance actions, the dance movement therapist gives form and meaning to these emerging expressions.

## PROMOTING HEALING PROCESSES

Certain aspects of dance movement therapy are thought to promote the healing process.

■ **Synchrony**—moving together in time and space—creates the initial social bond in a dance movement therapy group. As people move in unison, internal emotional states are expressed and thus can be explored and understood.

■ **Rhythm**—the recurring patterns of bodily movement—contains and organizes these expressions of emotional states.

Neither of the above could occur without the vitality inherent in dance. The liveliness of dance loosens muscular rigidity, diminishes anxiety, frees the impulse to act and provides the energy to do so. Through their participation in dance movement sessions, patients begin to feel whole, to integrate thoughts and expression, feelings and words, past and present. As they share in each other's dance they develop a sense of belonging to a group. They learn from their own experiences and the experiences of others, and they develop and participate in each other's symbolic expression. It is the shared dance symbol that illuminates intangible ideas, feelings and impulses that links the individual to society.

## VISITING A DANCE THERAPIST

All dance movement therapists, whether in private practice or in institutional practice, will carry out an overall assessment of the client's needs. In a verbal interview, the therapist gathers background information and the client's reasons for entering into treatment. Next, the dance movement therapist assesses the client's movement behavior. Using Labananalysis, the dance movement therapist notes, for example, the shape of the body—is the person erect or caved in, does the person reach out or keep to himself, are the movements fluid or restricted, can the person express tenderness or strength, etc?

Since personality is expressed in movement behavior this assessment serves as a diagnostic tool as well. Each person has been sculptured by his life experiences; some people literally disown parts of their bodies and the feelings associated with these parts. The dance movement therapist engages the client by tuning into his movements. Dance training allows the therapist to replicate the client's movements in her own body. Moving like and with the client—empathic mirroring—provides the dance movement therapist with very useful information while, at the same time, validating and accepting the client as he is.

This tuning into the client's emotional state, on a movement level, establishes rapport. The client feels this and responds to the therapist's interventions. The relationship between the client and the dance movement therapist is further developed by moving together. The dance movement therapist's movement interventions support the feelings, sensations, and interactions that emerge from these interactions. Verbal interpretations reinforce the therapeutic experience linking thoughts and feelings with actions. The dance and verbal dialogue are

## FORMS OF DANCE THERAPY

Dance movement therapy work takes many forms. How the sessions progress depends upon the client's background, needs and comfort level. The client may move alone or with the therapist. Music may or may not be used and techniques are adapted for specific ages and problems. Discussions and verbal interventions may occur during the dance actions or at the end of a session.

In group sessions, which usually take place in institutional facilities, the dance movement therapist explains what takes place during a session. Music is generally used and the dance movement therapist begins with simple, rhythmic actions that the entire group can follow. Each individual in the group is acknowledged for what he she is able to do. As people begin to express themselves, the dance movement therapist encourages the group to share and support the emotions that unfold.

entwined to intensify the patient's movements. Remnants of feelings are brought to their fullest intention, thereby helping the person to explore past experiences and to be brave enough to try new ones.

Walking into a dance studio for the first individual dance movement therapy session, a client will be asked to discuss his reasons for entering into treatment. The client might be asked to walk around the room, alone, or with the dance movement therapist, whichever is more comfortable. In this way, the dance movement therapist gleans information about the client's movements and interactive style. After this movement task, they discuss treatment goals and arrive at a contract regarding the duration and nature of the work. This contract is reviewed periodically to see if the goals are being met. The dance movement therapist then suggests that for subsequent sessions the client should bring some comfortable clothing in order to move freely.

## USES OF DANCE MOVEMENT THERAPY

Dance movement therapy is used with the mentally and physically disabled in hospitals in outpatient and inpatient programs, and also in educational, rehabilitative, and wellness programs. Mental disorders include psychosis, borderline and multiple personality disorders, eating disorders, depression, physical and sexual abuse and chemical dependency. Physical problems include brain injury, AIDS, arthritis, amputations, stroke and cancer.

Dance movement therapists also work with the imprisoned and the

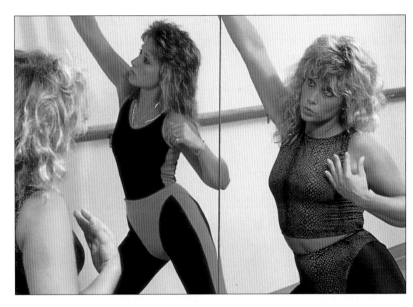

homeless. Much work has been done with children and with adolescents, particularly with the emotionally disturbed, learning disabled, sexually abused, depressed and suicidal, autistic, mentally retarded, asthmatic and the visually and hearing impaired.

Given the growing elderly population, dance movement therapists are now employed in some nursing homes and senior citizen centers where they work with the well elderly in addition to Alzheimer's Disease

and some other dementia patients.

Dance movement therapists are now working in managed care facilities, dealing with chronic pain, stress, hypertension and cardiac disease. In inpatient and outpatient facilities, dance movement therapists often run groups with art, music and drama therapists as part of a creative arts therapies team. In some facilities, dance movement therapists work in tandem with verbal group therapists meshing movement and words.

## THE BENEFITS OF DANCE MOVEMENT THERAPY

The principles inherent in dance movement therapy and the benefits derived from sessions are useful for all people. The sense of wellbeing, spontaneity and ease that come from moving alone and with others is something for which people strive. In dance movement therapy, people become aware of their habitual movement patterns—the first step toward change. They learn to recognize and trust their initial impulses, which gives them the freedom to express or to contain these urges. Knowing their bodily reactions to stress, they can use learned movement techniques to reduce tension in their shoulders, stomach and other areas of the body—to increase circulation and to deepen breathing. Likewise, when feeling sluggish they can become revitalized by re-enacting past movement experiences. In essence, the creative process implicit in the art of dancing opens up new ways of thinking and doing.

# YOGA

## CHAPTER FIFTEEN

*Yoga is understood to be both a process and a goal, a means and an end. The process is the consistent and intentional utilization of a set of formal and informal practices; the goal is an attainment, of which the description varies. A.G. Mohan addresses these dual aspects when he says that the goal of yoga is a "state of mind which is an end in itself" and adds that "whether we want to touch our toes or reach God, there must be movement. This movement is yoga." Joan Borysenko, co-founder with Herbert Benson, M.D. of the Mind/Body Clinic at New England Deaconess Hospital, says that the practice of yoga is*

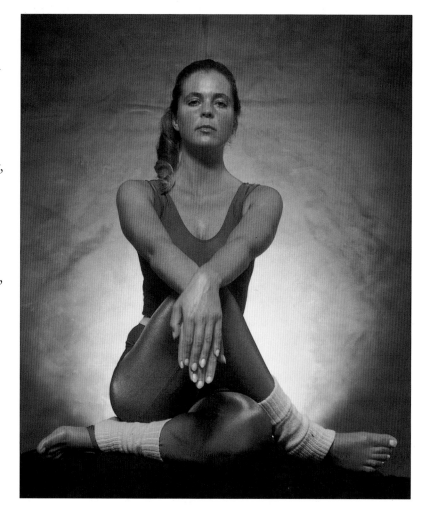

*"aimed at learning to quiet the mind and to direct it." She speaks of the practices as "centering" and asserts that the end result is an increase of awareness, honesty, confidence, competence and love. As you practice hatha yoga regularly and correctly you will feel, better, stronger, more balanced and flexible. Regular practice results in maintenance and restoration of health and wellbeing.*

## THE ORIGINS OF YOGA

Yoga has its origins in the ancient Vedas, scriptures sacred to all Hindus. The Vedas were passed down orally in story and song for many centuries and were first recorded between 1000 and 3000B.C. In the first half of each of the Vedas, ancient sages (rishis) express instruction in rituals and rules of conduct.

In the last half of each of the Vedas (which are collectively called *The Upanishads*) these sages express philosophical insights gained by their experiences of superconscious states, and offer encouragements to help readers achieve these insights through direct experience.

In the Vedas, Yoga is one of six equally valid systems described as paths to that experience. Later, *The Bhagavad Gita*, meaning "Song of God," was passed along and set down in writing to further help people understand and practice yoga. It is a section of the sacred epic scripture, *The Mahabharata*. In the *Bhagavad Gita*, Lord Krishna, as an incarnation of God, describes how one can carry on rightly in life. Krishna describes some of the paths in yoga which help one to achieve self-realization.

These paths include jnana yoga, bhakti yoga, karma yoga and raja yoga. Many versions of *Bhagavad Gita* are available, translated from the Sanskrit with commentaries by the teachers of various yoga traditions. Philosophical and practical approaches can vary widely depending on the translator's lineage and training.

## YOGA TEACHINGS

The wealth of teachings expounded as yoga can range from a specialized secular framework to a highly ritualized religious structure. Although yoga and Hinduism share common roots, people who practice yoga are not necessarily Hindu, and Hindus do not necessarily practice yoga. Hinduism, according to Houston Smith, is unique among most religions by holding that other religions "are alternate and relatively equal paths to the same God." However, it is also stated by other authorities that yoga is not wedded to any specific religious tradition, whereas others believe that yoga neither accepts nor rejects God. Yoga has been interpreted as being theistic, and it is certainly similar to religion in that it is based on ethical precepts, codes of behavior and established rituals and practises.

### ▦ RAJA YOGA

The Yoga Sutras is another text translated and interpreted by a wide variety of yoga teachers. They were compiled at some time between the third century B.C. and the fifth century A.D. by a man named Patanjali. Raja yoga is the study and practical application of the Yoga Sutras. The name was bestowed by Swami Vivekananda, a prolific writer who expounded on the "paths" of yoga, of which there are six (raja yoga, karma yoga, hatha yoga, bhakti yoga, jnana yoga and japa yoga).

The Yoga Sutras of Patanjali consists of four chapters which serve as a

## KARMA YOGA

Karma (karma means action and reaction) yoga is the path of yoga of dedicating one's actions to God. Any job or activity becomes an opportunity to serve a higher purpose, to engage in selfless service. All thoughts, words, and deeds are performed with love and care for the simple joy of doing and without any expectation of reward. When one realizes the connection to all life, one's actions express great care.

## BENEFITS AND PRACTICE OF HATHA YOGA

■ Exercise tolerance improves
■ Muscles gain strength and become more resilient
■ Flexibility and joint range of motion increase
■ Bones become stronger along with the structural integrity of joints
■ Circulation and respiration are more efficient, enhancing blood oxygenation
■ Healthy lipid and cholesterol metabolism are achieved
■ Sensitivity to insulin improves augmenting glucose metabolism
■ Normal bowel function results in regular elimination
■ Replacement of red and white blood cells occurs, stimulating the immune system
■ Reproductive organs and sexual function improve
■ Emotions become balanced, a sense of equipoise is experienced
■ Intellectual performance sharpens, increasing concentration

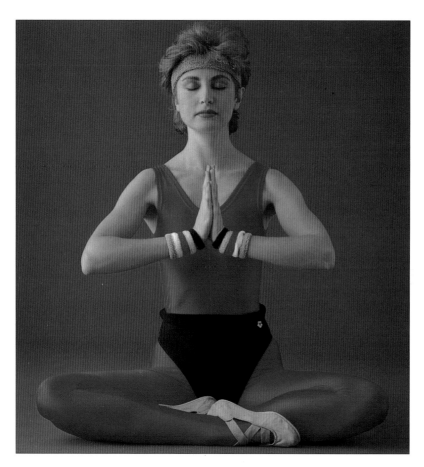

guide for exploration of the nature of the mind. The first chapter describes the goal of yoga (direct experience of true essence). Patanjali defines practice and non-attachment as two elements essential for achieving the experience

## READINESS STEPS FOR RELAXATION

- Allow for a 10-20 minute session
- Remove distractions
- Find a comfortable position
- Get quiet
- Relax the muscles
- Choose a focus point for resting the attention

of unity. He says that practice is persistence in making consistent efforts toward steadiness of the mind. maintained over time with trust in the goal; non-attachment is an acceptance of how things are in each moment. It is neither resignation nor disinterest; rather, it is an active effort toward non-judgement and flexibility of the mind. The rest of this chapter focuses on the nature of samadhi—the culmination of meditation. Samadhi is a complete absorption into the superconscious state of oneness with all that is.

### KRIVA YOGA

This consists of accepting pain as a purification, studying spiritual texts, and surrendering completely to Divine Will. Kriva Yoga is the name

Paramahansa Yogananda chose to describe the set of practices he developed for his followers. Each of these concepts takes a lifetime of applying them.

### ASHTANGA YOGA

These eight sequential building blocks mean "eight limbs." Ashtanga Yoga is the name Pathabi Jois uses for his teaching approach. These limbs are the cornerstones of raja yoga. They begin at ethical precepts (yama, niyama), move from physical practises (hatha, pranayama) to more inner-directed practises (pratyahara, dharana), leading to meditation (dhyana) and finally number eight, absorption (samadhi).

### HATHA YOGA

Hatha yoga is comprised of postures (asanas) and breath control (pranayama). "Ha" means sun and "tha" means moon, therefore hatha yoga means balancing opposites. Hatha balances movement and stillness, activity and rest. It balances forward bends with backward bends, standing poses with inverted poses, and inhalation with exhalation. Hatha is designed for relaxing and releasing deep body tension. It brings balance to the nervous system, and stimulates the internal organ functions. Breathing evenly, without strain, is one of the most important aspects of hatha yoga, both with stretching and with holding poses.

### PRANAYAMA

Pranayama means control of the prana. Prana is the life force, a subtle energy believed to be composed of waves and particles. It is called chi, ki or qi energy in the Orient. The breath, as the vehicle of prana, bridges the physical and the invisible realms. For this reason, it is of profound importance during hatha yoga.

Breathing practices are also used by themselves or prior to meditation. They help to control the mind. Yoga breathing practices increase tidal volume and vital capacity and have been found useful for asthmatics.

## ▪ JNANA YOGA

Jnana yoga is the path of yoga which actively uses the mind to get beyond the mind. Some people recognize traces of jnana yoga philosophy in humanistic psychology and psychohosynthesis. The Jnana yogi directs the intellect toward the big questions: Who am I? What is life? What is reality? What is permanent and unchanging?

Jnana means wisdom. By focusing the mind on the nature of the mind, the nature of nature, and the nature of reality, one can achieve highest knowledge. The yoga sutras recom-

## THE WITNESS CONSCIOUSNESS

This is a way of separating oneself from the activity of the mind where one steps back to observe it in action.

▪ To practice: cultivate a watchful attitude and frame of mind, become quiet and dedicate yourself to watching. Notice everything: what thoughts are passing through the mind; what sensations are happening in the physical body, what feelings are present. Just keep noticing. Simply observe and continue observing. If a judgment comes into the mind, notice it without judgment.

▪ Dharana means concentration. Here is the beginning of the meditation process, where the stream of awareness is directed inward from the senses.

▪ Many meditation teachers recommend that practitioners establish regularity in their practice and meditate at the same time and place daily, or two to three times a day.

▪ It is important that the focus for meditation is positive and appealing and elevates the consciousness.

mend use of viveka or discriminative discernment to remove ignorance and to provide understanding of the truth of universal oneness. Viveka means distinguishing what is real, permanent, and everlasting from what is temporary, transitory and changing.

## ▪ JAPA YOGA

Japa yoga is "communion with God through the repetition of God's name" according to Swami Satchidananda. He says that a mantra is a golden cord between the chanter and the cosmic force, which links a part

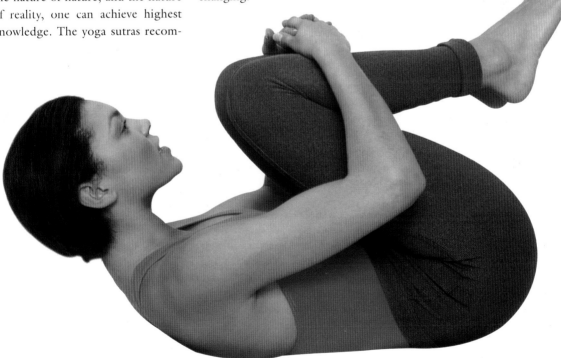

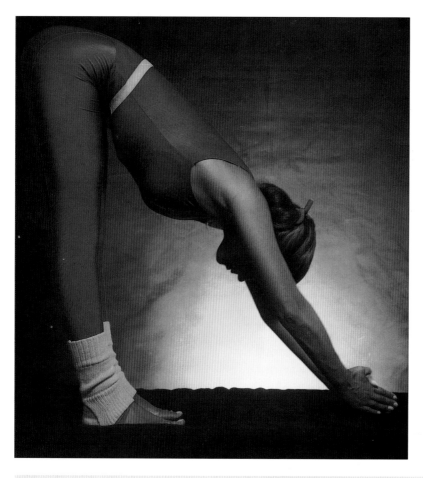

of the mind to God until, finally, the mind is absorbed and communion with God is experienced.

## YOGA AND MEDICINE

Yoga practices are being brought into mainstream medicine as a complementary healing modality for a variety of conditions and diseases, including asthma, arthritis, heart disease, cancer, AIDS, addictions and ageing. Patients with coronary artery disease (CAD) practice yoga as a stress management technique (one variable of a four-part comprehensive lifestyle adjustment) in Dr. Dean Ornish's Program for Reversing Heart Disease, at the Preventive Medicine Research Institute (PMRI) in Sausalito, California. The clinical trials that Dr. Ornish and his colleagues conducted (The Lifestyle Heart Trial) showed that the greater the adherence to the yoga practices, the greater the coronary artery block-

## NETRA VYAAYAMAM (EYE EXERCISES)

These are a practical application of yoga for stress management. Remove contact lenses before practicing this.

■ Sit with the head, neck and spine in alignment, shoulders relaxed and chest comfortable and expanded. Relax.

■ Breathe allowing the abdomen to soften so the lungs can take in a deep breath.

■ Exhale and contract the abdomen as the air leaves through the nostrils. Relax the breath and face.

1  Perpendicular movements: with the eyes open, lids relaxed and gaze soft, keep the head still and move the eyes up and down, following an imaginary perpendicular line. Do this several times without straining the eyes.

2  Close the eyes long enough for them to relax.

3  Horizontal movements: open the eyes, center them, then move them to the far right, making sure that only the eyes move, keep the head relaxed and centered. Then moving

straight across the center of vision, look to the far left. Avoid dipping the eyes. Continue several times, without straining.

4  Close and relax the eyes.

5  Circular movements: open the eyes, let them soften, then look far up (keep the head centered) and trace an imaginary circle with the eyes by gently moving them to the right, then down, then smoothly to the far left and finally up. Keep the movement deliberate and careful, moving as far to the periphery of vision as comfortable.

6  Repeat making circular movements to the left.

7  Close and relax the eyes until they feel rested.

8  Before opening the eyes, try another yoga practice called "Palming." Briskly rub the hands together until you feel heat in the palms. Then, keeping the eyes closed, cover them with the palms—no pressure on the eyeballs. Allow the warmth of the hands and the darkness to soothe and relax the eyes.

# Suuya namaskar (salutation to the sun)

The Sun Poses or Sun Cycle is a series of 12 yoga postures (asanas) which flow from one position to the next in a succession of movements (vinyasa) and provide a mini yoga practice which includes standing poses, forward bending, backward bending, slight inversion (having the head lower than the heart). The organs receive gentle internal massage. The Salutation to the Sun can be used as preparation or a warm up for asanas and other yoga practices.

Many variations exist: the series can be done slowly to calm the body or rapidly to give an aerobic benefit—for example, jumping from one pose to the next. As a start, try three repetitions, and as you become used to the movements, increase the number gradually.

1  Stand upright, feet straight, legs strong (avoid locking the knees), torso relaxed and lifted, shoulders broad, neck long, head balanced comfortably, face and eyes relaxed. Bring the palms of the hands together in front of the heart center. Breathe evenly: out and in, slowly, smoothly and with awareness.

2  Lock the thumbs and stretch the arms straight out in front, then bring them up over the head. Relax the shoulders away from the ears. Inhale. Look up and lift the heart center upward by bending slightly back.

3  Exhale as you bend forward from the hips, keeping the back straight. Knees can bend slightly to accommodate this forward bend, and to help keep the back in correct alignment to avoid strain in the lumbar area. Relax and breathe comfortably.

4  Bring the palms of the hands flat on the floor (bend the knees to accomplish this if necessary), then stretch the left leg and reach the left foot straight back to the flow, left knee to the floor. The right knee is bent with the lower leg perpendicular to the floor. Look up, breathe in.

5  Swing the right leg back parallel to the left. Hips can be high so the body forms an angle, or hips can be in line with the shoulders and heels forming a diagonal line, head to feet. Let the breath come out and in evenly.

6  Lower the knees, chest and chin to the floor. The body is in a zig-zag with the underneath of the toes, the knees, chest, palms of the hands, and chin to the floor. Hips are slightly raised. Exhale completely.

7  Pressing on the palms of the hands, push the body back to Position 5, with the hips high, palms of the feet and hands supporting the body. Breathe evenly.

8  Step the right leg forward back to the original starting position with the right foot between the hands, left knee to the floor and lifting the heart center, look up. Breathe in.

9  Bring the left leg forward next to the right foot. You are in the standing forward bend position as in Position 3. Exhale.

10  Keeping the legs strong (knees bent slightly as needed), allow the arms to stretch forward. Lock the thumbs, and extend the arms straight out. Upper arms will be alongside the ears. Relax the shoulders. Breathe in, and as if the arms and legs were the hands on a clock face, raise the arms to bring the torso up, back straight and comfortable.

11  Stretch the entire body upward, lift the heart center, look up, complete the inhalation as in Position 2.

12  Finish the cycle by bringing the palms together in front of the chest. Let the breath breathe by itself. Become aware of the effect of these movements on the body, breath, mind.

age reversal, regardless of age or other factors. PMRI's yoga includes gentle stretches and postures, breathing practises, deep relaxation, imagery and meditation.

At the Stress Management Clinic at The University of Massachusetts Medical School, in Worcester, Masachusetts, yoga, in the form of consistent, gentle stretching, is taught along with mindfulness meditation for pain management.

Herbert Benson, M.D., Associate Professor of Medicine at Harvard Medical School, and his associates have been researching the physiological benefits of meditation (one of the practises of yoga) since 1967. He and his colleagues reviewed secular and religious writings and concluded that most cultures and religions did indeed teach the use of some focus for the attention along with the prescription to passively disregard intrusive thoughts. They called the constellation of effects produced by their meditation research "the relaxation response." Benson's subjects have shown a reduction of the chemicals in the blood stream associated with anxiety. In addition, the basal metabolic rate (the amount of energy expended by the body at rest) lowers, i.e. the heart rate slows, muscle tension decreases and, for some people, blood pressure drops. The research also notes brain wave patterns shifting to those associated with relaxation. Benson found that many of these physiological relaxation responses could be triggered by other yoga practises as well, which he describes as active forms of meditation.

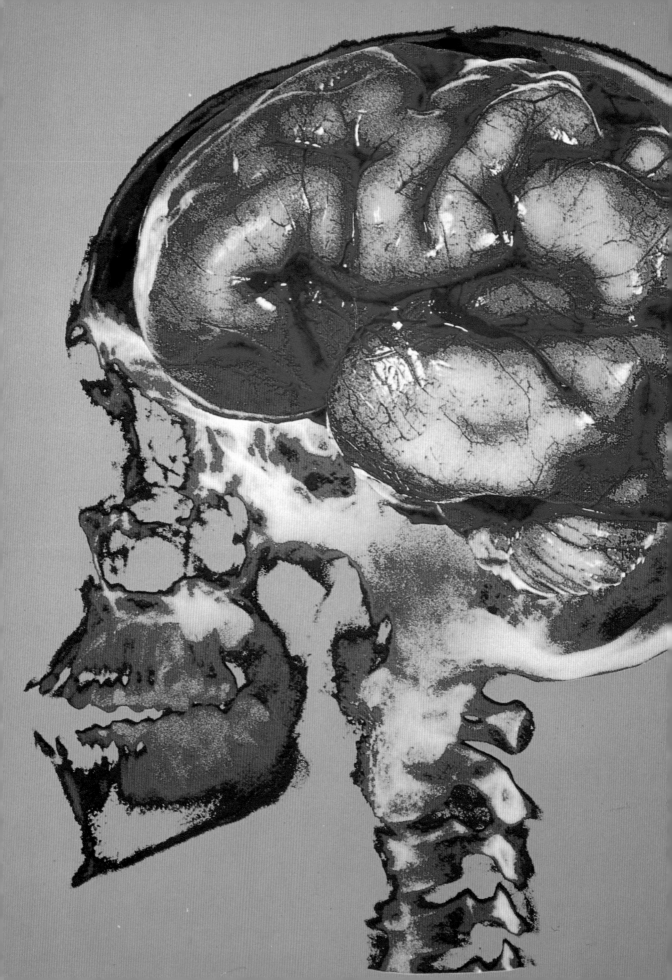

# THE MIND

## PART FIVE

*A*lternative medicine is a holistic approach to health care, which aims to treat not only the body but also the mind and the spirit. The symptoms of an illness or condition are perceived as the outward signs of an imbalance between the physical, mental and emotional levels as well as the vitality, or spirit, of the patient. In this section of the book are featured some of the therapies and practices that are concerned with the mind. These include psychotherapy, hypnotherapy, autogenic training, visualization therapy, meditation and music therapy.

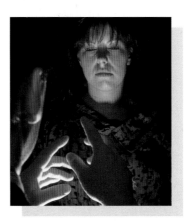

# PSYCHOTHERAPY

CHAPTER SIXTEEN

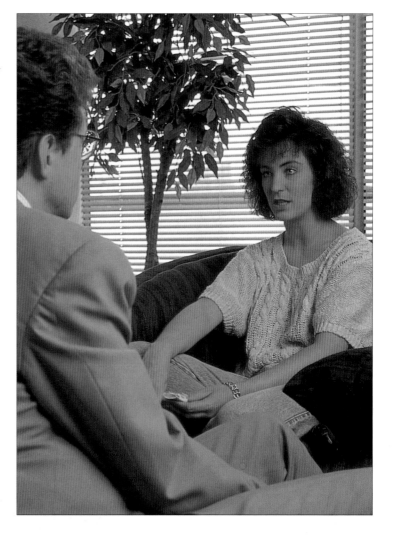

*P*sychotherapy is the systematic,
disciplined and ethical
application of psychological knowledge
and techniques which have been
shown to be effective in changing
mood, behavior and consciousness.

Anyone who has ever tried to
calm down an agitated child, help
a friend through a bereavement,
or simply distract themselves from
unpleasant thoughts, has practiced
a form of psychotherapy. As an
organized healing practice, the
psychotherapy family tree has its
roots in the eighteenth and early
nineteenth centuries when Anton
Mesmer discovered the age-old
shamanic wisdom that when
individuals suffering from a variety
of mental illnesses are put into a
hypnotic trance or under "animal
magnetism," their symptoms

disappear. Although eventually dismissed as a "quack," Mesmer's discovery was later rediscovered
by Sigmund Freud, who showed that, in the presence of a caring, attentive and trusted listener,
when people focused upon their experience, recalled long-forgotten traumatic events, and
re-experienced the mind states that had accompanied the original traumas, neurotic and even
psychotic symptoms could be cured. With this simple but profoundly significant observation, the
"talking cure," or psychotherapy, was born.

# MEDICAL PSYCHOTHERAPY

In its earliest days, psychotherapy was considered as a medical treatment for the brain/mind and was practiced by physicians, psychiatrists, some of whom were highly authoritarian and anything but respectful of a person's own natural healing potential.

The first psychiatrists had at their disposal behavioral management—unlearning maladaptive behaviors and re-learning more adaptive ones, biological treatments which were aimed at directly altering the brain. These included surgeries, electroshock and medications, and psychotherapy aimed at identifying unconscious drives and changing emotional responses.

Medical psychotherapy was originally based in Freud's psychoanalytic theory which posits that the basic driving forces within the human psyche are the self-centered and anti-social impulses for sex and aggression. If mismanaged, these powerful and largely unconscious forces produce anxiety or psychic pain, which leads to neurotic and even psychotic symptoms. Trauma in childhood, such as physical and sexual abuse, neglect, serious illness, loss or abandonment, are common reasons why some children fail to develop healthy self-management mechanisms.

Healing requires that past traumas and repressed urges should be acknowledged by the patient, who then experiences release or catharsis of pent-up feelings. Through a process of re-parenting, with the psychotherapist in the role of the parent, healthy mechanisms for coping with stress and anxiety can be developed. To facilitate the creation of a strong parent-child-like bond between the analyst and patient, psychoanalytic patients usually lie on a divan with the therapist out

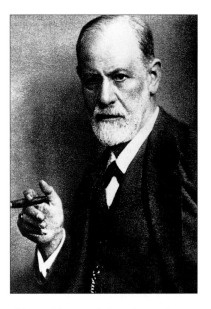

*Above: Sigmund Freud was the originator of psychoanalysis. Through his work, psychotherapy was born.*

of sight behind them. In the early days of medical psychotherapy, psychiatric patients were frequently subjected to invasive treatments, such as aversion therapy, shock therapy, insulin treatments, lobotomies, and physical restraints, and were routinely given massive amounts of mind-numbing tranquilizers. Because of this, by the 1940s, the general public image of medical psychotherapy was distinctly negative. It was widely regarded by the public as a paternalistic and sometimes oppressive form of social control for people whose unconscious urges were either neurotically repressed or psychotically out of control.

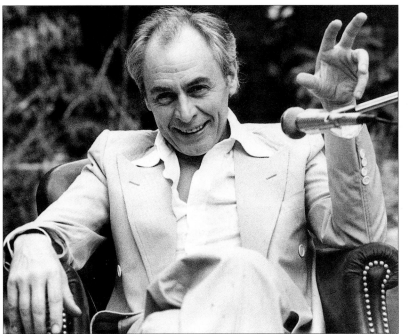

*Left: R.D. Laing was a leading exponent of radical psychiatry, which echoed the healing model of humanistic psychology.*

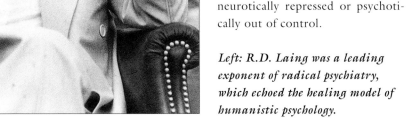

# HUMANISTIC PSYCHOLOGY

Humanistic psychology begins with three basic assumptions:

■ From infancy to old age, human beings strive to actualize their highest potentials and establish and maintain close mutual connections with others.

■ People, including psychotherapy clients, possess enormous inner resources for self-regulation and self-healing which can be accessed in the service of recovery, growth and self-transcendence

■ Healing and self-actualization are facilitated by participation in relationships characterized by a few key interpersonal conditions, namely mutual respect, warmth, acceptance, genuineness and empathy.

With these simple yet profoundly radical and controversial ideas, a revolutionary new psychology was created and within a decade it had changed the face of psychology and counseling.

The movement quickly expanded and almost at once acquired a psycho-spiritual branch which incorporated the ideas of American psychologist William James about altered consciousness states, parapsychology, and religious experience. It focused its interests on the higher reaches of consciousness associated with mysticism, ritual, Far Eastern disciplines, such as Yoga, Zen Buddhism, Taoism and other non-Western paths to wholeness and transcendence, and it drew heavily from the more mystical psychology of

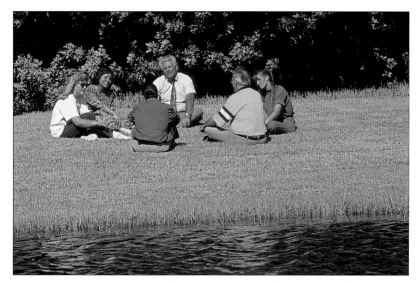

*Above: group counseling sessions can be held indoors in a formal setting or outdoors as shown here on the river bank.*

Carl Jung. This movement became Transpersonal Psychology.

In the 1970s, Radical Psychology made the connection between sociopolitical issues and psychological distress and brought new perspectives from women, people of color, working classes and sexual minorities into

## ALTERNATIVE PSYCHOTHERAPIES

In the 1950s, Brandeis University Professor of Psychology Abraham Maslow began corresponding with a group of fellow psychologists, the most notable among them being George Kelley, Rollo May, Clark Moustakas, Kurt Lewin, Henry Murray and Carl R. Rogers, who held more positive and life-affirming views both about the nature of the psyche and about psychotherapy. A new movement was gaining momentum within American psychology which was to revolutionize psychotherapy.

At the outset there was debate about what this new psychology should be called. Maslow favored the term "Eupsychology" to signify its focus on health rather than pathology. Others wanted to call it "Existential Analysis," to reflect the influence of European Existentialism. The name "Humanistic Psychology" was finally chosen to acknowledge indebtedness both to the classical humanism of ancient Greece and to the great humanist scholars of the Renaissance. Humanistic psychology rejected the medical sickness model and embraced a growth and emancipation model of healing. These ideas were echoed in the radical psychiatry of R.D. Laing and the anti-psychiatry movement led by David Cooper in the United Kingdom and Thomas Szaz in the United States.

the psychotherapy mix. These three alternatives to medical psychotherapy share a perspective which puts growth and transformation at the center, and while there are important differences among them, there is so much overlap in the actual practice of psychotherapy that it is useful to think of them together as the humanistic approaches.

## A NEW PARADIGM

Humanistic psychotherapies are distinguished from both Freudianism and Behaviorism in their underlying philosophical beliefs about the nature of reality and the nature of human knowledge. Influenced both by twentieth-century physics and Eastern philosophical traditions, the paradigm of humanistic psychology is holistic and relational rather than mechanistic and causal. Humanistic psychologies acknowledge multiple world views and accept that in human affairs, at least, truth is always personal and in part social construction.

## WHAT DOES A HUMANISTIC THERAPIST DO?

### A THERAPEUTIC RELATIONSHIP

Humanistic psychotherapists do not cure or heal their clients; clients heal themselves. Because of this, no parent-child or doctor-patient dependency is needed. Therefore, the humanistic psychologist's office is likely to be informal and relaxed, no couch is to be seen. Therapists and clients meet face to face, like people anywhere meeting to have an important conversation. Humanistic psychologists are trained to facilitate

## THE CONCEPT OF "SELF"

Humanistic psychology does not see the mind or Self as a permanent structure—a machine carried around in our heads—but as a fluid, always in process "holographic creation" which changes continually as a result of millions of interactions between a deep inner organismic awareness and the almost infinite number of possible contexts in which we participate. Humanistic psychologists believe, therefore, that it is meaningless to make generalizations about human beings. Every person must be understood in the here and now, in his or her own terms and particular circumstances.

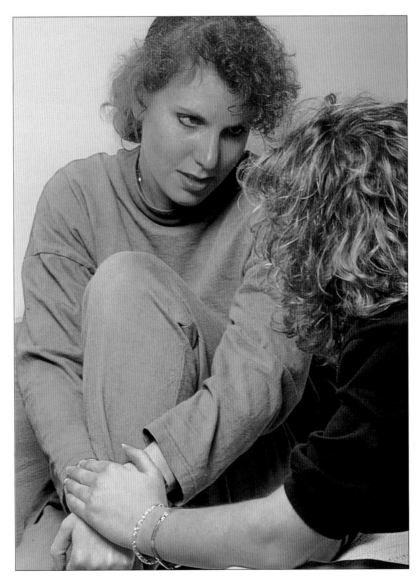

the creation of relationships in which it is safe for clients to access their own awareness, powers of self-regulation, growth and self-healing potentials and put them to use in the service of their own (within reasonable limits) self-set aspirations.

Relationships that are therapeutic are characterized by certain conditions, which were first identified by Carl Rogers sixty years ago, and which are essential for all healing. These are:

■ The relationship is non-authoritarian and the therapist and client meet in a collaborative, I-Thou relationship.

■ The client is seen as essentially competent.

■ The client sets the therapeutic agenda, and solutions to problems are sought which are consistent with the client's deepest sense of reality and values.

■ The client experiences the therapist as authentic, respectful, accepting, empathetic, warm and engaged.

■ The psychotherapist positions himself or herself as an ally to the basic life force or actualization tendency.

For many clients, the psychotherapy relationship might be the first time in their lives when they have been truly listened to deeply by a non-judgmental caring person.

## THE PROCESS OF PSYCHOTHERAPY

Humanistic psychotherapists and counselors do not usually offer advice but seek to assist clients find their own solutions to problems. A typical psychotherapy process of whatever

# ORIGINS OF PSYCHOLOGICAL DISTRESS

All schools of psychotherapy have their own view about what creates illness and pain. The humanistic view is that people experience pain when spontaneous movement towards self-actualization and successful connections with significant others becomes cut off, blocked, violated or exploited. If these disconnections or violations occur early in life, or persist over long periods, people develop defensive psychological routines or coping mechanisms which cut them off even more from the deeper organismic flow of life.

Self-awareness becomes interrupted and authentic interactions with others become impossible. When this happens, vital life satisfactions become unavailable, causing further distress and alienation which then may spiral into deeper difficulties which frequently result in a crisis.

approach has five more or less clearly identifiable stages:

### 1 Making contact
The best way to choose a therapist is to ask someone you know and respect—ideally a mental health professional—for the name of someone whom they would recommend. Referrals can also be obtained from the organizations listed in the Useful Addresses section at the end of this book. However it is possible to do a preliminary screening about the therapist's personal warmth, therapeutic orientation, his or her training and credentials, experience with your kind of problem, and fees over the phone.

### 2 Identification of problem and building a therapeutic alliance
Therapy begins with identification of the problem. The therapist might ask, "Could you tell me in your own words what brings you here?" for instance. As the client tells his or her story the therapist helps keep focus by asking clarification questions, picking up on vague references that seem to invite further exploration, and so on. At this stage the client's own characterization of their problem holds the greatest potential for showing the way to a solution.

In this initial phase, both parties are checking each other out. The therapist looks for where to best help, the client to see if he or she feels comfortable with the therapist and the process. Emphasis is on establishing the ground rules of therapy and building trust. Ground rules include the cost, frequency and schedule of visits, and explanation by the therapist of what the client can expect in the way of techniques.

Throughout this process, the therapist will be attempting to build an empathic bond with the client and to create a close and respectful relationship with therapeutic potential.

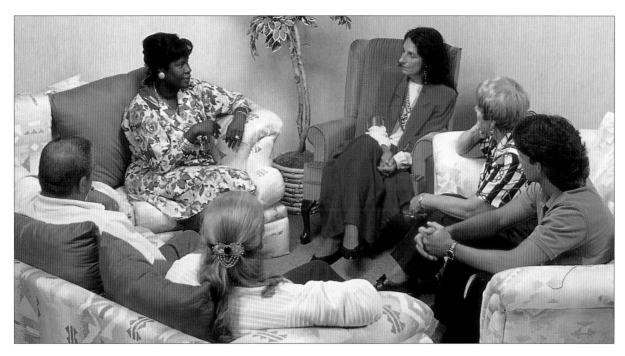

*Above: group therapy is now an accepted form of psychotherapy. This group counseling session involves five patients.*

### 3 The working stage

The therapist helps the client explore conscious and unconscious aspects of the problem, resolve internal conflicts, access his or her own subjective truth, and learn to act in new, healthy and empowered ways. Therapeutic techniques might include nothing more complicated than honest conversation, but more likely will be augmented by experiential focusing, work with symbols, role-playing, dream-work, psycho-drama (acting out important and problematic scenes), guided imagery, relaxation, active fantasy, cognitive therapy (learning to interrupt troublesome thoughts and substitute positive thoughts and images), body work such as bioenergetics, expressive arts, dance and movement, meditation, awareness exercises, rehearsing new expressive options, such as assertiveness skills, and learning problem resolution and negotiation skills.

### 4 Praxis

As therapy progresses, the therapist will encourage the client to put what he or she is learning in therapy into practice in the rest of their lives. Therapists might offer suggestions for home-work, such as keeping a feelings journal, meditating, recording dreams, attending workshops or seminars on psychological subjects. Connections between lessons learned in therapy and life in the hurly burly of daily life are evaluated. Sometimes, at this stage, therapists will suggest that a client should attend a psychotherapy group, to enlarge the circle of people with whom they can be their emerging healthy self. The goal of this stage is to risk trying a

## THERAPEUTIC GOALS

The twin goals of psychotherapy are to relieve suffering and optimize joy. These are achieved through:

■ Helping clients to become more fully aware of their own experience, to identify their psycho-spiritual blocks, and liberate their own healing potentials.

■ Facilitating renewed access to clients' own deeper organismic wisdom.

■ Helping clients make existential choices which respect their inner truth.

■ Helping clients move towards ways of being in the world which places the flow of life at its center and expanding possibilities for "right action" in co-operation with the wider interpersonal, cultural and ecological worlds.

new "way of being" as Carl Rogers called it, which is more consistent and congruent with one's own felt sense of reality, and then to realistically assess the consequences.

## 5 Progress review, consolidation, closure

Eventually the original concern which brought the person to therapy either becomes resolved or the person decides to discontinue working on it. The focus of therapy then shifts to termination—ending the relationship and achieving closure. When well handled, this stage permits review, finishing unfinished business, and consolidation of lessons learned. It also provides an important opportunity to face one of the most challenging human experiences—loss.

Unsatisfactory or premature termination can be very upsetting long after the therapy stops. It is important for clients to find another therapist with whom to address unresolved issues from psychotherapy that ends too abruptly.

# CONCERNS THAT PSYCHOTHERAPY ADDRESSES

People of all ages benefit from psychotherapy for many issues; most commonly these are:

**▩ Relationships**
Marriage enrichment and therapy, creating relationships, sexual problems, parenting, work relationships.

**▩ Trauma and loss**
Death, divorce, loss of a love, severe illness, trauma recovery, violence, abuse, rape, childhood sexual abuse.

**▩ Identity**
The existential questions, Who am I? What does my life mean? Am I crazy? How should I live? Sexual identity; vocational and motivational questions.

**▩ Psychological pain**
Depression, anxiety, compulsivity, phobias, impulsivity, stress, addiction, anger, delusions and hallucinations.

**▩ Personal development**
Love, intimacy, creativity, self-transcendence, spirituality and wholeness.

**▩ Sports psychology**
Performance, teamwork, motivation.

**▩ Physical illness**
Heart disease, cancer, chronic fatigue, stress-related illness, ulcers, arthritis, premenstrual distress, diabetes, headaches, allergies asthma, lower back pain, all have psychological dimensions and psychotherapy can aid in recovery.

### RESOURCES REQUIRED

Occasionally resolution can be accomplished in one or two sessions or in an intensive weekend growth workshop. More commonly, for a simple or surface problem, psychotherapy takes several weekly visits. Deeper, long-standing issues, or a serious commitment to a personal growth process may take months and even years. Humanistic psychologists usually trust that clients are the best judges of how much therapy they need, although they will make suggestions based on their experience with other clients.

The cost of psychotherapy varies depending on geographical region, the level of training and experience of the therapist. Many therapists will often work on a variable fee scale that reflects the financial realities of both the client and therapist. Do not be afraid to ask. Group work is often much less expensive.

### INTERACTION WITH OTHER THERAPIES

Humanistic psychotherapies are frequently practiced in conjunction with

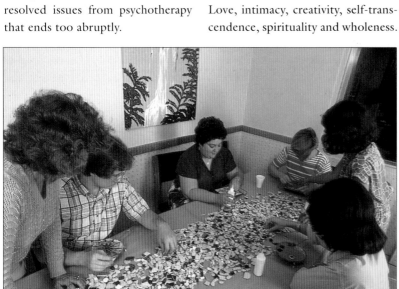

*Left: there are many forms of psychotherapy and counseling, including group art therapy as shown here.*

both traditional medicine and alternative therapies, especially somatic and nutritional therapies. When psychological suffering is severe it may interfere with a person's ability to participate fully in psychotherapy, in which case anti-depressant medication or anti-anxiety medication prescribed by a psychologically minded psychiatrist may prove helpful, as may nutritional changes, exercise and meditation.

## TRAINING AND CERTIFICATION

Psychotherapy of whatever tradition takes several years of intensive training to master. In the United States, most therapists have Master's or Doctorate degrees in Counseling, Psychology Pastoral Counseling or Social Work. Legal practice of psychotherapy is limited to practitioners who have been licenced by the individual States. To obtain a license, practitioners must undertake up to 3000 hours of supervised training beyond their degrees and sit for a licensing examination.

In Britain the situation is different. Psychotherapists usually have Bachelor's degrees in psychology, counseling or social work and postgraduate training and certification in a particular psychotherapy approach. Training programs are accredited by the United Kingdom Counsel for Psychotherapy. The Association for Humanistic Psychology Practitioners also accredits psychotherapists. At

present no certification is required for counselors in Britain although the British Association for Counseling does accredit some qualified counselors. Accredited counselors subscribe to a code of ethics and code of practice. Most have post-graduate training in counseling.

All the professional organizations have ethical and practice standards which guide the activities of their members. Should any consumer believe that they have received substandard care from a licensed or accredited psychotherapist they can complain to these professional organizations.

A quick word about "eclectic" psychotherapists—"Jacks Of All Therapeutic Trades, Masters of None." Eclectic usually refers to therapy which combines techniques from different approaches. When this integration is done by a therapist who has immersed himself or herself in one systematic approach and then over time has introduced wisdom from other systems, this probably represents the best of all possible worlds. But too often under-trained therapists, who pick and choose from different systems but master none, call themselves "eclectic."

Consumers should be cautious about working with psychotherapists who are not affiliated with any one of the professional organizations for psychotherapists. Psychotherapy is a complex, subtle and potent intervention when practiced by people who have received

## SOME BETTER KNOWN HUMANISTIC PSYCHOTHERAPIES

There are hundreds of "name brand" psychotherapies. Some of the best known are:
- Client- or Person-Centered
- Gestalt
- Transactional Analysis
- Transpersonal
- Existential
- Self-psychology
- Feminist
- Narrative
- Constructivist
- Self-in-Relation
- Experiential/Focusing
- Mythopoetic/Jungian
- Psychodrama
- Expressive Arts
- Eriksonian
- Primal-Integration
- Family Process
- Bioenergetics
- Ethno-cultural.

All of these can be done individually, with couples and families, or in groups.

good training from a recognized institute. However, because it is so powerful it can also do harm when practiced naively by under-trained therapists. To determine the credentials of a psychotherapist contact one of the organizations listed in the Useful Addresses section.

# HYPNOTHERAPY

## CHAPTER SEVENTEEN

*H*ypnotherapy is an increasingly accepted technique in which hypnosis is used as a tool to treat a wide variety of psychological, behavioral and medically related problems.

Although hypnotism has at times been misunderstood and even feared, the greater understanding in modern times of this valuable tool has led to receptiveness to hypnotherapy by the general public and more widespread use by medical and other practitioners.

Today, hypnotherapy is used extensively by physicians, dentists and therapists treating psychological problems. Practitioners of the technique now can cite many success stories that have further enhanced its acceptance in such varied instances as relieving pain in surgery and helping people to stop smoking or lose weight.

In the United States, hypnotism has been accepted as a treatment modality since 1958, and hypnotherapy is now widely used to treat many common medical conditions, ranging from asthma and allergies to heart disease, as well as an adjunct to anesthetics in dentistry, and as a behavior modification tool. It has even been used as an experimental technique in treating cancer.

# HYPNOTISM

To understand the history of hypnotherapy, we must first understand hypnotism and its origins. In simplest terms, hypnosis is an artificially induced sleep-like condition in which an individual is in a high state of concentration and extremely responsive to suggestions made by a hypnotist.

To be hypnotized is to be in an alpha state, one in which the critical factors of mind can be bypassed and a person is more receptive to suggestion. A hypnotic state can be induced by a wide variety of techniques, ranging from simple verbal suggestion to an eye fascination method, perhaps induced by a moving object.

## ORIGINS OF HYPNOSIS

Hypnosis itself is an ancient technique. Various visual depictions and hieroglyphics have led historians to conclude that the ancient Chinese and Egyptians used hypnotism in religious rituals and medical treatment. It is believed that the Egyptians used hypnotism as an anesthetic in surgery.

In more recent times, a score or more of individuals can be credited with playing key roles in advancing hypnosis and laying the foundation for the emergence of modern hypnotherapy. Among the more notable are the following.

■ **Franz Anton Mesmer** (1734-1815), was an Austrian physician, the father of modern psychiatry and hypnotism, which he called "animal magnetism." Mesmer incorrectly believed that a magnetic fluid emanated from his hands, making the process possible.

■ **James Braid** (1795-1860), a noted British physician who coined the word "hypnotism" in 1842. Braid used hypnotism to relieve pain during surgery. Not only was it successful for this, but it also reduced bleeding and hastened healing in many of his patients. Through the use of hypnotherapy, Braid recorded a drastically reduced mortality rate in surgery among his patients, which was not matched until many years later, when more modern techniques became avail-

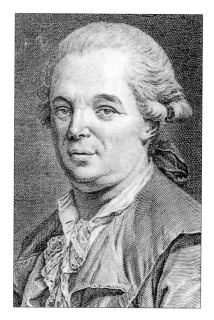

*Above: Franz Anton Mesmer is the father of hypnotism.*

able to physicians.

■ **Ambrose-Auguste Liebeault** (1823-1904), French physician and founder of the Nancy School of Suggestive Therapeutics.

■ **James Esdaile** (1808-1859), was a Scottish physician who performed 300 major operations and more than 2,000 minor ones using the hypnotic principle.

■ **Sigmund Freud** (1856-1939). Although he later turned to traditional psychoanalysis, Freud spent time at the Nancy School and contributed greatly to the scientific study of hypnotism. He had some difficulty in inducing the hypnotic

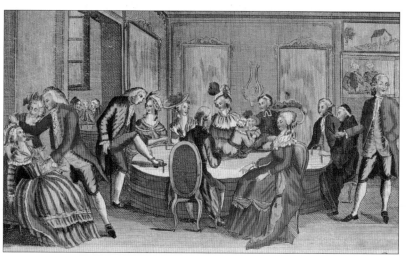

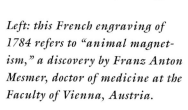

*Left: this French engraving of 1784 refers to "animal magnetism," a discovery by Franz Anton Mesmer, doctor of medicine at the Faculty of Vienna, Austria.*

## PHILOSOPHY AND OBJECTIVES

To understand hypnotism is to understand that there are different states of human consciousness. In hypnotism, the alpha level, a state of high concentration between sleeping and waking, is induced. In this relaxed state, critical factors of mind can be bypassed and a person becomes more receptive to suggestions, such as the reduction of pain or to eat less.

Also in this state, a person can be more receptive to recalling earlier life events that might have had a traumatic impact. These events can be dealt with in therapy. The hypnotherapist can help a patient replace negative thought processes with positive ones.

In essence: when critical factors of mind are bypassed in hypnosis, patients can more easily accept their ability to achieve desirable, positive behaviors—"Can't do" becomes "can do." Hypnotherapy is a testament to the power of the mind to bring about positive behavior and help heal the body.

hypnotherapist of modern times. He used hypnotism as a behavior modification technique with numerous patients.

**Note:** In a great breakthrough from the days when hypnotism was shrouded in superstition or seen as stage entertainment, in 1958 the American Medical Association accepted hypnotism as a treatment modality.

## TREATABLE CONDITIONS

Hypnotherapy can be used to treat many conditions, including depression, multiple personalities, anxiety, bi-polar disorder, problems in concentration, impotence, anorexia, insomnia, panic, fear of flying, stress and neuroses.

state in his subjects but always felt that the technique would be extremely valuable if used by more skilled practitioners than he.

■ **Karl A. Menninger** (1893-1990), the leading American

psychiatrist and also the founder of the famed Menninger Clinic, where hypnotism is being practiced both clinically and experimentally.

■ **Milton Erickson** (1901-1980), often called the most influential

■ Medical doctors use hypnotherapy to treat a variety of ailments, including allergies, arthritic pain, heart disease, hypertension, nervous tension, headaches, colitis and asthma. In one case, a hypnotherapist regressed a patient back to birth, at which time the patient had almost been strangled by his mother's umbilical cord. That experience had caused later asthma-like symptoms, which disappeared after the hypnotherapy.
■ Some oncologists, including Carl Simonton, have used hypnotism as an experimental technique in the treatment of cancer. This involves

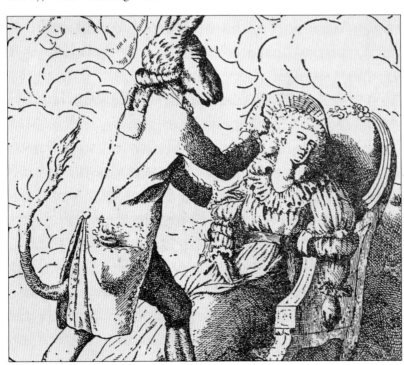

*Left: this caricature shows an ass mesmerizing a woman. This form of hypnotism was developed by Mesmer, who called it "animal magnetism."*

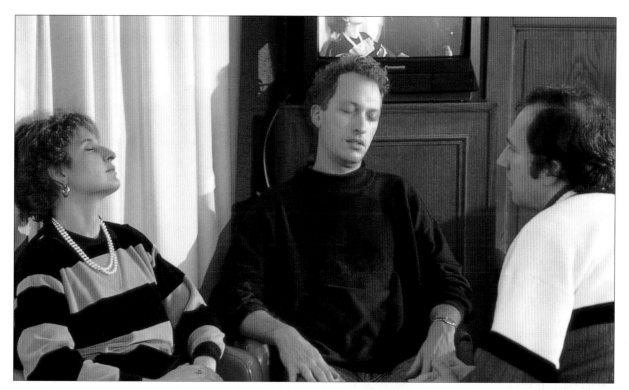

*Above: these trainee therapists
are undergoing instruction in
hypnotism.*
*Right: hypnotherapists use hypnosis
as an accepted tool to treat a wide
range of psychological, behavioral
and medically related problems.
The hypnotherapist induces a state
of high concentration, the alpha
level, in the patient.*

visualization in the hypnotic state in
which patients are asked to imagine
their bodies successfully battling the
cancer cells.

■ Many dentists use hypnotism as
an adjunct to traditional anesthetic
and to help control bleeding and
salivation. They also use it to help
relax patients.

■ The use of hypnotherapy as a
behavior modification tool to help
people stop smoking or lose weight is
widespread and extremely successful.

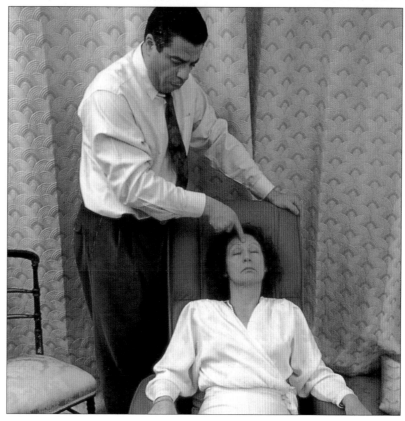

## CHOOSING A HYPNOTHERAPIST

In choosing a hypnotherapist it is a good idea to choose one who is licensed in the healing arts or who works under the supervision of someone who is licensed. Beware of practitioners who make what seem to be exaggerated claims. Although hypnotherapy works faster than many other modalities, it is not a miracle cure.

A reputable hypnotherapist will first talk with a client to determine what, if any, previous experience they have had with hypnosis. What have they heard about the technique? Have they ever seen a person being hypnotized? What are their fears in regard to hypnosis? Have they read any books or articles on hypnosis? Have they ever been hypnotized before?

A hypnotherapist might choose to demonstrate a hypnotic induction on a third party initially, to put the patient further at ease. The patient must be told that he or she will not do anything against their will while in hypnosis. The sensations that will be experienced while in the hypnotic state also need to be explained to the patient to further allay any fears or suspicions.

A hypnotherapist, for example, might tell clients that he or she is going to help them accomplish something that they very much want to do but have been unable to do by themselves. The difference between the delta (deep sleep), theta, alpha and beta (normal, waking, average levels of consciousness) states would be explained. The client might be given a chart that shows different brain wave frequencies and it would be explained where on the chart hypnosis takes place.

The alpha state is very similar to the state that we experience when we begin to awaken in the morning.

We can't quite open our eyes yet we are very aware. We can hear the birds singing outside or sounds in or outside our house. Our eyes remain closed, and we feel as though we either can't or don't want to wake up and open our eyes. This is the alpha state, and it is what many people experience when they go into hypnosis; it is a very suggestible state of consciousness.

## SELF-HELP MEASURES

Unlike many other treatment techniques, patients can easily be taught to practice self-hypnosis and experience the resultant benefits from the treatment. They can learn to place themselves in a hypnotic state, implant positive suggestions and leave the hypnotic state.

A hypnotherapist might give a client material that will help induce a state of self-hypnosis. One example of this type of material is:

"For your first experience, choose a time when there is no possibility of disturbance and all is absolutely quiet. Placing yourself in your usual, most comfortable position and without hurrying, you should concentrate on yourself to bring about the most completely relaxed physical and mental condition that you are able to create.

"When perfectly sure that this state has been reached, turn your attention to one of your arms,

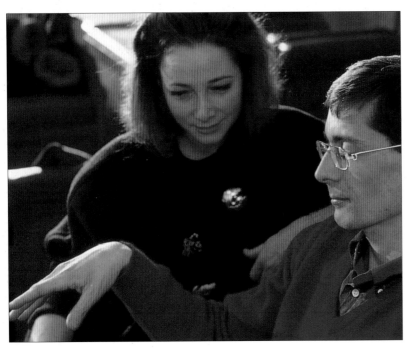

*Left: qualified hypnotherapists have to undergo comprehensive training. Hypnotherapy is used widely by physicians, dentists and therapists to treat many medical and psychological conditions.*

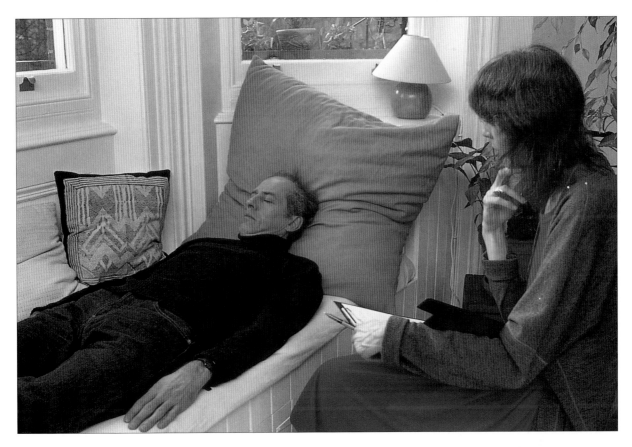

concentrate on it and proceed to think to yourself:

" 'I am thoroughly relaxed. I am more relaxed with every second that goes by. My lower left or right (whichever you choose) arm from the elbow to the fingertips is now so relaxed that it feels light and weightless. With each breath I take, the lower left arm feels lighter and lighter. The lightness is filling my fingers, moving up, from the hand to the wrist, and without conscious effort, it is lifting away from the top of the couch, lap or armchair etc. As I continue to relax even more deeply, my arm rises higher and higher, lighter and lighter, rising up, lifting. My lower left arm is floating. With each movement it makes, it becomes lighter and lighter, and causes me to

relax more deeply. Completely, without any conscious effort.'

"Be certain that there is no conscious direction to the arm itself to lift, but that the thoughts are directed solely to the unconscious mind. When contact with the unconscious has been made, the arm will rise automatically and involuntarily, its speed and sureness depending on the quality of the contact.

"Usually, and quite slowly, the muscles on the arm will seemingly contract of their own accord, pulling the arm jerkily upward. Remember that as soon as the arm begins to lift, a probable state of hypnosis does exist; as the unconscious is obeying suggestions directed to it."

The individual then is in a hypnotic state, where he or she may

give and receive positive suggestions, to create more desirable behavior, for example.

## THE FUTURE OF HYPNOTHERAPY

Although hypnosis is an ancient technique, the scientific use of hypnotherapy is still relatively recent. Already it has come into much greater use and acceptance by many people who once were skeptical of it, including many physicians and doctors in the medical establishment.

As more time goes by and more success stories are credited to hypnotherapy, the modality will become more accepted and widespread, and many more people will benefit from its great healing value.

# MEDITATION

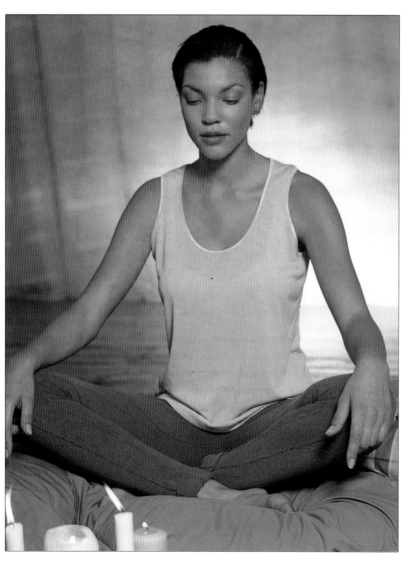

## CHAPTER EIGHTEEN

*M*editation is a commonly used word but, most often, it is used incorrectly. Meditation is a state of being in the same way that sleep is a sense of being. One cannot practice meditation any more than one can practice sleeping—one is either in a state of sleep or one is not as any insomniac knows. When a person sits down to practice meditation, he is really practicing concentration. He engages in the continuous activity of directing the mind to a single point of focus. By drawing the attention to one point in a gentle, persistent way, the mind may become empty of thoughts and the person may drop into a state of meditation. This practice requires a conscious effort to refocus the attention whenever the mind has wandered. It is not unusual for beginners to become frustrated by the process, assuming that everybody else has amenable, cooperative minds which are willing to be silent upon request.

For the sake of accuracy, some teachers refer to meditation as "sitting" in the sense of "I sit for an hour each day." Saying "I sit" instead of "I meditate" may relieve expectations of accomplishment which could interfere with the process. Regular practice acts to reinforce the goal and helps bring about a readiness for stillness, which is the fertile soil for the state of meditation.

# THE HISTORY OF MEDITATION

The history of meditation coincides with the development of mentation in human evolution. The awareness of consciousness allowed human beings to learn how to control thoughts, breath and the physical body—to realize God, experience unalloyed Truth, know the Clear Light, what IS, etc. Meditation is natural, easy to learn and safe. Its benefits are chronicled in all of the world's great spiritual traditions, and examples of meditation techniques can be found cross-culturally. In the literature of the yoga tradition, much detail is provided for instruction and inspiration in meditation. Varieties of meditative practices exist in Zen and Tibetan Buddhism, Taoism, Christianity and Islam.

# ENGAGING THE SENSES

Sometimes it is helpful to engage one of the senses in the meditation process. For a person who is visually oriented, holding a picture in your mind of someone or something which evokes positive feelings may be the best focusing tool. The picture should be seen as a single unit and not as a scene. This is because the mind could take the scene and use it to wander into imagination and fantasy.

Visual imagers could focus on an object such as a light, a candle, a specific design, the face of someone dearly esteemed, or some image from nature such as a flower, a stone, the

## CAUTIONS OF MEDITATION

Here is some cautionary advice that you should consider before you meditate.
1 Always avoid meditating immediately after a meal.
2 Never force yourself to meditate or to prolong the practice uncomfortably. This can be dangerous and unpleasant.
3 If visions, sounds or other extra-sensory perceptions occur, be careful not to let them distract you or mislead your efforts. Often what many people consider to be psychic powers may present themselves, and these can be misleading.

4 Keep alert during meditation. Do not meditate when you are feeling tired or fatigued. Sometimes people fall asleep instead of meditating. This habit is very difficult to break once established.
5 Do not get discouraged. The yoga sage Patanjali, who first codified yoga practices in the "Yoga Sutras," explains that "practice becomes firmly grounded when tended to for a long time, without interruption, and in all earnestness."

sky or the ocean. One common focus for meditation is to simply watch the natural flow of one's own breath.

# MANTRAS

People who are more auditorially oriented could choose a sound for a focus, such as sounds from nature—the wind in the trees or the lapping of the ocean waves. In Sanscrit, the word mantra means "sound vibration." Many meditators recite mantras to generate vibratory frequencies.

Common mantras include: Om, hari om, om shanti, ram, hari ram, om namah shivaya. Many people prefer to use words from their own language such as "Peace," "Love" or "Joy." Even a meaningless syllable may be a useful meditation tool if it helps to focus the mind. People who are kinesthetically oriented may prefer to focus their attention on a sensation such as the touch of the wind against the skin, the feeling of motion as the breath flows in and

out, or the sense of height one feels from being on the summit of a mountain.

# A SIMPLE MEDITATION EXPERIENCE

This meditation experience can focus and calm the mind.

## ▮ GETTING READY
By putting aside a few moments for preparation, your meditation practice will be more comfortable and you will gradually find that the length of time you sit will increase, along with your ability to concentrate.

## ▮ TO BEGIN
Allow yourself about 20 minutes of undisturbed time. Turn off the telephone, put your pets in another room and open a window for ventilation. Go to the bathroom and empty the bladder and bowel. Wash the hands and face. Check your clothing to loosen any constrictions. Sit on a firm chair with your feet flat on the

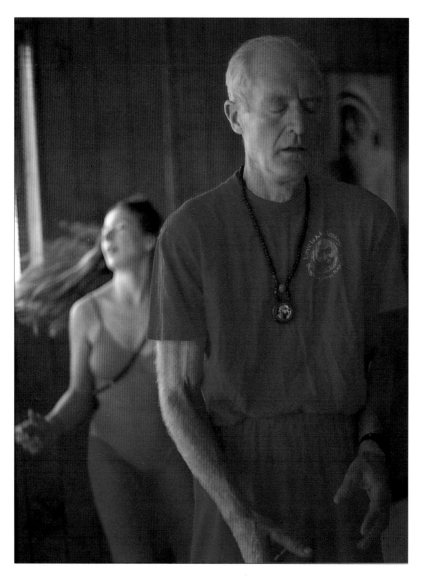

the rhythm of the breath be even, smooth and unbroken with no jerks or breaks in the stream of air. Remember to avoid any strain and discomfort. Eventually you will notice that the breath breathes by itself.

### ■ CONCENTRATE ON THE FLOW OF BREATH

Concentrate the mind on the observation of the flow of breath. As thoughts, feelings and other mental activity come, notice them. Let them remind you to bring the focus of attention back to the breath. Feel the touch of air in the nose, the gentle out and in of the flow of exhalation and inhalation, and keep the awareness on the experience of the breath.

### ■ INTERNAL SILENCE

Increasingly, you will realize that the body is calm, the mind focused and a feeling of peaceful alertness remains. There will be an internal silence as the process of meditation becomes more familiar.

## MEDITATION POSITIONS

There are many positions that you can adopt for meditation. They range from the yogic lotus position to the shavasana position. You can use almost any comfortable position in which you can still your body and your mind. Two of the most commonly used postures are the half lotus and shavasana.

### ■ HALF LOTUS

This is a simple cross-legged position, affording balance and stability, which

floor. Alternatively, you can sit on the floor in a more traditional cross-legged position as long as your body is comfortable. Allow yourself to relax completely.

### ■ THE PROCESS

Sit your head, neck and spine straight. Relax your shoulders. Allow your arms to rest on your lap with your hands still. Bring the awareness to the "place" your body occupies. Note the environment, consider where you are, and close your eyes.

### ■ YOUR BREATHING

Become aware of the "space" your body occupies. Bring your attention to the breath by exhaling through the nostrils. As the breath returns through the nose, fill the lungs completely, always avoiding any strain or exertion. Concentrate on the flow of air in the nose, and feel the temperature of the breath—the warm exhalation, the cool inhalation. Let

you can use for meditating.

1 Sit on the floor with your knees bent and the soles of your feet together. Gently press your knees toward the floor and then release them.

2 Holding on to your ankles, press forward, trying to get your face as close to your feet as possible. Return to the upright sitting position.

3 Now go into the half lotus itself. Sit on the floor with both legs outstretched. Bend the left leg, bringing the left foot beneath the right thigh. Bend the right leg and bring your right foot on top of your left thigh. Both knees should be touching the floor and your back should be straight.

### ▓ SHAVASANA

1 Lie flat on the floor with your legs apart and relaxed, and your arms relaxed at the sides of your body.

2 Keep your body relaxed and still without becoming rigid with ten-sion. If you start feeling tense, stop immediately and try again later. Start off by trying to stay still for three minutes, and then gradually extend the time as you improve with practice.

## BREATH AWARENESS MEDITATION

These techniques will serve as an introduction to breath awareness meditation.

### EXERCISE 1

Sit comfortably in your chosen position, eyelids lowered or eyes closed. Breathe naturally, counting your breaths either on the inhalation or exhalation, from one to ten. Concentrate on the numbers and don't let your thoughts drift. Just keep focusing on the numbers and your breathing. This helps you to concentrate and stay alert.

### EXERCISE 2

Sitting in the same position, breathe naturally. Focus your attention on the tips of your nostrils where the breath flows in and out of the body. Feel the sensation and focus on this. Don't let your attention wander.

### EXERCISE 3

Sitting as before and breathing naturally, focus on the space between breaths—the space outside the body where the exhalation ends and the space inside the body where the inhalation ends. Notice the stillness of the breath. Keep practicing this breath awareness meditation and eventually it will help still the mind. You will find that the space between breaths increases with practice.

**Note:** you might like to try combining these breathing techniques with the half lotus posture.

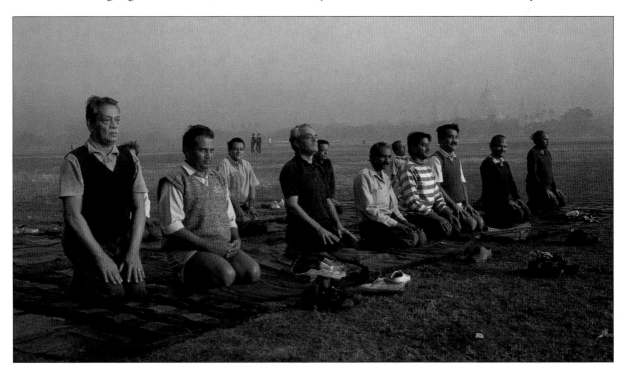

# TRANSCENDENTAL MEDITATION

## WHAT EXACTLY IS TRANSCENDENTAL MEDITATION?

Transcendental Meditation is a very simple, natural, effortless technique practiced for 15 to 20 minutes twice a day, sitting comfortably with the eyes closed. During the practice, the mind settles down experiencing finer levels of thought, until it transcends the finest level of thought and experiences the source of thought, pure consciousness, the source of the unlimited creativity and intelligence of both man and nature. The Transcendental Meditation technique does not involve concentration or control of the mind and is not a religion, philosophy, or change of lifestyle.

## WHAT DOES TM DO?

The mind profoundly influences the body and vice versa. As the mind settles down during the TM technique, the body naturally gains a unique and very profound state of relaxation, far, far deeper than ordinary eye-closed rest.

During the past 25 years, more than 500 scientific research studies have been conducted on the effects of the Transcendental Meditation technique at 210 independent universities and research institutions in 33 countries. The studies—many of which have been published in leading scientific journals—have shown that the Transcendental Meditation program may do the following:

- Reduce stress
- Increase both creativity and intelligence
- Improve memory and learning ability
- Increase energy
- Increase inner calm
- Reduce insomnia
- Increase happiness and self-esteem
- Reduce anxiety and depression
- Improve relationships
- Improve health
- Promote a younger biological age

## CASE STUDY: HIGH BLOOD PRESSURE

High blood pressure is a critical health epidemic in all industrialized nations (e.g. in the U.S., over 43 million people suffer from the "silent killer"). The main treatment for high blood pressure is drugs, but these do not cure high blood pressure. In fact, they even produce serious side-effects in some people, such as diarrhea, fatigue, dizziness, depression and insomnia

The American Heart Association's journal, *Hypertension*, published a study in November 1995 showing that the Transcendental Meditation program can be as effective as medication sometimes in reducing hypertension, without its hazardous side-effects. The study also

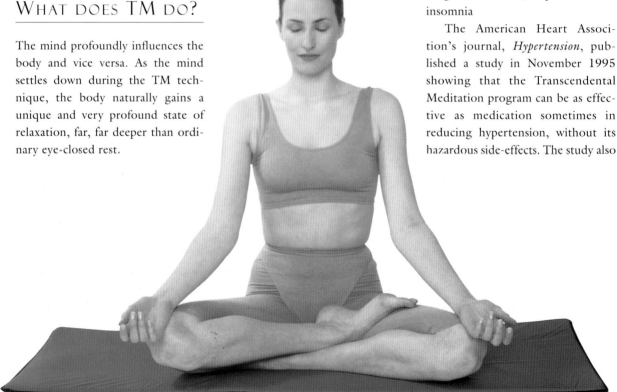

showed that 20 minutes of TM might be seven times as effective in reducing high blood pressure compared to changes in diet and exercise.

## CASE STUDY: HEALTH CARE COSTS

Health care costs are spiraling out of control and threaten to bankrupt many businesses, even governments. Increasingly, experts recognize that the solution is not in finding ways to cut costs on expensive medical procedures, such as coronary bypass surgery, but rather to make people healthier.

A large study of the insurance statistics of 2,000 Transcendental Meditation participants over a five-year period found that the TM group had 50 percent less medical care utilization, both in-patient and out-patient, compared to controls matched for age, gender and occupation. The TM group had lower sickness rates in all categories of disease, including 87 percent less hospitalization for heart disease and 55 percent less for cancer. The difference between the TM and non-TM groups was greatest for individuals over 40 years of age.

## ARE ALL MEDITATION TECHNIQUES THE SAME?

This is the most frequently asked question about meditation now that interest in the practise has gone mainstream. For years the answer appeared to be "Yes, all meditation techniques are basically the same." But in the past few years, scientists have drawn another conclusion. Four studies compared findings of research on different meditation and relaxation techniques. These studies are called "meta-analyses".

### ▧ Reduced anxiety

This meta-analysis of 146 studies indicated that compared with every other meditation and relaxation technique tested to date, Transcendental Meditation may be more effective in reducing anxiety, the most common sign of psychological stress.

### ▧ Increased self-actualization

This meta-analysis of 42 studies found that Transcendental Meditation was more effective in increasing self-actualization than other meditation and relaxation techniques.

### ▧ Reduced substance abuse

This meta-analysis of 198 studies found that Transcendental Meditation was more effective in reducing drug, alcohol and cigarette abuse than were standard treatment and prevention programs, including relaxation.

### ▧ Improved psychological health

This meta-analysis of 51 studies showed that compared with every other meditation and relaxation technique tested to date, Transcendental Meditation may be far more effective at enhancing psychological health and maturity. The studies showed that Transcendental Meditation promotes greater overall self-actualization, as indicated by increased self-regard, spontaneity, inner directedness, and capacity for warm interpersonal relations.

## HOW ARE THE TECHNIQUES DIFFERENT?

Meditation techniques have traditionally fallen into two groups: those involving concentration and those involving contemplation. Concentration attempts to control or subdue thoughts and contemplation gives the mind something inspiring to evaluate on the level of the meaning of thoughts. Transcendental Meditation involves neither concentration or contemplation. It is an effortless procedure that makes use of the natural tendency of the mind to move towards a field of greater happiness, or bliss. TM systematically leads the mind to deeper, quieter, more blissful levels of the thought process until the finest level of thought is transcended and the source of thought, pure bliss consciousness, the Self, is directly experienced.

## HOW DO YOU LEARN TM?

The process of transcending thought is simple, effortless, and enjoyable, but properly learning the process is exceedingly precise and individual. For this reason, throughout the ages, learning to meditate has always involved personal instruction from a qualified teacher. Therefore, those who are interested in meditating should have access to a complete follow-up program that provides proper guidance throughout life.

The Transcendental Meditation program is taught through a seven-step course of instruction offered through hundreds of Maharishi Vedic Universities and Schools throughout the world.

# AUTOGENIC TRAINING

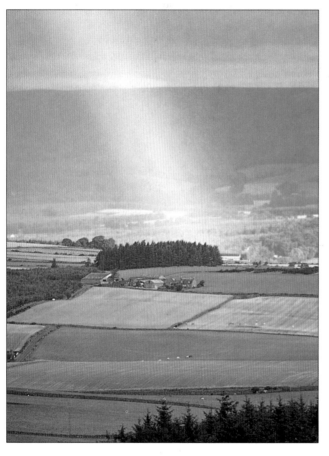

## CHAPTER NINETEEN

*S*tress is one of the biggest bug-bears of the modern era which affects our health detrimentally and leads to enormous amounts of chronic ill health and even death. Although it is not entirely a modern phenomenon, it tends to spiral dangerously out of control, more recently for a great many people if they do not control and manage it by some form of relaxation. The probable reason for this perception of immensely increased stress is the fact that a combination of a number of stressors are bombarding us simultaneously.

However, it is important to remember that the main chemicals, adrenalin and nor-adrenalin, which are released in the body whenever we are stressed, are also produced in situations that are associated with excitement, pleasure and enjoyment, such as sport, competitions or sexual activity. Therefore, life without any form of stress or stressful situations would be extremely boring. It is only when the level of stress goes beyond a certain threshold level, which varies in different individuals, that it becomes problematic and starts affecting the physical, emotional, mental and even the spiritual wellbeing of the individual. These are the times that the symptoms which are associated with anxiety, depression and disturbed sleep as well as those of other psychosomatic (stress related) diseases become apparent and the affected person starts seeking help for the removal of the unpleasant symptoms of the over-stressed situation.

Furthermore, stress also plays a very important role in progression and exacerbation of any serious illness which might already be present. For instance, in those individuals suffering from multiple sclerosis, ME (chronic fatigue syndrome), cancer or AIDS to name but a few, the progression and spread is faster in those who are unable to control or manage their stress level.

## HOW DOES STRESS AFFECT US?

Despite the awareness of most individuals that they become much more susceptible to illnesses, including simple things such as colds and flu, when they become stressed, tired or when they are under pressure for any reason at all, it was only in the early 1970s when the subject started being taken really seriously, following the publication of scientific reports from the American space agency, NASA. It was found that the immune system of even the super-fit astronauts was detrimentally affected by the stress of what they were doing, and their immune systems only returned to normal after a variable time following the cessation of the stressful events. The immune system consists of a complex system of cells, tissues, organs and chemicals which are widespread throughout the body. Its integrity and proper functioning is absolutely essential for perfect health and wellbeing.

It was following the publication of scientific papers from NASA and the confirmation of their results following experiments with many groups of healthy individuals which enabled the science of psycho-neuro-immunology or mind-body-immunity to be born.

Apart from the correlation between the altered immune state, the onset of many serious and potentially fatal diseases and various stresses such as bereavement, loss of work or any other important or life threatening situation which is now well documented, it has also been found that an individual under stress is much more likely to sucumb to disease, if he or she has also got the sort of personality which is unable or unwilling to deal adequately, effectively and satisfactorily with the so-called negative emotions such as the feelings of rage, anger, depression, guilt and frustration, and can only cope with these either by repressing or denying them.

Early childhood deprivations might also play a part, as may loneliness, lack of social support and feelings of hopelessness and helplessness. Not only is the inception of disease commoner in those individuals who have a combination of these factors, but also the prognosis as far as its progression or deterioration is concerned is much poorer in those who accept their diagnosis blandly and without expressing any strong feelings or emotions, or putting up a fight against the diagnosis, once the initial shock and denial stages have been worked through. On the other hand, it has also been shown that the

## REDUCING STRESS AND RELAXATION

The first step in reducing the stress levels in our lives is to identify their possible source for us as individuals, as they are different for each and every one of us. Not only that, they also tend to vary from time to time, depending on the combination of the stressors. For example, a racing driver finds what he does exciting whereas most of us would find that pursuit extremely stressful. The stressors for most people come under the headings of "environmental;" "social," which includes the lack of loving and caring support leading to loneliness and feelings of hopelessness and helplessness; "housing"; "personal," which includes the relationship with family members and friends; "sexual"; "work and unemployment." There may, of course, be others which may be specific to your own unique situation. Include these in your list as well. Often by identifying our stressors, we can start eliminating some of them at least and thus reduce our stress levels.

However, even with doing this, the majority of individuals under stress need to learn a technique to control and manage their stress levels. There are a number of different forms of relaxation from Jacobsen's progressive muscular relaxation, various forms of meditation (from simple breathing techniques to transcendental and Zen), yoga, hypnosis, biofeedback, healing and autogenic training. Here, we are going to confine ourselves to discussing autogenic training, which is among the most effective of all of them and satisfying the criteria for relaxation, dealing with the negative emotions and stimulating individuals' creativity for the enhancement of their health. As will become apparent, this is much more than just another relaxation technique. Autogenic training helps to institute change in all the levels of body, mind, emotions and spirit which is the true essence of a holistic approach. What is probably one of its most important functions and which is often overlooked and understated is its ability to be an exceptionally powerful preventive tool which can mitigate the onset of many of the stress-related diseases.

use of positive emotions such as love, fun, humor, laughter and creativity are effective in enabling and empowering the individual to deal with and combat disease and disability much more effectively.

As important as the effects of stress and the negative emotions and other factors already enumerated are in weakening the immune system, it must be remembered that there are other factors which also contribute towards the inception of disease and feelings of unwellness. These include lack of exercise; consumption of unhealthy foods and inadequate nutritional supplements, as well as large amounts of drugs and chemicals, especially excessive amounts of unwarranted antibiotics, the use of recreational stimulants such as alcohol and caffeine-containing drinks and, of course, more potent drugs, and finally multiple sexual partners without the use of safe-sex practices. It is so much easier to prevent disease rather than try and fight it once it is established. Therefore, it is well worthwhile looking after all the aspects of your body, mind, emotions

## WARNING

Being such a powerful technique, autogenic training is not suitable for everyone. Individuals suffering from epilepsy, insulin dependent diabetes, active alcoholism, drug addiction and any psychotic illness such as schizophrenia should not undergo autogenic training, unless supervised closely by a highly qualified trainer who specializes in these diseases.

and spirit in this truly holistic way on a regular basis.

Tranquilizers can have an immediate, dramatic and marked effect on the control of the symptoms of stress. However, in so doing they have no effect in helping to control or eradicate the underlying causes of what actually precipitated the stress related crisis. The fact that thousands of tons of tranquillizers are consumed yearly on a world-wide basis is an indication that their use on their own is not the answer, particularly since they can bring about their own problems, such as habituation, addiction, acute rage and other withdrawal symptoms. This is why many people, including the members of the medical profession, have become very alarmed at the astronomical increase in the consumption of tranquillizers, and have started looking for alternative methods of trying to control and manage stress; better still to try and utilize it to the best advantage and for the benefit of the individual affected by it.

## WHAT IS AUTOGENIC TRAINING?

Autogenic training is a simple, powerful and effective method of mental relaxation which leads the body's physiology and inner workings towards normalization and healing. It is particularly appealing to the Western mind, because unlike many forms of meditation and yoga, it has no cultural or religious overtones, and requires no special clothing or unusual postures or positions. Most important of all, the physical and mental relaxation, as well as feelings of peace and tranquillity are generated from within oneself and are not

dependent on any external values, philosophies or therapists. All the beneficial effects which ensue go on accruing so long as the individual goes on practicing the technique. Furthermore, it can be used anywhere or any time, unlike certain other forms of relaxation.

## HISTORY AND PHILOSOPHY

The technique was devised by a German neuro-psychologist called Dr. J. Schultz in 1932 and was later perfected by one of his co-workers, Dr. Luthe, in Canada prior to the onset of World War II. It consists of a series of simple mental exercises designed to turn off the stressful "fight-flight" mechanism in the body which causes the release of adrenalin, and turn on the restorative and recuperative rhythms associated with profound psycho-physical relaxation and healing. It is a method, which when practiced daily brings about results comparable to those achieved by Eastern forms of meditation on the mental level, and the chemical and physiological body changes associated with those people who train hard for physical or sporting activities on the physical level. It also enables the trainees to get in touch with their deeper feelings of repressed emotions if that is relevant, and deal with them effectively through specific additional practical exercises, so that the deep states of peace and tranquillity which are achieved can be maintained on a prolonged basis.

Passive concentration is the most important and the simplest concept in autogenic training, but for some individuals who are particularly stressed or used to active concentration, it can sometimes be the most difficult part to achieve, though everyone always manages to get there eventually. Most of the time we concentrate actively, i.e. our concentration is aim-oriented. However, in passive concentration, the individuals sit or lay back and just observe what is happening to their mind, body and emotions. They don't try and do anything with it. Therefore, they accept and acknowledge any distracting thoughts that may creep in. This is the way in which the conscious, for reasons best known to itself, tries to block the relaxation process. However, the trainees eventually learn to dissociate from them. It is these intruding thoughts which are often the product of active concentration in other techniques which help to make them less effective by creating in the individuals the feeling that they are not doing it correctly, and hence the reason why they are having the distractions.

The simple commands that are used in autogenic training consist of concentrating on a series of normal, physiological and physical sensations, such as heaviness, warmth and cooling, starting from the limbs and gradually working through to deep within oneself, going through to breathing, heart and circulation and eventually to the solar plexus, which is situated beneath the soft area just below the junction of the ribcage. This is the nerve center for all the so-called automatic functions of the body, such as blood pressure, bowel movements, pulse rate, breathing, etc. By learning to affect and control the solar plexus, the

## WHAT HAPPENS DURING THE TRAINING?

Autogenic training can be learned from a qualified trainer. When attending a trainer, it is usually taught either individually or, preferably, in small groups of six to eight over a period of eight consecutive weeks. Each session usually lasts between one-and-a-half to two-and-a-half hours. During the first session, the three main sitting, as well as lying down, positions are demonstrated and practiced. Then in the following sessions, the progressive exercises are taught, during which the trainees are taught to concentrate passively on normal physical sensations such as heaviness, warmth and cooling in the mental exercises. The focus of attention starts in the limbs and gradually and gently shifts to the heart and circulation, breathing and the nervous system through the solar plexus. The trainees are also taught the off-loading exercises which can be used to deal with emotional problems. The whole process leads to a profound state of relaxation. The ability to do this and achieve "passive concentration" at will, breaks through the vicious cycle of excessive stress and tension, whatever its origin. Motivation to perform the exercises regularly on a daily basis is of utmost importance in order to gain the maximum benefits from the training course.

individual learns to control the functions of the brain indirectly through the various nervous connections between the two. Thus one can learn to control indirectly the functions of the brain which include the immune, glandular and reproductive systems of the body to name but a few.

There is no magic about it. All that we learn to do is to use the body's own normal mechanisms and sensations to bypass the conscious and try to get into the unconscious and the so-called silent parts of the brain. Thus, we can utilize their enormous powers and energies for the benefit of our health.

Although autogenic training is a particularly powerful technique, it is not an answer to everything, but it can be conveniently and harmoniously combined with a great many other techniques and therapies, both conventional and complementary, as part of a holistic approach to health and disease. It can be used both as a starting point to get you in the right frame of mind to receive the treatment, or to help enhance its beneficial effect and potential.

## WHAT DOES IT TREAT?

Autogenic training can be used as part of holistic (looking after the body, mind, emotions and spirit) management, prevention and treatment of numerous conditions including the following; AIDS and HIV infection, angina, anxiety, arthritis, asthma, aviation and flying, backache and neck ache, blood pressure control, blushing, cancer, cholesterol and lipids, circulatory problems, colitis, concentration improvement, constipation, depres-

# KEY BENEFITS

These can be divided into the clinical (health related) and non-clinical ones. Although autogenic training has specific benefits in each one of the non-clinical situations, the benefits are summarized jointly.

**Benefits in education, sport, business and industry**
1 Improvement in concentration and ability to learn new concepts and skills.
2 Improvement in self-discipline and standard and quality of homework.
3 Improvement in the ability to study for much longer periods without getting tired as the students could regularly refresh themselves by doing AT.
4 Marked stabilization of personality and reduction in unnecessary

emotional problems interfering with the studies.
5 Improved sleep patterns and ability to cope.
6 Reduction in anxiety including that associated with examinations.
7 Better and friendlier relationships with other students, their parents and teachers.
8 Increased flexibility.
9 Reduction in psychosomatic symptoms, such as headaches, stomach aches, or nervous tics, etc.
10 Improved ability to achieve. Even the so-called under-achievers were found to perform much better, and gain much better marks than expected, compared with their past performances.

sion, dieting, education, eczema, headache, herpes infection, hiatus hernia, irritable bowel syndrome, indigestion, industry, infertility, insomnia, ME (chronic fatigue syndrome), menstrual problems, menopause, migraine, multiple sclerosis, muscle problems, obesity, pain control, palpitation, Parkinson's syndrome, PMS (premenstrual syndrome), pregnancy, labor and delivery, recovery from accident, illness and surgery, sciatica, sexual problems, skin diseases, sleeping problems, stuttering, thrush, thyroid problems, torticollis, tranquillizer addiction treatment, ulcers (stomach and duodenal), urinary problems.

## ADDICTIONS
Autogenic training can also be used in many cases to help people lose weight, stop smoking, come

off addictive tranquillizers and sleeping tablets.

## SPORTS PERFORMANCE AND JET LAG
Autogenic training is also taught to sportspeople to try and improve their performance, and to airline staff to help them fight the effects of jet-lag and insomnia in strange surroundings.

## WORK AND INDUSTRY
Autogenic training is also being used some in industries to enable both the management and the work force to cope with the progressively increasing stressful demands of modern living which are being imposed upon them.

## EDUCATION
It is also used education to improve

concentration and performance of students.

# CLINICAL AND HEALTH BENEFITS

Some of the many clinical and health benefits of autogenic training are listed below:
■ Autogenic training is a simple, powerful and effective method of mental relaxation.
■ The basic and essential premise of "passive concentration" removes the anxiety and fear of not carrying out the technique properly.
■ It leads the body's physiology towards normalization and healing.
■ It can be used anywhere and at any time, and the longer it is used, the more powerful it becomes.
■ It can be used in conjunction with orthodox or complementary therapies, both to enhance their effects and to reduce the possibility of side effects.
■ If used during the day, it can be very refreshing. But when used at night it helps the trainee to fall asleep quickly and peacefully.
■ It is non-religious, although it can lead to spiritual awakening.
■ The power, peace and tranquillity are self-generated and are not dependent on any external therapies, philosophies or values.
■ It allows the individual to become aware of feelings, emotions and negative behavioral patterns which could be holding them back.
■ Additional practical exercises enable the individuals to deal with these safely and effectively and convert them to positive patterns of behavior.
■ It enables the individuals to deal

with the back-log of stress and un-resolved emotions.

▓ It balances the two halves of the brain, and thus enables the individuals to become aware of their full potential for creativity and positive attributes which can be used as additional tools for healing.

▓ Autogenic training advances positive affirmations, visualizations and autogenic meditation to enable the individuals to maximally direct their healing energies to the affected sites.

▓ It enables individuals to become aware of their own immense innate healing power and potential.

▓ It enables individuals to become aware of alternatives, choices and possibilities.

▓ It helps individuals become aware of hopeless/victim/loser behavioral patterns, and enables them to transform their attitudes to enable and empower those with serious diseases or disability to improve their condition and quality of life.

## AUTOGENIC MEDITATION

The relaxation exercise below is an abbreviated and simplified version of one of the autogenic meditations. It is very easy and anyone can do it in order to try and relax and get the flavor of what it is like. However, it is important to realize that when you first start doing it, especially if you have never done anything like this before, you may not feel or see anything. Furthermore, you may actually become aware of more distracting thoughts. Don't worry about that. It is very common. Just acknowledge the distractions and continue with your meditation.

**Note:** to find out more about autogenic training, you can read one of the many books available, or turn to the Useful Addresses section.

## HEALING LIGHT MEDITATION

Sit in a comfortable chair, making sure that your legs and arms are not crossed and that your feet are firmly on the ground. Take a few deep breaths in and out. As you breathe in, breathe in peace, light and love and as you breathe out, let out as much of the tension, stress or pain that is possible. You can also do this meditation while lying down. However, you may fall asleep if you do it that way, especially if you are tired.

As you breathe in and out, imagine great big roots forming from your feet and base of your spine (coccyx) growing deep into the ground until they hit an energy source. Then imagine the Earth's energies coming up through your roots into your legs and gradually take it right up through your body to the top of your head. As the energy is coming up, imagine the following light and color changes are happening, making sure you take the color or the light that is appearing right the way through the whole of the indicated part of your body.

■ It goes red through your legs and up to your lower abdomen (bladder region).

■ Then is goes orange at your belly button region.

■ Imagine it going golden yellow at the top of your tummy (solar plexus region).

■ It goes green at your chest and arms.

■ Then it goes blue at your throat region.

■ It goes purple in your forehead.

■ Finally it goes white at the top of your head (the crown region).

Now, imagine an enormous source of silver/white light above you, connecting with the white light at the top of your head. Bring this white high-energy healing light into you from the top of your head, overtaking all the other lights and colors to your feet and into your roots. The energy cycle is now complete. Earth to sky, sky to earth.

As you bring the white light into you, concentrate more of it on those parts of your being that are in a state of distress, pain, discomfort or disease. You can spend as long as you like doing this exercise. However, it should be for at least five minutes twice a day—the more the better. As you get more proficient at it, you can prolong the duration.

Once you have mastered the technique, then you can also incorporate positive affirmations into it at a point where you feel most relaxed. You can make up your affirmations to suit your needs. An example is "I am calm and confident." Or "I am calm, confident and without pain." They must be short, snappy and positive.

Continue doing this and you will improve your quality of life and that of those around you and you will be able to achieve whatever you wish.

# VISUALIZATION THERAPY

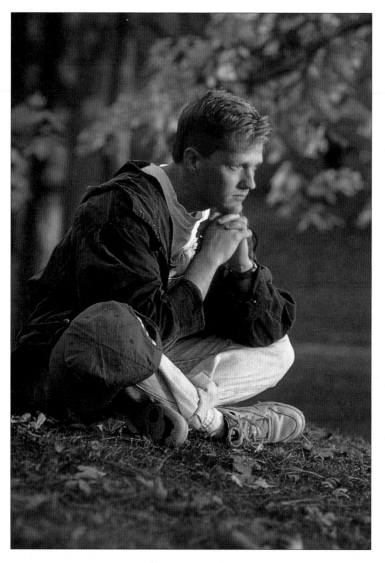

## CHAPTER TWENTY

*Visualization or imagery is the thought process that invokes an inner mental picture usually using all the senses which include vision as well as hearing, smell, touch, taste, position and movement. However, in a great many forms of visualization the sense of vision seems to be the one that is predominantly used. It can be self- or therapist-directed. One of its greatest benefits and advantages is the fact that once an individual learns how to utilize the technique, it can be used to great advantage on a regular basis. Literally, the sky is the limit, as the boundaries of imagination in the majority of people is limitless.*

*Altering or changing an image within our minds positively alters our expectation and perception of a disease or disability that may afflict us, and this is probably the principal reason why visualization can be such a powerful tool in altering the course and outcome of any disease. The positive images that we perceive can have a powerful and fundamental impact on our physical body, down to the tissues and even individual cells.*

# HISTORY

The use of images and imagination in healthcare is almost as old as Western medicine itself. Although it has lost its popularity in traditional medical practice in the last 200 years, imagination has continued being used by the shamans (traditional folk healers who were also political and social advisors to the local tribes and communities) in the various cultures around the world. Surprizingly, the way in which the shamans worked seems remarkably similar irrespective of whether they were working in America, Australia or Europe. Fortunately the beneficial effects of visualization and image work have been rediscovered and appreciated again more recently and have started being used once again in the conventional medical settings for improvement of health and wellbeing.

During the ancient Greek civilization which formed the basis of modern medicine as we know it, Asclepius, Hippocrates, Aristotle and Galen were all great advocates of the use of the art of imagery and imagination as part of the holistic (looking after the body, mind, emotions and spirit as a whole) management of disease as known in those days. Their legacy was fully utilized by the creative Christian physicians of the Renaissance.

Asclepius (circa 1000 B.C.) was believed to have been a physician, warrior, healer and the son of the god Apollo, whose wife was a mere earthly being. He was therefore attributed as being the god of medicine and healing. His healing powers, especially through the use of "dream and

imagination therapy," were so well known that, following his death, over 200 healing temples were erected all over Greece, Italy and Turkey utilizing his principles. These temples, which were known as "Asclepia," were really the first ideal examples of holistic treatment centers; the sorts of ideal centers we are striving to create again today.

The temples were located in beautiful settings and contained baths, spas, theaters and places of worship and recreation. Everyone who came for treatment was accepted irrespective of whether or not they could pay. The use of dream or imagination therapy during the "divine sleep" as it was known at the time (later it was called "incubation sleep" by the Christian practitioners), reached a state of the art perfection as a healing tool.

The patients, who were usually extremely ill and had failed to respond to other forms of known treatments, would be starved of food for one day and of wine for three days, so that they would be in a perfect state of spiritual awareness to accept the healing that would be imparted to them during the sessions. They would then be taken to the inner temple or buildings in the evening to await the arrival of the god Asclepius and after his death, his representatives on earth.

The healing took place during that special state of consciousness before sleep when the imagination is particularly active. During this sensitive and susceptible period, there would be soft gentle music playing and incense burning. The physician/priest/healer would then appear dressed in white in the guise

of Asclepius with a retinue of other healers, patients' relatives as well as animals, such as geese and serpents, which were purported to have healing gifts and properties. They would move from patient to patient and the physician/healer would then either give direct healing or advocate treatment which would include the use of known medical practices of the time, such as herbal mixtures, surgical interventions and magical rites.

Surrounded by the magnificent and magical shrines, in the semi-darkness, with gentle music playing in the background, and with the earthly representatives of the healing deities, the innate healing ability of the patient was thus greatly stimulated and enhanced. It was a perfect opportunity for the imagination to get to work and apparently it did with positive results judging by the number of "cures" reported. The conditions that were treated successfully

## RESEARCH

There is now a large body of scientific research showing the effects of visualization and imagery on the body, mind and emotions. Some of its negative aspects have already been covered in the section on "stress" in the chapter on autogenic training relaxation. Some of the more recent research has not only shown that individuals can learn to affect their general state of health positively by using visualization, but they can also learn to influence specific parts of their bodies, tissues, the immune system and even single cells within that system.

varied from impotence, headaches, boils and varicose veins to the recovery of the blind, the deaf and the lame. These, and the cure of a variety of other diseases, were recorded on the temple walls and were attributed to the Asclepian techniques of healing.

Aristotle, Hippocrates and even Galen were trained in the traditions of Asclepius and were great believers in the power and use of imagination. Aristotle believed that the emotions did not exist in the absence of images, and that these images caused changes in the bodily functions which, in turn, affected both the production of disease as well as its cure. Hippocrates, who was considered to be the father of medicine, believed that the physician's role was

## DEEP RELAXATION

The essential prerequisite for any form of visualization to work effectively is a complete state of deep relaxation, preferably leading to an altered state of consciousness which can be achieved by techniques such as autogenic training. The other important factor about the type of relaxation used is that only the minimum amount of talking is required to allow the conscious thought and active parts of the mental process to be by-passed and to access the unconscious. Excessive amounts of speaking or verbal content in the relaxation or meditation keeps the individual in the conscious mode and can thus reduce or even inhibit or block the creation of beneficial images by the mind.

to assist nature in healing in the spirit of love, concern, gentleness and dignity, by being aware of man's relationship to food, drink and occupation, and how each of them would interact with the other. Galen (A.D. 131-200) was the first person to record and describe fully the effects of imagination on health and the relationship between the body and mind in the context that we view it today.

## WHAT HAPPENS DURING A SESSION?

Many forms of relaxation techniques have been used for getting the individual into a state of readiness for the fantasy journey of imagination which visualization really is. These include simple breathing techniques, self-hypnosis, biofeedback, meditation and autogenic training. This latter technique is probably the most effective as far as the visualization work is concerned as the individuals using the technique enter a deep and passive state of relaxation as well as altered state of consciousness. They are therefore in the ideal state of readiness to carry on with the visualization or image work.

As mentioned earlier, visualization can be self- or therapist-directed. It has often been found that spontaneous self-directed images can be the most effective as healing tools. Apart from being used as a healing agent, visualization can also be used for rehearsal of whatever the individual wishes to achieve or do. This mode of its use is particularly useful in acting, sporting and educational activities, preparing for interviews, giving lectures and so

on. For instance, it has been shown that when a golfer visualizes his action in hitting the ball, all the relevant muscles are activated in the same sequence that they would have been if the player was actually using his body on the course. The movements of the muscles during visualization are almost imperceptible to the individual, but they can be detected by the use of sensitive instruments.

The effectiveness of imagery for this sort of purpose is enhanced if it is combined with autogenic positive affirmations. By adopting this technique, sports people can not only keep their minds sharp and focused, but also practice their craft and keep themselves in top training condition in situations where the sport is inadvertently interrupted. A prime example of this is during an outdoor championship tennis match, when it is interrupted by the weather.

## SELF-DIRECTED VISUALIZATION

In the self-directed version, the individual enters a deep state of relaxation using whatever technique he knows or suits him best. Then either some of the common standard images can be used or one can concentrate on the issues, i.e. the diseased or problem areas, and allow the imagination to roam freely until an appropriate healing image turns up.

This may not happen immediately and sometimes it can take a great many sessions before a useful image appears. It may be worth using a standard image which has either been suggested by the therapist or which the individual has read about, while waiting for the spontaneous images to come up. Once this happens, the individual can then exchange it for the older image. Both images can, of course, be used in conjunction if that seems appropriate.

One of the commonest standard images is that of the white cells, which are responsible for the defense of the body, being like sharks wandering around the body and eating up any infected or cancerous cells. Although this form of imagery is useful for people with infections and cancer, it can be counterproductive or even dangerous in certain other diseases. A particular example is in HIV infection and AIDS. As the infection is in one of the fractions of white cells responsible for the immune system (CD4), if the same form of imagery is used it can actually lead to the destruction and dangerous diminution of these cells.

In one case, in which an original eye condition was leading to blindness, the main problem was the destruction of the retina (the vision sensitive back layer of the eye). This left black scars which interfered with the vision. The patient had many spontaneous images which helped him with his recovery over the years, but one of the very useful and enjoyable ones was that the black scars were bubbling away from the retina and being absorbed into the fluid of the eye and then drained away by the blood vessels. The bubbling effect was a bit like the bubbles of champagne bubbling up from the bottom of the glass and then disappearing from the top.

## CASE HISTORY

A client with multiple sclerosis had

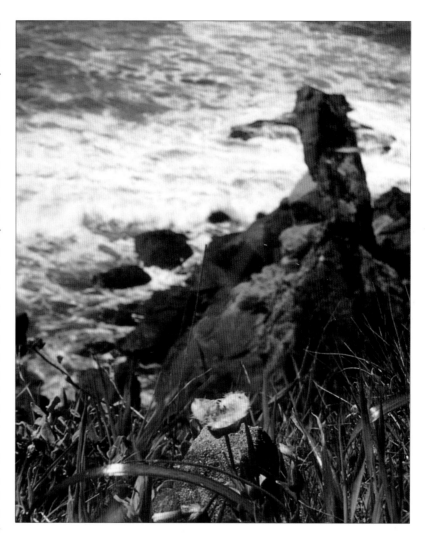

the spontaneous image, during his autogenic training relaxation, of a decorator going round his nervous system and brain filling in the gaps formed by the destructive aspects of the disease, and then going round with a paintbrush, painting all over them to make the nerves smooth. He found that this image was of tremendous value to him.

If the visualization is to be used for rehearsal of a particular activity or event, then the individual would get into a state of deep relaxation and then visualize the activity or the result they wanted to achieve in great detail;

*Above: focusing on an image of natural beauty can be positive and beneficial when you are practicing visualization therapy.*

exactly as if they were doing it in reality. This would need to be done repeatedly for maximal benefits, just like any other form of visualization or image work.

## CUTTING THE TIES

Apart from self-healing, self-directed visualization can also be used for releasing, letting go and trying to deal with any people, situations or memories, present or past, that are causing problems for the individual and thus preventing him from moving on, changing and healing. This is called cutting the ties using visualization. There are many ways of doing this. The easiest way of doing this is by proceeding as follows.

■ Get yourself into a deeply relaxed state, using whatever method you usually employ. Imagine a figure of eight which may be in light, color or a lightweight material that comes into your mind easily.

■ Then imagine yourself in one section, and the offending person, memory or situation in the other. Cover yourself completely with pink or any other light that comes to you easily. Then cover whatever is in the other half of the figure-of-eight separately in the light as well.

■ Consciously and deliberately cut the waist of the figure-of-eight and imagine the section that does not contain you drifting up towards the sky and eventually disappearing.

■ While that is happening, you repeat to yourself a phrase such as "I release and let go of whoever or whatever." It is important to name whatever you are working with, especially if you are working with a person. Sometimes doing this once can do the trick. At other times, especially if the hurt or attachment is very deep, you may have to repeat this exercise on a number of occasions before it works.

## THERAPIST-DIRECTED VISUALIZATION

This can be used in a number of different ways depending on the needs of the client. Here are three of the commonest forms.

1 The therapist takes the client (patient) through a simple but powerful relaxation technique and then asks him a number of questions in order to try and elucidate the individual's perception of his disease. The questions will depend to some extent on the disease and the therapist's knowledge of the individual. The following are a few examples:

■ What does it look like? What color is it?
■ What does it feel like? Is it hard or soft? Is it solid or not?
■ What does it smell like?
■ What does it sound like?
■ What does it taste like?

Once the questions have been answered by the client, some therapists ask the client to draw the disease as described. However, that is not essential.

The client is relaxed once more and is then asked, step by step, how the various properties of the disease which have thus been elucidated can be altered so that it disappears and the damaged tissue etc. returns to normal. The therapist writes down the client's answers and once the visualization is concluded, discusses all the questions and answers with the client just in case there are any additional comments he would like to make. The client is then asked to work on the visualization on a daily basis, using the disease as visualized and the answers to try and get rid of it and return the damaged tissues to normal. This is particularly helpful in patients with cancer.

2 This is a variation of the previous exercise. Once again, the client is taken through a relaxation process. He is then asked to imagine that he is lying by the foot of a tree. Then he imagines another part of him, often referred to as the "higher self," climbing up the tree and looking down on himself lying below. While looking down, the client is then asked to observe where the disease is and go through a variety of questions similar to the first method. Once the answers to the questions are elucidated, then the client is asked what tools are needed to remove the disease or disability. Once that is established, then the "higher self" climbs down the tree and enters the body once more. At the end of this visualization the client is given the tools to work with and asked to continue working with them at home through the visualization on a daily basis.

3 Guided visualization with positive affirmations can be custom made and used on an individual basis, but most therapists tend to use this method for group sessions, during which the clients are taken on an imaginary fantasy journey following the induction of a state of relaxation. Throughout the journey, positive affirmations and images are incorporated. These are absorbed directly in the unconscious and help to release the clients' negative conditioning as well as reinforcing their positive and healing attributes. Ideally, at the end of the guided visualization, once the clients have been brought back to reality, they discuss their experiences in pairs or small groups depending on the time available.

# VISUALIZATION EXERCISE

Here is a simple exercise which can be done either sitting or lying down. Imagine yourself somewhere outside on a beautiful warm sunny day. Choose a place where you feel comfortable, confident and secure. It can be either imaginary or real. It can be in a garden or a meadow, for example.

■ Having chosen your place, give yourself a few moments to fix the scene well into your mind. That done, look around you slowly and deliberately. Are there any plants about? Any shrubs? Any trees? Any flowers? Look at the colors and the textures. Feel the plants or anything else in the vicinity if you wish. Are there any smells? Any sounds? Perhaps the sound of birds singing? Flowing water? Or gentle rustling of the wind? Any other sounds at all?

■ You can feel the warmth of the sun on your body and that makes you feel even more relaxed, content and happy. Allow the rays of the sun to permeate through you, and as this happens, feel any fear, anxiety or apprehension that you might have felt being burnt away by the warmth and the glow of the rays of the sun.

■ You are now feeling extremely relaxed, and comfortable, calm and confident.

■ As you walk around your garden or meadow, you come across a little pond with a fountain in the middle. It is incredibly beautiful. The pond is full of the purest, cleanest healing water. You drink a handful of this heavenly healing water.

■ Feel it going deep inside you and particularly to those areas within your being which are in the greatest need of healing.

Take as long as you like, and really feel the healing energy doing you good and healing your disease or disability.

■ Now move away from the pond and find yourself a comfortable place to sit.

■ While you are sitting down, feel the healing energy spread from deep inside you and fill your entire body, mind, emotions and spirit. Imagine this energy converting into light and radiating out from you, forming a circle of light in front of you. Imagine anyone else or any number of people, animals, plants or any other situations which you feel need healing in that circle of light in front of you. Concentrate on them for as long as you can. They will benefit as much as you do yourself from this distant healing energy directed towards them.

■ When you are ready, gently allow your circle of light to empty. Stand up and walk back to the part of the garden or meadow where you started this journey.

■ As you have now come to the end of this short imaginary journey, bring your attention to the present and become aware of what you are sitting on, and your presence in the room where you started the visualization.

■ Clench your fists tightly. Stretch your arms out. Take a deep breath in and open your eyes. You have now come to the end of this short journey.

■ It is important to think about any other images that may have come during this visualization, as they can be symbols guiding you and leading you to other things that you may need to do in order to complete your process of healing.

## GROUP HEALING

The actual visualization can be extremely varied as it is entirely dependent on the vivid imagination of the therapist or the material being used. Some therapists also incorporate soft relaxing background music during the process of visualization, as well as burning incense sticks or scented candles, in order to try and stimulate as many senses as possible. Some sessions are short and simple, while others are longer and more complex, depending on the available time and the purposes for which the fantasy journey is undertaken. There are now numerous visualization tapes on the market which can either be bought from specialist book/record stores or by mail order from specialist catalogs.

The members of the group can be given continuous healing throughout the duration of the visualization. Consequently, the power and the beneficial effects for the individual members become much more profound as a result.

## WHERE TO GO?

There are no specialist centers that just use visualization. The technique is used extensively by most relaxation therapists, especially those working with patients with serious diseases, including cancer and AIDS, as part of their general armory of healing tools. Some therapists run regular day workshops on stress management and healing during which they use guided visualization extensively.

# MUSIC THERAPY

CHAPTER TWENTY ONE

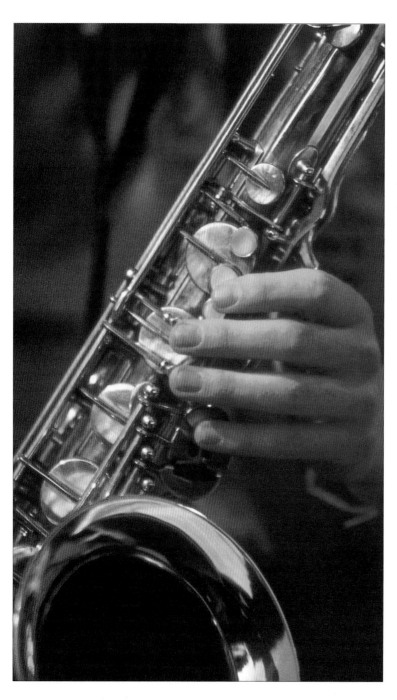

*M*usic therapy is the planned use of music to accomplish therapeutic goals. Music therapists draw from a wide range of music-related activities and musical elements when designing programs for specific clients. Music therapy goals address needs associated with motor, cognitive, communicative, social or affective areas of function. Integral to music therapy is the dynamic relationship between the therapist, the client, and the music. Therapeutic change occurs within this relationship, including the potential for generalization outside of the music therapy environment.

Today there are over fifty professional organizations for music therapy worldwide. Such organizations continue to work toward the advancement of music therapy, including the establishment of guidelines for music therapy education, training, research, program development, and public awareness.

## ORIGINS OF THE THERAPY

Music therapy originated and continues to evolve today in view of four considerations well-rooted in history.

First, as has been reported in such disciplines as anthropology and ethnomusicology, music and healing are considered one of the many uses of music found in all societies, historical or current. For example, in preliterate or indigenous cultures, music may facilitate trance states experienced by either the medicine practitioner or the patient when engaged in healing rituals.

Second, with the emergence of civilizations, written philosophical, magical or religious accounts of music and healing indicate music was perceived as having general therapeutic value and influence over one's soul, emotions, thoughts, or physical condition. For example, ancient Chinese texts assigned to music such attributes as moralistic virtue, a means of spiritual expression, and a way to link ancestors and descendants (DeWoskin 1982).

Third, as civilizations embraced rational thought, music became increasingly associated with having influence over particular medical conditions and states of mind, either as a curative or preventive power. Through Antiquity, the Middle Ages and the Renaissance, music was thought to cure plagues, alleviate mental disorders, balance the four cardinal humors, improve respiration, and reduce melancholy and depression (Davis & Gfeller 1992).

Fourth, the movement toward specialized areas of medical practice in recent history contributed to the emergence of modern-day music therapy. Beginning in the late 1800s, music therapy treatises and dissertations first appeared in medical journals. Efforts were underway to investigate empirically its effectiveness, to identify methods of practice according to specific kinds of disabilities, and to define its role as an adjunct to other forms of medical treatment. Throughout the first half of the twentieth century, particularly in the United States, hospital music programs, professional organizations, and educational training programs were established, furthering the growth of music therapy as its own discipline.

## PHILOSOPHY AND OBJECTIVES OF MUSIC THERAPY

The philosophical orientation for any one music therapist typically depends on training, assessed needs of the client, and the mission of the institution in which service is provided. Hence, approaches to music therapy are far ranging. In determining music therapy goals, whether attempting to rehabilitate, restore, maintain, or improve a client's condition, two frameworks are provided.

They are not intended to be mutually exclusive, and both perspectives have contributed to efforts to construct theoretical constructs specific to music therapy in terms of explaining the nature of practice and as the basis for research.

■ **Foundations based on the principle of normalization**: norms of behavior established by the society-at-large are used as points of

## MUSIC THERAPY WORLDWIDE

Music therapy continues to progress worldwide as a result of individual and collective effort, as well as gradual acceptance among the various systems of healthcare. Overall, music therapy is becoming increasingly scientific in its approach, with both quantitative and qualitative research represented in its literature. Foundations of music therapy practice continue to evolve not only in relation to naturalistic, cultural, and societal perspectives, but also in relation to advances in medical science.

reference in establishing objectives. For example, the music therapist may use music as a way to teach skills for daily living, including self-help skills or social interaction skills. Normalization may also include establishing objectives in the context of current understanding of developmental theory, whether working with children or adults. For children, objectives may be established based on developmental expectations according to chronological age across the areas of communication, cognition, motor, social, or emotional functions. For adults, objectives may be established based on expectations of behavior across one's life span.

■ **Foundations based on integration with a particular psychotherapy:** Music therapists may borrow from among the extensive list of modes of psychotherapy, their theoretical constructs and methods of practice currently in use by psychologists and other related disciplines and adapt them to music therapy practice. For example, music therapy literature includes efforts to combine music therapy with such approaches as Gestalt Therapy, Rational Emotive Therapy, and Transactional Analysis. In some instances integration with a previous established perspective results in highly specialized and even unique forms of music therapy practice. One example is Creative Music Therapy, a type of improvisational music therapy well grounded in Humanistic Psychology.

# HOW THE THERAPY WORKS

In understanding how music therapy works, consideration is given below to three areas: neurology and music, the nature of the music experience, and the role of the music therapist.

Musical activity engages several senses simultaneously. For example, when playing a musical instrument several senses are activated, including hearing, vision, touch, balance and movement. By taking advantage of the multi-sensory nature of music, neurological responses are likely to increase. This is particularly important if damage to a specific area of the brain is evident. Neurological processes are further enhanced as sensory input is evaluated in relation to cognitive functions, including thinking and memory. The summation of this activity engages the limbic system and related physiological responses, resulting in feeling or mood states. The underlying assumption for the music therapist is that music provides direct access to the emotional state of the client, and that it is this state that must be positively engaged if therapeutic change is to occur.

Music, according to Sears (1968) offers three distinct kinds of experiences that music therapists are able to utilize in their work. First, musical structures, including rhythm, melody and form, provide points of reference for behavioral responses. For example, the rocking behavior of a child with autism may be matched rhythmically by the music therapist. Once a relationship is established in terms of pulse, the therapist stops, starts, or varies the tempo, modeling additional choices for the client as ways to musically interact.

Second, music serves as the stimulus for responses that are not readily observable, including thoughts or feelings about issues related to oneself, other persons, things, or events. A carefully constructed music therapy program provides the means by which the realization, understanding, expression and resolution of such issues is possible.

# VISITING A THERAPIST

**What to expect and diagnosis**

For clients referred for music therapy, the music therapist first conducts an assessment to determine need for services. It is common for a music therapist to observe positive behaviors not observed in other kinds of assessments due to the general attractiveness of music. The final decision to provide music therapy is usually done in collaboration with other members of the treatment team. A written music therapy program plan is constructed, stating the course of action to follow over an extended period of time. Depending on the philosophical orientation of the music therapist and facility, the goals for treatment progress are documented and periodically evaluated to determine if the goals are being met, if they should be revised, or if services should be discontinued.

Depending on assessed needs and availability of staff, clients may receive music therapy services in individual or small group sessions for one to two sessions per week. Sessions are approximately 30 minutes to one hour in length. For each session the therapist constructs a specific objective to be accomplished in view of the long-range goals previously established. Sessions may begin with a simple, music-based activity for the purpose of engaging the client both physically and mentally within a musical structure. The main body of the session follows in which specific therapeutic outcomes are derived. The primary concern here is that extra-musical needs are being addressed while engaged in music, including anesthetic or performance-related values that may also be evident. Finally, a music-based activity may be used to bring the session to a close.

## CONDITIONS WHICH IT CAN BE USED TO TREAT

"Music therapists serve a wide range of disability-related conditions. Music therapists have become increasingly specialized according to the type of disability served. Several broad areas are described below, including music therapy in special education, gerontology, long-term care, and medically based acute care. Music therapists are employed across all areas of special education, serving at "risk infants" and young children, students with developmental disabilities, learning disabilities, autism, speech disorders, physical disabilities, behavioral problems, and visual and hearing impairments. In each instance the music therapist contributes to the accomplishment of special education goals. For some students, such as those with mental retardation or physical disabilities, sheltered workshops and vocational rehabilitation programs provide employment and training opportunities beyond the school setting. Music therapists assist here also, enhancing skills related to social interaction and concentration.

Music therapists are employed at all levels of service to the elderly, including day programs, residential programs and nursing homes. Music is used to encourage reminiscence, reality orientation, physical activity, and social interaction.

Music therapists are well-established in long-term care settings, including institutions for psychiatric conditions and adults with mental retardation. The primary role of music therapy is to enhance the resident's quality of life. Music therapy goals focus on appropriate use of leisure time, enhancement of self-esteem through success-oriented music activities, and positive group interaction through music ensemble experiences. Music therapists also facilitate the residents' participation in musical experiences common to the society-at-large, ultimately contributing to their sense of identity.

Individual services are also offered to assist in maintaining appropriate behavior. For psychiatric patients music may be used in conjunction with medications to reduce depression or psychotic behaviors.

Third, a musical environment offers the participants the opportunity to engage in relationships that are mutually supportive and conducive to therapeutic growth. Expressions of goodwill and cooperation in the accomplishment of a group-related music task typically bolsters the client's positive sense of self.

Ultimately, music therapists play a central role in constructing and maintaining musical and extra musical conditions in which progress is likely to occur. Music therapists take full advantage of the range of possible ways to be musical, from a simple strike on an instrument to virtuosic skill, from identifying the title of a song to self-expression through lyric writing, as a way to reach and guide clients according to their needs.

## PRACTICAL APPLICATION

The range of music activities used by music therapists includes listening, moving, playing, singing, lyric discussion, lyric writing, guided imagery and improvisation. Client preference plays a major role in the choice of actual music or musical styles to use. Musical instruments used are typically those that promote social interaction, such as the guitar, piano and rhythm instruments. The manner of use for the client often facilitates musical expression quickly, without extensive rehearsal or practice. Regardless of the method or instrument used, the music therapist must be ready to apply techniques commonly used in psychotherapy or special education in order to facilitate the desired responses from moment to moment.

Publications with information to assist the work of the music therapist are increasing. Yet, music therapists tend to be creative and resourceful in the design of their programs and in the manner in which materials are used. In using the art form of music in a systematic manner to address disability-related needs, musical expression will necessarily differ from client to client.

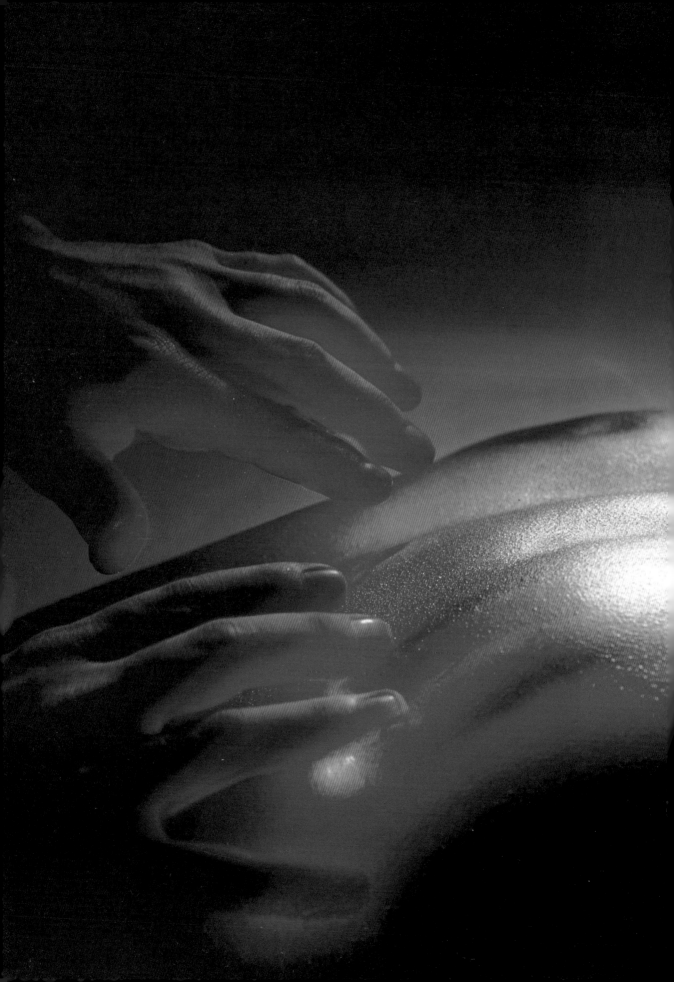

# MASSAGE AND TOUCH

## PART SIX

*T*he laying on of hands has long been accepted by many cultures as a powerful means of healing. Alternative medicine employs many "hands-on" therapies and modalities, including massage therapy, aromatherapy and reflexology. These ancient therapies date back over thousands of years and can help to improve health, relieve stress, promote relaxation and prevent disease. There are practical illustrated step-by-step photographic guides at the end of each chapter in this section to demonstrate the techniques involved.

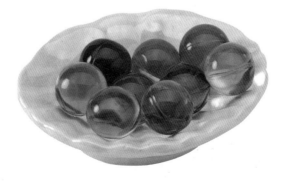

# MASSAGE THERAPY

## CHAPTER TWENTY TWO

*M*assage therapy is one of the oldest existing disciplines in the pantheon of health care practices. References to massage are found in Chinese medical texts which are over 4,000 years old. Massage has been advocated in Western health care practices in an almost unbroken line since the time of Hippocrates, "the Father of Medicine." In the fourth century B.C. Hippocrates

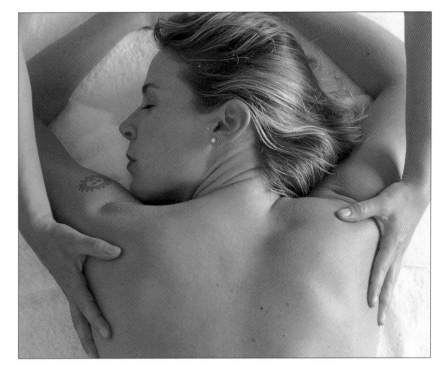

wrote, "The physician must be acquainted with many things and assuredly with rubbing" (the ancient Greeks and Romans referred to massage as rubbing).

Some of the greatest physicians in history recommended massage, including Celsus (25 B.C.-A.D.50), who wrote De Medicinia, an encyclopedia of Roman medical knowledge which dealt extensively with prevention and therapeutics using massage; Galen (A.D. 131-200), the most influential physician in the ancient, medieval, and renaissance worlds, who addressed techniques and indications for massage in his book De Sanitate Tuenda (which is translated as The Hygiene, meaning prevention); and Avicenna (980-1037 A.D.), a Persian physician who wrote extensively about massage in his Canon of Medicine, which was considered the authoritative medical text in Europe for several centuries. A sampling of other noted advocates includes Ambrose Pare, who wrote the first modern textbook of surgery; William Harvey, who discovered the circulation of the blood; and Herman Boerhaave, who introduced the clinical method of teaching medicine.

## MODERN METHODS

Modern, scientific massage therapy was introduced in the U.S. in the 1850s by two New York physicians, brothers George and Charles Taylor, who had studied in Sweden. The first massage therapy clinics in the U.S. were opened by two Swedes after the Civil War. Baron Nils Posse ran the Posse Institute in Boston and Hartwig Nissen opened the Swedish Health Institute near the Capitol in Washington, D.C. Several members of Congress and U.S. presidents, such as Benjamin Harrison and Ulysses Grant, were among the massage therapy clientele.

As the health care system in the U.S. began to be more influenced by biomedicine and technology in the early part of the 1900s, physicians began assigning massage duties, which were labor intensive, requiring much time to be spent with patients, to assistants and nurses (who together were the forerunners of physical therapists), In turn, in the 1930s and 1940s, nurses and physical therapists lost interest in massage therapy, virtually abandoning it. However, a small number of massage therapists carried on, removed from the medical field, until the 1960s, when a new surge of interest in massage therapy, which continues to this day, revitalized the field, albeit in the realm of complementary health care.

The latter 1960s saw the rise of the human growth movement and the emergence of humanistic psychology. A significant outgrowth of this movement was the notion that one could benefit from being involved in a therapeutic process even

## DESCRIPTION OF MASSAGE THERAPY

Massage therapy is the scientific manipulation of the soft tissues of the body for the purpose of normalizing those tissues and consists of a group of manual techniques (using primarily the hands and sometimes other areas such as the forearms, elbows, or feet) that include applying fixed or movable pressure, holding, and/or causing movement of or to the body. These techniques affect the musculoskeletal, circulatory/lymphatic, nervous, and other systems of the body. The basic philosophy of massage therapy encompasses the concept of *vis Medicatrix nature*, which is aiding the ability of the body to heal itself, and is aimed at achieving or increasing health and wellbeing.

Touch is the fundamental medium of massage therapy. While massage methods can be described in terms of a series of techniques performed, it is important to understand that touch is not used solely in a mechanical way in massage therapy. There is also an artistic component in massage. Because massage usually involves applying touch with varying degrees of pressure, the massage therapist must use touch with sensitivity in order to determine the optimal amount of pressure to use for each person. Touch used with sensitivity also allows the massage therapist to receive useful information about the body, such as locating areas of muscle tension and other soft tissue problems. Because touch is also a form of communication, sensitive touch conveys a sense of caring, which is an essential element in the therapeutic relationship for the person receiving massage. Using the wrong kind of touch, sometimes thought of as "toxic touch," is counterproductive and will render a technique ineffective and/or cause the body to defend or guard itself, which introduces greater tension.

though one might be considered not to be sick, or "normal." In other words, one did not have to be ill to benefit from therapy. Massage represented many of the values extolled by the growth movement, infusing the field with new interest.

The 1970s saw the rise of the term "lifestyle." Massage fits well into the quest for improving the quality of one's life. The wave of interest grew even more in the 1980s as the popularity of the notion of fitness and taking responsibility for one's health took root. Massage was recognized for its stress reduction and relaxation effects. Those who maintained a personal fitness plan found massage to be an excellent complement to an active lifestyle.

The resurgence of interest in forms of complementary health care in the 1990s provided massage with another burst of interest. Massage therapy is now used in a variety of ways ranging from simple relaxation to stress reduction to sports and treating specific maladies. Massage therapy is practiced in settings ranging from doctors' offices to massage clinics to health spas.

# KEY BENEFITS AND EFFECTS OF MASSAGE THERAPY

Massage therapy can be an important part of a personal health and fitness program. Massage has powerful healing qualities that can help counteract the debilitating effects of the twin nemeses of modern life—the underuse and overuse of our bodies—by mobilizing the body's resources. While it can be an aid in restoring health and recovering from injury, massage is also the perfect wellness medicine because you do not have to be sick or hurt to use it. Regular massage, in combination with exercise and good nutrition, can be a wonderful way to maintain health.

Massage increases the circulation of the blood and movement of

## KEY EFFECTS

Massage primarily affects the body as a whole. Taking a look at the key effects of massage gives insight into how massage works and what the benefits of massage are:

- Reduced muscle tension
- Improved blood circulation
- Better lymph movement
- Increased mobility and range of motion of joints
- Stimulated or soothed nervous system
- Enhanced skin condition
- Better digestion and intestinal function
- Relief of acute and chronic pain
- Reduced swelling
- Reduced stress
- General relaxation

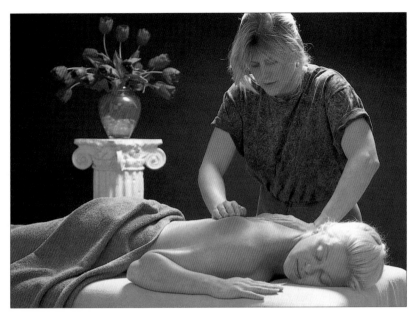

lymph. The direct mechanical effect of rhythmically applied pressure, along with the stimulation of nerve receptors, can increase the rate of blood flow.

Lymph is a milky white fluid that drains impurities and waste away from the tissue cells. This is vital because a component of these wastes is toxins which are the by-products of metabolism. Muscular contraction has a pumping effect that moves lymph, so exercise helps best. However, massage is the next best way to move lymph.

For the whole body to be healthy, the sum of its parts, the cells, must also be healthy. The individual cells of the body are dependent on an abundant supply of circulating blood and moving lymph because these fluids supply nutrients and oxygen and carry away carbon dioxide and wastes.

Massage affects the muscles and other soft tissues throughout the body. It can help to loosen contracted, shortened, hardened muscles and

*Above: massage is a powerful healing tool, helping the body to heal itself and increasing health and wellbeing.*

can stimulate weak, flaccid muscles. Tense or spasmed muscles not only can cause discomfort, but they also consume much energy and lead to many other problems, such as postural and muscle imbalances which can lead to injury. Chronic muscle tension also further reduces the circulation of the blood and movement of lymph in an area.

Massage does not increase muscle strength, but it can promote recovery from the fatigue and minor aches and pains that occur with exercise. In this way, it can be possible to do more exercise, which may in the long run strengthen muscles. In turn, all the systems of the body will benefit from better circulation and efficient functioning of the musculature and other soft tissues.

Another effect of massage is that it either soothes or stimulates the nervous system depending on the needs of the person receiving it at that particular time. If someone is very overstimulated, massage can provide a calming effect. On the other hand, if someone is very listless, massage can be stimulating and raise energy. It also enhances skin condition by improving the function of the sebaceous and sweat glands, which keep the skin lubricated, clean, and cool. Internal organs and the immune system also benefit. There can be an overall improvement in physical health and the quality of life.

Another reason massage therapy can have such a broad effect on the body is the interrelationship between structure and function in the body. The musculoskeletal structure of the body affects function, and function affects structure. Massage therapy works with both aspects. For example, massage therapists will work with structure by both relieving trauma or stress and influencing muscular patterns that affect posture. In turn, this will allow greater ease of movement, wider range of motion, and more flexibility.

The relationship between stress and illness is of great interest to anyone maintaining their health. We have stress in our daily lives relating to work, family, environment, and social demands and pressures. Mental tensions, frustrations, and insecurity are among the most damaging. Stress causes the release of hormones that

*Right: a soothing therapeutic massage can be extremely effective in relaxing tense shoulder muscles and relieving back pain, leaving the patient refreshed.*

make blood vessels narrow and constrict, resulting in less blood flow. Affected by stress, the heart works harder, breathing becomes more rapid and shallow, and digestion slows. Every body process becomes degraded. Studies show how stress factors can cause headaches, hypertension, depression, etc. It is now estimated 80 to 90 percent of illness may be stress induced. Massage is a non drug intervention that can help counteract the effects of stress and increase relaxation. The risk of stress

induced illness can be decreased.

Massage can also have a psychological effect that is based upon the interaction or interconnection of the mind and body. Simply put, the mind affects the body and the body affects the mind. In this sense, mental tensions can manifest physically as muscular tension or other physical conditions. Similarly, physical tensions can have an impact on mental and emotional states. To demonstrate this effect, try clenching your fists for an extended period of time, perhaps

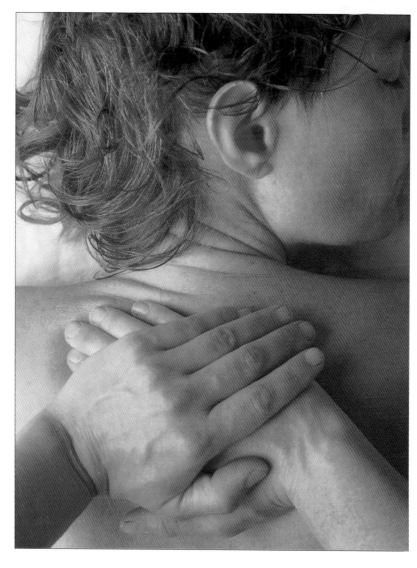

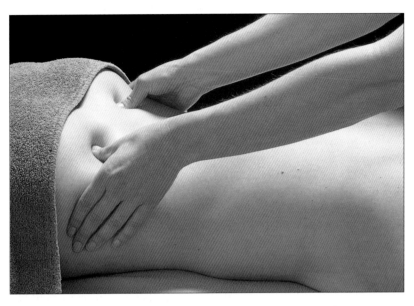

*Left: most contemporary Western massage is based on Swedish massage.*

10 minutes. The chances are you will begin to feel angry or irritable. From a therapeutic point of view, dealing with a fixed pattern or habit in one realm may affect the other. Sometimes loosening chronic muscular tension patterns will lead to an emotional release and result in improved awareness of feeling. Massage also improves body awareness, which, in turn, promotes better personal

## THE TACTILE SENSE

Massage also animates the tactile sense, which is the body's primary sense. This has another psychological effect of bringing people in the here and now and away from a constant preoccupation with problems and the tension generated by mental hyperactivity. This has a centering effect that often leaves people feeling mentally refreshed and restored. Massage therapy recipients often describe this as a "mental vacation."

insight. Consequently, massage therapy and psychotherapy complement each other, and massage therapists and psychotherapists will work with the same clients.

## THE FIELD OF MASSAGE THERAPY

There are over 100 different methods that may be classified under massage therapy. Most of them, about three-quarters, are less than twenty years old. This can be confusing for the consumer, so this section will help you to sort out these many methods and will focus on the most prevalent.

There are several reasons why so many methods exist. The period of the 1930s to the mid-1960s was a relatively dormant one for the massage therapy profession. Little standardization was established within the field. Then in the 1970s, stimulated by changes in society that included a greater interest in fitness, healthier lifestyles, personal improvement, and alternative methods of health care to complement biomedi-

cine, a steady boom of renewed interest in massage therapy began. An influx of new practitioners brought with them a wave of new ideas and creativity regarding ways to use "hands-on" techniques along with the established ones. Since there was little standardization, these techniques sometimes developed into free-standing methods, rather than being incorporated into an existing system of classification.

Another source of new techniques was the many forms of massage native to most cultures around the world, many of which are not readily linked with each other. For example, many of the forms of massage that come from Asia are based on concepts of anatomy, physiology, and diagnoses that differ from the Western ones.

This proliferation of methods has slowed. It is expected, as has similarly happened in the development of other professions, that as the development of standards and credentials continues, there will be some consolidation and integration of these methods.

Most of these methods can be organized into five basic categories; Traditional Methods, European, Contemporary Western, Structural/ Functional/Movement Integration, Oriental and Energetic (nonoriental). In practice, many massage therapists use more than one method in their work and sometimes combine several in an integrative manner. As a result, quite a variety of technique repertoires can be presented by massage therapists.

■ **Traditional European Massage** includes methods based on traditional, conventional Western concepts of anatomy and physiology. Five basic categories of soft tissue manipulation techniques are used: effleurage (long flowing or gliding strokes in the direction of the heart), petrissage (kneading, lifting or rolling stokes), friction (rubbing on the underlying structures beneath the surface), tapotement (percussion-tapping, cupping, hacking), and vibration.

■ **Swedish Massage** is the main form of Traditional European Massage and is probably the most widely practiced method in Western countries. It was developed by Per Henrik Ling (1776-1839), a Swedish fencing master who wanted to develop a method that provided benefits similar to exercise. He designed manual techniques and movements to both maintain health and treat illness. Ling's method was the first modern Western systematization of massage.

Swedish massage uses a system of long gliding strokes, kneading, and friction techniques on the more superficial layers of muscles, generally in the direction of blood flow toward the heart because there is an emphasis on improving blood flow to the soft tissues, and sometimes combined with active and passive movements of the joints. It is used to promote general relaxation, improve circulation and range of motion, and relieve muscle tension.

A massage therapist doing Swedish massage usually uses oil as a lubricant to facilitate the rubbing action of the massage strokes. Sometimes a lotion or talcum powder is substituted. Swedish is fairly vigorous and usually used as a complete, full body treatment, though sometimes only a part of the body is worked on when one area needs extra attention. Swedish massage is the most commonly used form of massage.

■ **Contemporary Western Massage** includes methods based on modern Western concepts of human functioning, including anatomy and physiology, using a wide variety of manipulative techniques that go beyond the original framework of Swedish massage. These may include broad applications for personal growth, emotional release, and balance of the mind, body, and spirit in addition to traditional applications. These methods include Neuromuscular massage, "Sports massage," Deep Tissue, Transverse or Cross-fiber Frictioning, Myofascial Release, Myotherapy, Bindgewebsmassage, Esalen, and Manual Lymph Drainage. Many of these methods were developed since the later 1960s, with a few exceptions.

■ **Deep Tissue Massage** is used to release chronic patterns of muscular tension using slow strokes, direct pressure, or friction directed across the grain of the muscles using the fingers, thumbs, or elbows. It is applied with greater pressure, to deeper layers of muscle, and with greater specificity than Swedish, which is why it is called deep tissue. In many areas of the body, the muscles are arranged in layers and sometimes the deeper layers need to be worked on. Deep tissue massage techniques are designed for massaging these deeper muscles or deeper portions of thick muscles that have greater depth. For example, if someone has upper back and shoulder soreness, it could be necessary to massage the rhomboid muscle which is located beneath the trapezius muscle. Using deep tissue massage, the deeper layer of muscle will also be worked on.

*Below: massage improves blood circulation and helps lymph drainage.*

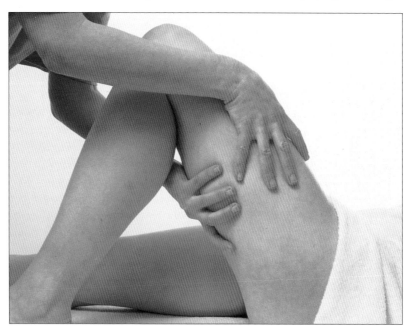

**Sports Massage** uses techniques which are similar to Swedish and Deep Tissue, but are specially adapted to deal with the effects of athletic perfomance on the body and the needs of athletes. Sports massage is used before, during, or after events, as part of an athlete's training regimen, and to promote effective healing of and recovery from injuries. Before an event it is used as an adjunct to an athlete's warm-up routine and gets the athlete ready to perform. After an event sports massage is used to aid recovery from the event. Sports massage can be equally beneficial for high-level athletes, fitness enthusiasts, or "weekend warriors."

Sports massage therapists are being included in the medical services program provided at the 1996 Olympics at all the Olympic venues. A number of professional and collegiate teams have sports massage therapists on their staffs.

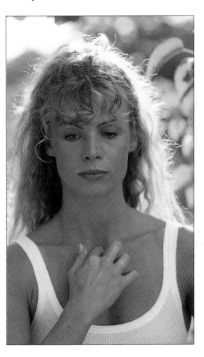

**Neuromuscular Massage** is a relatively detailed form of deep massage that is applied specifically to individual muscles. It is used to increase blood flow to specific areas that are considered to be ischemic, i.e. lack blood flow; release trigger points, which are intense knots of muscle tension that refer pain to other parts of the body; and release pressure on nerves caused by soft tissues. It is often used to reduce pain. Trigger point massage and myotherapy are methods similar to neuromuscular massage.

**Manual Lymph Drainage** improves the flow of lymph using light, rhythmic strokes. It is primarily used for conditions related to poor lymph flow, such as lymphedema and neuropathies. For example, it has been shown to be effective for the lymphedema that commonly follows mastectomy surgery (removal of cancerous breast tissue).

**Esalen Massage** is named after the growth center where it was developed, the Esalen Institute in Big Sur, California. Its focus is more on creating deeper states of relaxation, beneficial shifts in states of consciousness, and overall wellbeing, rather than on relieving muscle tension or increasing circulation. Compared to Swedish, Esalen is more slow, rhythmic, and hypnotic-like, and focuses on the mind-body as a whole. Swedish and Esalen complement each other well and some practitioners will combine them.

*Left: it is natural to rub or press on areas where you feel discomfort or pain to alleviate them.*

**Structural, Functional and Movement Integration** approaches place an emphasis on body structure and movement. This grouping includes methods that organize and integrate the body in relationship to gravity through manipulating the soft tissues and/or through correcting inappropriate patterns of movement. These methods seek to bring about a more balanced use of the nervous system through creating new, integrated possibilities of movement. Examples are Rolfing, Hellerwork, Aston Patterning, the Trager approach, Feldenkrais method, and the Alexander Technique.

**Rolfing** (also known as Structural Integration), developed by Ida Rolf, uses techniques intended to realign the body in the field of gravity through manipulation of the fascia (connective tissue) of the body, which allows the body to function more effectively and efficiently. The technique loosens or releases adhesions in the fascia, the pliable connective tissue that wraps around muscles and muscle groups. This is intended to result in a rearranging of the body structure's major segments into a more correct vertical alignment. Rolfing consists of a series of 10 sessions, each one dealing with a different area of the body.

**Trager,** developed by Milton Trager, uses light, rhythmic, rocking and shaking movements to loosen the joints, ease movements, and release chronic patterns of tension. The Trager practitioner, while working in a meditative-like state, moves the client's trunk and limbs in a gentle, rhythmic way in order to foster a sense of freedom and lightness. After the hands-on portion of the session, the client is often given instruction in the use of Mentastics, a system of self-directed movement sequences to support and reinforce the work done on the table.

■ **Feldenkrais,** developed by Moshe Feldenkrais, takes two forms. In individual one-on-one sessions, the practitioner's touch and passive movement are used to improve awareness of movement patterns. In a series of classes, exercise lessons consisting of sequences of slow body motions organized around various human funtions are used for "relearning" proper body movement.

■ **Alexander Technique,** developed by F.M. Alexander, involves learning simple, efficient movements based on body alignment, designed to improve balance, posture, coordination, and relieve pain. It intends to work with unconscious patterns of thinking and the resultant movements or postures that become set in the musculature. The relationships among the head, neck, and back are of particular importance. The Alexander teacher uses both verbal and hands-on guidance to help the student experience new ways of moving.

■ **Oriental Massage** includes the methods based on Traditional Oriental/Chinese Medical principles for assessing and evaluating the life energy in the body that is believed to flow through invisible channels. Treatment using strong or very light pressure and manipulation is applied by finger or thumb tips to predetermined points in order to affect and

balance the energetic system. These methods may also be used in conjunction with acupuncture and herbs. Some examples are Tuina, Shiatsu, Acupressure, AMMA, Jin Shin Jyutsu, and Jin Shin Do.

■ **Energetic Methods** include approaches that work with the energy of the body, but are not based on the Oriental/Chinese system. These are methods that intend to affect the biofield that surrounds and infuses the human body, by pressure and/or manipulation of the physical body, or by the passage or placement of the

hands in, or through, that energetic field. These methods are based on Traditional Ayurvedic (Indian), Eastern or Western Esoteric, or other systems of healing. Examples are Polarity Therapy, Therapeutic Touch, and Reiki.

**SUMMARY**
Massage can be used for a number of conditions and generally will help any condition that would

*Below: this Reiki therapist, who is working with the energy of the body, is "cupping" the eyes of a patient.*

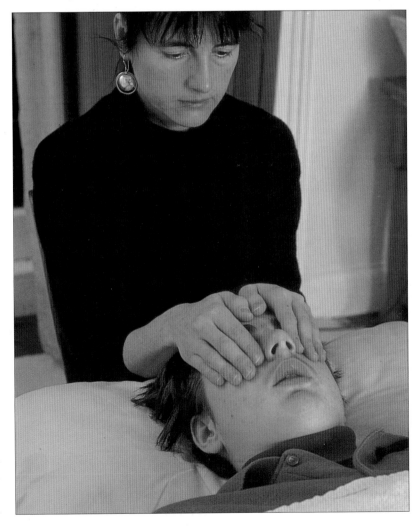

benefit from improved circulation and reduction of tension. From the psychosomatic point of view, the ability of massage to reduce anxiety, depression and stress is a logical counter to the strain of any malady. Some of the conditions listed below are affected directly by massage, particularly soft tissue injuries. Other conditions are affected more indirectly.

Massage is also highly complementary to all other medical tradition. The effectiveness of other forms of treatment in most cases can be enhanced by inducing relaxation and promoting circulation. Massage can also help one tolerate more in-vasive approaches and handle the side effects of other treatments. For example, massage is being used in some hospitals to ease the suffering of cancer patients. Massage is not expected to directly treat the cancer, but it may help the patient to deal better with the effects of the disease and/or the treatment. It may also have an indirect effect by supporting the body's functions, including the immune system.

## COPNDITIONS HELPED BY MASSAGE

Here is a listing of some of the most common conditions that massage can be used for:

■ **Strains, sprains, and other soft tissue problems**—massage is particularly effective for soft tissue injuries, especially muscle strains, commonly called muscle pulls or cramps, and sprains, which involve the tissues around joints. Some other conditions helped by massage are tendinitis and tenosynovitis.

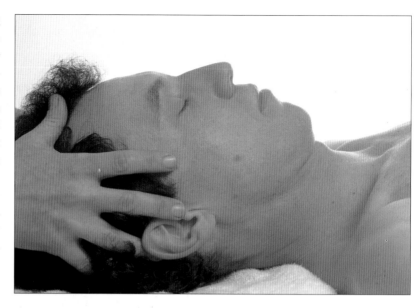

■ **Arthritis**—massage can help relieve the pain and stiffness associated with osteoarthritis, and swelling caused by rheumatoid arthritis.

■ **Anxiety**—a number of scientific studies show that massage consistently reduces anxiety.

■ **Back pain**—massage can help relieve muscles spasms that typically accompany and often cause back pain and restore circulation, which is often reduced in the afflicted area.

■ **Carpal Tunnel Syndrome and other repetitive motion disorders**—massage can help to the extent that the problem may be caused or aggravated by muscle tension and poor circulation.

■ **Fatigue**—massage can help recovery from fatigue due to vigorous activity through removing the byproducts of metabolism. Massage also helps the type of fatigue that results from stress.

■ **Headache**—massage can help relieve headaches, especially tension headaches.

■ **Pregnancy**—massage can help the expectant mother recover from the physical and emotional stress caused by pregnancy. Infants also love massage.

■ **Sciatica**—massage can help relieve muscle spasms that may either cause or be the result of sciatica. It can be especially useful if muscle tension is placing any pressure on the sciatic nerve.

## MASSAGE WARNING

Remember, massage therapists do not diagnose illnesses, so do not hesitate to see a doctor in order to receive a diagnosis and medical treatment. Injuries that involve considerable pain and loss of function should be referred to a doctor first. There are some conditions and situations for which massage should not be used, such as certain skin conditions, unhealed wounds, later stage osteoporosis, certain circulatory conditions and bleeding disorders.

■ **Swelling**—massage can reduce swelling around joints or injuries.

■ Massage can also be used for the following: acute and chronic pain, asthma, bronchitis, chronic inflammatory bowel diseases (ulcerative colitis and Crohn's Disease), chronic lymphedema, cerebral palsy, colic, congestion, constipation, depression, diabetes, eating disorders, eyestrain, fibromyalgia syndrome, fibrositis syndrome, gas, insomnia, irritability, menstrual cramps, post traumatic stress disorder, premenstrual syndrome, restless leg syndrome, scars, scoliosis, shin splints, sinus problems, temporomandibular joint disorder, and tennis elbow.

## FINDING A MASSAGE THERAPIST

One of the best ways to find a massage therapist is by a recommendation from someone you trust, such as a friend. You may also get a suggestion from another health professional, such as a physician or chiropractor. However, their familiarity with massage therapy can vary widely, so not all doctors may be helpful.

You can also locate a massage therapist by getting a referral from a credible professional association. The largest and oldest professional association for massage therapists in the United States is the American Massage Therapy Association (AMTA). The AMTA is the largest and oldest national association, with over 24,000 members. For further information, consult the Useful Addresses section at the back of this book. AMTA members practice many of the techniques discussed in this chapter. There are also smaller orga-

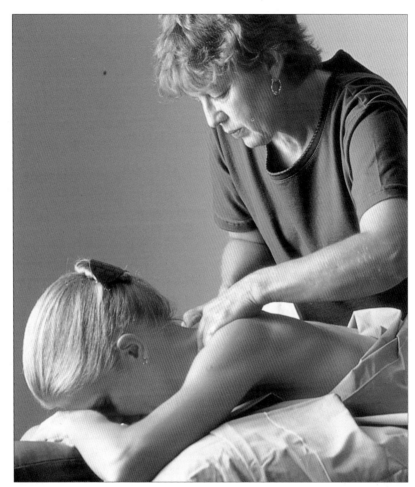

nizations that represent specific methods only.

Feel free to inquire about a potential massage therapist's qualifications. Look for a minimum of 500 hours of education, preferably from an accredited school. For example, in the U.S., 62 programs are accredited/approved by the Commission for Massage Training Accreditation/Approval (COMTAA), which accredits training programs based on stringent educational standards. Another credential to look for is if a massage therapist is nationally certified by the National Certification Board for Therapeutic Massage and Bodywork (NCBTMB). One must

pass an exam to earn certification by the NCBTMB.

You can also ask if someone belongs to a credible professional association, such as the AMTA. Be aware that there are some groups that sound like associations, but are actually privately owned businesses. To be an AMTA member, for example, a massage therapist must have graduated from a training program which is accredited or approved by COMTAA, or hold a license in a state that meets AMTA standards, or pass the National Certification Exam for Therapeutic Massage and Bodywork. If someone specializes in a specific method, such as Rolfing or Trager, ask them if they have a credential for that particular method.

A license may also be a helpful credential, but not all states regulate massage. Currently 21 states and the District of Columbia and various localities regulate massage.

## WHAT TO EXPECT

Before your session, it is best to eat lightly in the two hours before your appointment. Make time to relax before and after your session. The more slowed down you are going in to your session, the looser you can get. A hot shower is usually a good prelude. Leave yourself some time afterwards to enjoy the after effects and/or integrate the results.

Most often, your therapist will ask you to disrobe while he or she leaves the room. You should only remove as much as you feel comfortable taking off. The purpose for disrobing is that most massage tech-

niques depend on direct contact with the body. You will be covered or "draped" with a sheet or towel so that only the part of your body that is being worked on is uncovered at any particular moment during the massage. Your massage therapist will be sensitive to respecting your privacy and comfort. Some forms of massage, such as seated massage, do not require removing clothing. It is a good idea to remove jewelry and contact lenses before a massage.

Before the session begins, your therapist is likely to ask if there are any areas that are especially tense or tender, and about any medical conditions. The massage therapist will be trying to find out particularly if there are any reasons why you should not be massaged.

Depending on the techniques used, oil may be used for lubrication to facilitate the massage movements. Massage oils are generally vegetable based. Mineral oil is not used for massage. Some massage oils are scented, so if you are sensitive to scents or some oils, be sure to tell your massage therapist. Sometimes lotion or talcum powder can be substituted. Some massage therapists like to play soothing music during the massage; some do not.

Communication between your massage therapist and you is essential. You should feel free to speak up if the therapist is using too much or too little pressure, or if anything else is a problem for you. It is your right not to do anything that you are not comfortable with.

*Left: massage therapy aims to improve balance, posture as well as relaxation.*

## EFFECTS OF MASSAGE

Generally, a person feels relaxed and an afterglow of peace and calm following a massage. However, sometimes the change process naturally causes temporary discomfort, which needs to be accepted, so that expectations of feeling good are not always appropriate. Similarly, sessions that emphasize therapeutic work on chronic areas of tension and recovery from injury may involve some discomfort. This is because unhealthy or damaged tissues are more sensitive, not necessarily because the massage technique was bad. Sometimes tense muscles will feel sore a day or two following a massage, which is common and usually clears up in a day or two, and is a little like what happens when unused muscles get exercised. It can help to drink lots of water after a massage.

As far as conversation goes, it depends on what is appropriate for you during your massage. There is a wide variation among practitioners and approaches concerning how much verbal exchange takes place. As far as the recipient is concerned, sometimes people need to talk as a form of release, but at other times talking can be a distraction and it is better to have silence. Keeping talk to a minimum can help you focus your full awareness on the massage experience. If your mind tends to be overactive during the massage, try focusing on the massage therapist's hands and/or your breathing.

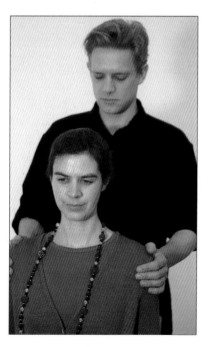

# INTRODUCTION

A full body massage is featured in the following step-by-step illustrated photoguide to some basic massage strokes and techniques. Remember not to eat a heavy meal in the two hours before a massage session—if you are hungry, just have something light to eat.

You do not have to disrobe completely unless you feel comfortable doing so. You will be draped with a towel while you are being massaged, and only the area of your body that is being worked on at any particular time will be uncovered.

## MASSAGE GUIDE

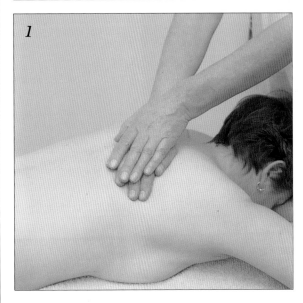

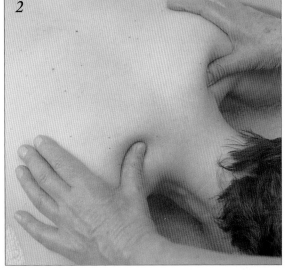

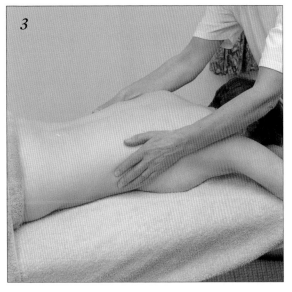

*1 The massage begins by working on the shoulders to ease out tension and relax the upper back. The hands move round each shoulder blade, tracing them to soften up the area and relieve the tension.*

*2 Next, the thumbs are used around the shoulder blades to work deeper, especially on any sore or tender areas.*

*3 The whole upper body area is stroked (effleurage) to warm and relax the body and to stimulate circulation. This warm-up routine can be interspersed with other massage strokes, if wished. Then the therapist pulls back to stretch out the sides of the body, starting from the hips and pulling slowly upward to the shoulders.*

# MASSAGE GUIDE

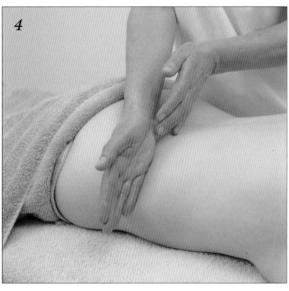

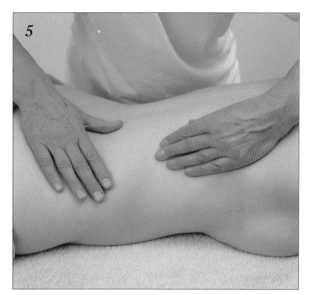

4 *After stroking the area to warm up the muscles, the therapist traces round the ilium, the uppermost part of the hip bone, with the sides of the hands. This helps to ease muscular tension.*

5 *The therapist kneads the lower back and ilium areas with each hand, working gently initially and then working a little deeper to ease out tension, aches and pains.*

6 *Using her body weight, the therapist then uses both hands to double knead the area. This sequence is repeated on the other side of the patient's body.*

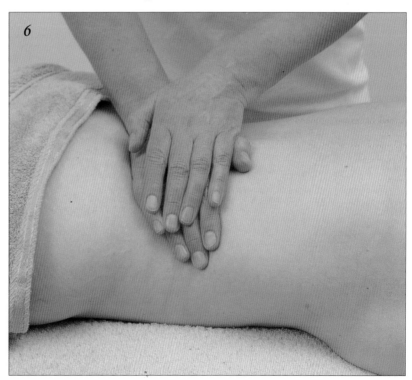

7 *The therapist works on the trapezius muscles, which cover each side of the back and shoulders, and rotates the shoulder blades. The aim is to ease out any tension and knots in this area and relax the shoulders.*

8 *Leg massage: both hands are used to sweep up and down the legs. This increases circulation as well as being very soothing.*

9 *Effleurage (stroking movements) are used along the sides of the legs. Often the therapist will use a scented massage or aromatherapy oil to facilitate movement and to make the massage a more soothing and pleasurable experience for the patient.*

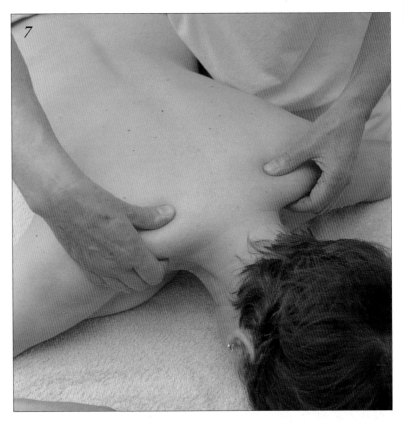

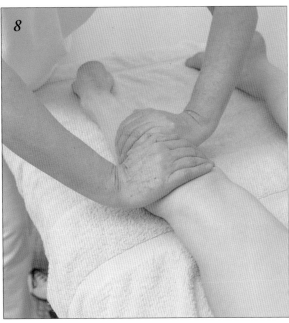

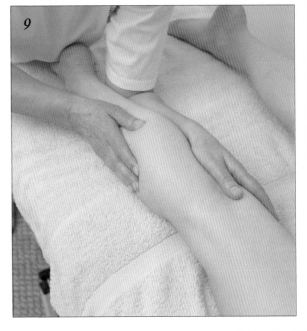

# MASSAGE GUIDE

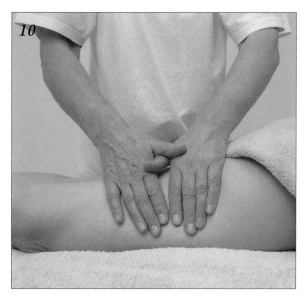

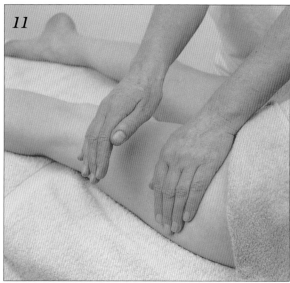

*10 Rolling is another technique which is often used in massage. With the thumbs crossed for additional stability, the flesh is lifted and rolled.*

*11 The therapist cups her hands and, using the cupping movement, moves her hands rhythmically up and down with a cushion of air beneath them. This helps encourage blood flow and brings blood to the surface.*

*12 With fingers between the ribs, the therapist works on the intercostal muscles, gently easing them out.*

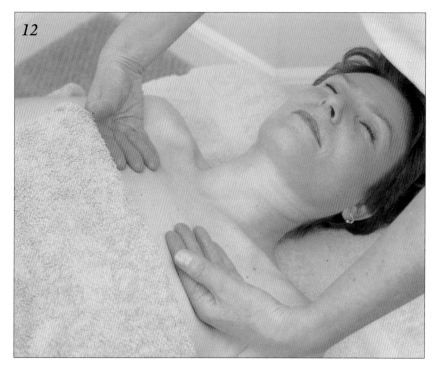

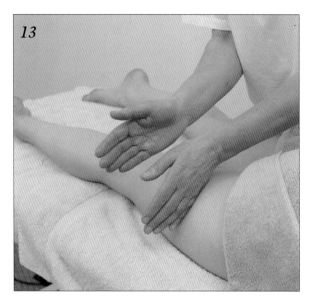

13 Hacking is a stimulating form of massage which brings the blood to the surface and leaves the skin feeling tingly. It should be very light and relaxed without chopping.

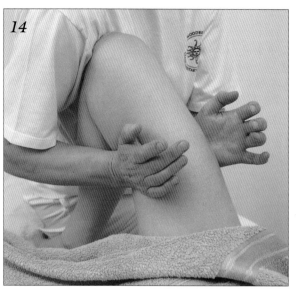

14 The heels of the hands are used to work on the quadriceps muscles on the front of the thighs. The hands work evenly and deep up the sides of the thighs to ease out any tension.

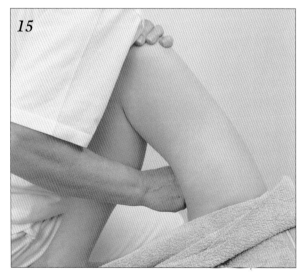

15 Next the therapist works down the back of the hamstrings, running down the thighs behind the knees. These areas can get very tight, especially in athletes, and massage can be beneficial.

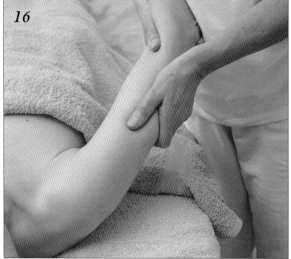

16 The muscle is literally picked up and lifted away from the bone. The session ends with some gentle stroking along the length of the body to leave the patient feeling refreshed and relaxed.

## SELF HELP

### DE-STRESS BREAK ROUTINE

**1** Place your fingertips on your scalp and make small circles over the entire area of the scalp. You should press in slightly with your fingertips so that you are moving the top layer of the scalp over the underlying layers, rather than rubbing or sliding over the surface of the skin. About 30 seconds.

**2** Place your fingertips on your temple area on the side of your head and make firm, slow circles. Work upwards onto the area just forward of the tops of your ears. About 30 to 60 seconds.

**3** Place your thumbs on your jaw just in front of your earlobes. Press in with your thumb tips into your jaw muscles. Hold for five seconds and slowly release. Continue down your jaw to just below the level of your mouth.

**4** Interlace your fingers and firmly knead your thumb into your opposite palm. Massage the entire surface of the palm. Be sure to work the muscular area at the base of the thumb. Then squeeze and lightly pull and squeeze each finger; 30 seconds for each hand.

**5** Place your right hand on your left shoulder. Press your fingers firmly into the muscle. Hold for 5-10 seconds and release. Then repeat, but this time tuck your chin in toward your chest while you press. Then grasp and squeeze the muscular area on top of your shoulder and release. Repeat on other side. Don't tense your shoulders while doing this.

**6** Place all your fingertips on your forehead just above your eyebrows. Press in slightly and move your fingertips up and down, inching up until you reach your hairline. About 15 seconds.

**7** Cup both eyes with your palms, resting the heels of your hands under your eye sockets. Using light pressure, make circles in both directions for about 30 seconds.

### FOOT MASSAGE

**1** Place your foot on the edge of a chair. Squeeze the foot lightly with both hands, moving your hands to cover the entire foot. If any spots are especially stiff or sore, squeeze them for about 10 seconds.

**2** Place the middle finger of each hand on the sole of your foot, just below the ball of the foot. Press for about 10 seconds. Repeat along the whole area of the ball of the foot.

**3** Touch either side of your ankle with your fingertips and make small, gentle circles around the round, bony projections on either side of the ankle.

**4** Grasp each toe between your fingers and thumb. Squeeze and pull lightly.

**5** In a sitting position, place one foot over your other knee, so the sole is facing you. Hold your ankle with one hand. Starting at the base of your heel, press in with your thumb and move it in a straight line toward your toes. Make several of these "stripes" along the surface of your sole.

### HEADACHE ROUTINE

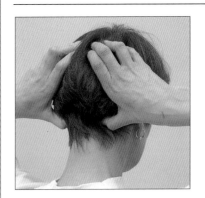

*1 Place your fingertips on your scalp. Press in slightly and move your scalp back and forth over your head. You should feel the scalp sliding back and forth almost like a cap. Do not slide your fingertips over the surface of your scalp. Repeat this over the entire scalp area.*

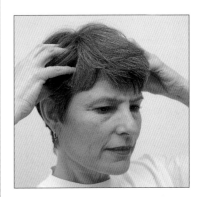

*2 Place your fingertips on your forehead. Press in and move the skin on your forehead like you moved your scalp, working from your eyebrows to hairline. Do not slide your fingertips over the surface of your forehead.*

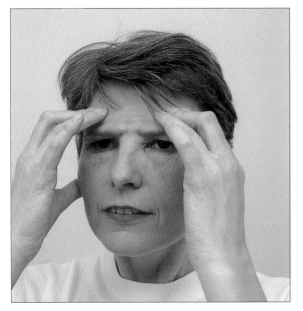

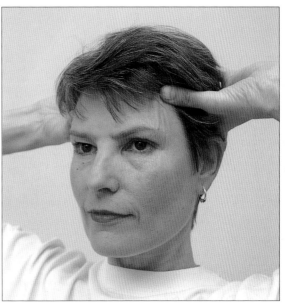

3 Place your thumb tips at the base of your skull where your head meets your neck. You may feel a bony ridge there. Press in with your thumb tips and make small circles along the base of your neck.

4 Place your thumb and fingers on either side of your head so that they are circling your entire head. Alternate moving your hands in a clockwise, then counterclockwise direction, back and forth, as if you were unscrewing your scalp or opening and closing a jar lid.

5 Use the middle and index fingers of each hand to press gently up underneath your cheekbones, directly below your eyes. Hold this position for about 30-60 seconds. Take some long, deep breaths while you are doing this.

6 Press your thumb tip into the webbing between the thumb and index finger of your opposite hand, pushing against the bone that connects with the index finger. Hold for 30-60 seconds. Repeat for the other hand.

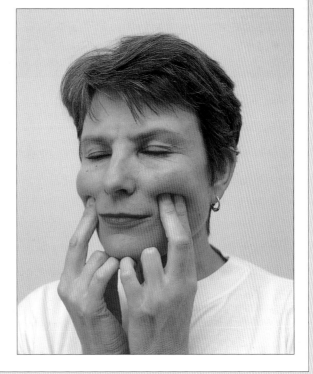

# AROMATHERAPY

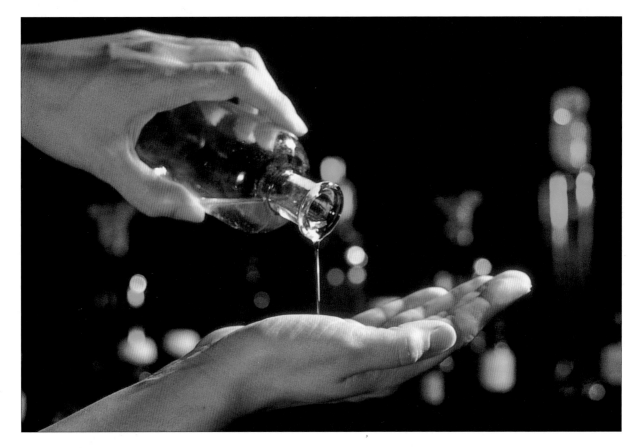

## CHAPTER TWENTY THREE

*A*romatherapy is the use of essential oils and hydrosols to promote personal health. The concentrated essences are extracted from plants, usually by a process called distillation in which plant materials are heated with water in a pot called a still, so that their aromatic oils are released from the plant, vaporize, and rise with the steam of the heated water.

The steam and vapor move through a tube to a condensing coil, where they are cooled and return to a liquid state. The essential oil, which is an easily evaporated (volatile) liquid having the characteristic odor of the plant, floats on top of the water or, in rare cases, sinks below the water. The resulting water contains water-soluble parts of the plant and micro-molecules of essential oil and is termed the hydrosol. Both of these products of distillation are considered to be valuable therapeutic substances in aromatherapy.

## A HEALING ART AND SCIENCE

Aromatherapy combines the sciences of chemistry, botany, and physiology with the art of essential oil blending and is thought to achieve physical, emotional and mental balance and harmony. Healing effects of organic chemical components are achieved by inhalation or direct application of essential oils and hydrosols. Central themes of the practice of aromatherapy include:
■ The connection between mind and body.
■ The powerful effects of botanical remedies on human health.
As a part of nature, essential oils are both tools of a healing art, and chemical components of healing science. By application and inhalation, they seem to affect the entire being to promote vital health and wellness.

## HISTORY OF AROMATHERAPY

The term aromatherapy was coined by the French chemist René Maurice Gattefossé in *Aromatherapie,* published in 1937, although the aromatic properties of plants had been recognized and in use for health and wellbeing for many centuries. Before methods of distillation were perfected, aromatic herbs were burned as incense, drunk as tea, used externally in both unguents and ointments, internally in medicine, and for personal adornment.

Egypt has a particularly rich history of using aromatics in everything from daily dress to the embalming process. Resins of plants such as frankincense, myrrh, and galbanum were commonly used by the Egyptians. Although distillation was invented around 3000B.C., the earliest products of this process were not the essential oils.

Aromatic ointments were made by soaking aromatic plants in washed animal fat until the fat took on the fragrance of the plant. Fragrant plants have been an important part of the medicinal and cultural histories of China, India, the Far East, the Middle East, Central America and the native Americans of North America throughout history. Greek and Roman medicine also incorporated the use of aromatic herbs and both cultures practiced widespread use of perfume unguents based on plant fragrance. The gift of frankincense and myrrh to the newborn Jesus from the Wise Men indicates the value of these aromatic substances at that time.

In the year A.D.1000 an alchemist by the name of Avicenna greatly improved the art of distillation and his method was used in Europe until the invention of the condensing coil in the early fifteenth century.

Finally, around 1500 the art of distillation for essential oils commenced, and essential oils were widely used from that time forward throughout Europe for the production of perfumes.

In 1576, the Swiss alchemist Paracelsus wrote the *Great Surgery Book* in which he suggested that the main role of alchemy was to develop medicines, especially "*quinta essenta*" (the healing extracts from plants), claiming that essential oils were the most highly desirable part of a plant. Essential oils continued to be used in mainstream medicine throughout the sixteenth and seventeenth centuries, especially for treating the Bubonic plague. Many people believed that the wearing of plants and essential oils disinfected the air, giving them protection against the plague. However, in the late eighteenth century, as chemists began to isolate and

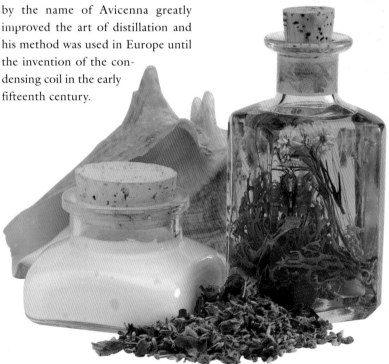

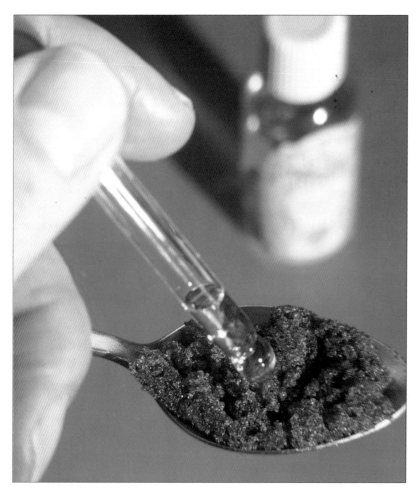

*Above: aromatherapy essences can be used to treat a wide range of medical conditions, both physical and psychological.*

somed. As with all forms of science, the more it is practiced, the more discoveries are made and questions raised. Recent developments in aromatherapy include numerous schools and courses of certification for aroma-therapists, research into the use of essential oils for various illnesses, and a number of aromatherapy organizations developing standards of education, certification, and practise for aromatherapists.

## THERAPEUTIC PROPERTIES

■ **Alcohols**, such as linalool, are strong bactericides, anti-infectious, antiviral, stimulating, warming, good general tonics, and circulatory decongestants. They are also gentle, non-irritating components.

■ **Phenols** have strong effects and are antiseptic and bactericidal. They are thought to stimulate the immune and nervous systems and can be skin irritants. Thymol, found in essential oil of Thyme, is an example.

■ **Aldehydes**, such as citral found in Lemon oil, can tend to be skin irritants and are used with discretion. They are anti-inflammatory, anti-infectious, tonic, hypotensive, and calming to the nervous system, and temperature reducing.

■ **Ketones** are quite harsh, can be neurotoxic, and are not found in the majority of essential oils. Those ones that do contain ketones are used occasionally in a highly diluted form for short periods of time for their calming and sedative properties and for their ability to break down fat and mucus, and to encourage the formation of scar tissue. They can also be digestive, analgesic, stimulant, and

synthesize the components of essential oils in the laboratory, the use of essential oils and herbs declined.

### ORIGINS OF MODERN AROMATHERAPY

During World War I, René Maurice Gattefossé experimented with the use of essential oils for the treatment of war wounds. In 1910 he had burned his hands in a laboratory explosion and after rolling in grass to extinguish

the flames, gas gangrenous sores began to appear. He applied essential oil of terpene-free Lavender to the burns and documented an abrupt arrest of the gasification of tissues and subsequent rapid healing of the wounds.

In the late 1950s, Marguerite Maury, the wife of a French doctor and homeopath, worked with essential oils for medicinal and cosmetic purposes, and aromatherapy was introduced to Britain through the practises of estheticians and massage therapists. Since that time, the use of essential oils in other healing methods and the practice of aromatherapy as a mode of healing have blos-

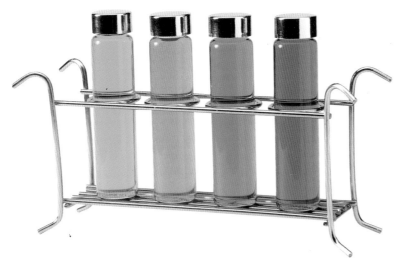

expectorant. Carvone, found in Caraway essential oil, is an example of a ketone.

### ORGANIC ACIDS

These are found in essential oils, usually in combination with esters, which are the product of a reaction between organic acids and alcohol. Esters, such as linalyl acetate, are known for their balancing, anti-inflammatory effects and, since they are found in gentle, essential oils, esters are often used for skin conditions. They are both calming and uplifting and are balancing to the nervous system.

### OTHER COMPONENTS

These include ethers which are anti-depressant, anti-spasmodic, and sedative; and oxides which can be mucolytic, yet are used with caution as they are skin irritants. Lactones such as coumarins, which are sedative, appear in essential oils which are obtained by other means rather than distillation.

**Note:** the chemical components of essential oils have a powerful healing capacity, whether inhaled directly into the limbic system, or therapeutically applied. Ideally, aromatherapists have a good understanding of the chemical composition of essential oils, and their healing or toxic effects.

## UNDERSTANDING ESSENTIAL OILS

Since essential oils are from plants and are not scientifically constructed according to a chemical recipe, an understanding of chemistry alone does not provide the aromatherapist with the depth of understanding necessary. The holistic aromatherapist must also have an awareness of the element of nature in essential oils. For example, two plants of the same species grown side-by-side in the same field, given the same amount of sunlight, water, and fertilizers, will not necessarily have the same percentages of the characteristic components.

Also, there are components within essential oils that exist in minute amounts but which may be as important to the healing properties of the oils as the main constituents. Likewise, essential oils are often labeled with the common name of the plant, rather than the scientific Latin binomial. All of these factors leave much room for misuse of essential oils unless the aromatherapist has a firm understanding of botany, and the organic nature of essential oils and hydrosols.

### ESSENTIAL OIL QUALITY

The percentages of chemical components found in an essential oil often depend on factors, such as the age of the plant, the time of year at which it

## SCIENCE AND ART

Aromatherapy is both a specific science and a deeply complex art. The practice of aromatherapy requires familiarity with the scientific fields of chemistry, botany, and physiology. Chemical components are the building blocks of essential oils and are the basis of their healing properties. Responsible use of the essential oils requires an understanding of Latin binomials used for naming botanicals as well as characteristics of plant growth and life cycle. Ideally, aromatherapists are ever conscious of the connection between a plant and its essential oil. Finally, an understanding of the human body and the interrelated functions of all its systems allow the aromatherapist to apply the potent organic chemistry of essential oils to encourage a balanced state of mental, physical, and emotional health.

was harvested, the soil and weather conditions, and the expertise of the distiller. While it may not be necessary for an aromatherapist to be familiar with these details for each essential oil in order to practice, it is vital that the grower, distiller, and marketer of essential oils is reliable and takes such factors into consideration.

Essential oil quality is based not only on the chemical components present in the oil, but also on its purity. In recent history, the most common use of essential oils has been in the flavor and fragrance industry in which oils from plants are used to flavor mass marketed food products and as perfume ingredients. Sometimes the chemical make-up of essential oils are changed and these standardi-

## HYDROSOLS

It is important that hydrosols are fresh, and must be the water collected from the condenser after the process of distillation. Other products, such as essential oils added to distilled water, are sometimes mistaken for hydrosols. The best hydrosols are from locally grown organic plants.

**Key points**

■ Hydrosols are perishable and

sensitive to heat and light. Store them in a cold, dark environment, such as the refrigerator.

■ The use of hydrosols from plants which are grown and distilled locally eliminates some of the concern of perishability.

■ Hydrosols for aromatherapy use should be from organically grown plants to eliminate the presence of harmful chemicals.

zed or adulterated oils are unsuitable for aromatherapy. Most aromatherapists agree that as aromatherapy is a practice that is based on the healing properties of nature, only pure, natural, unmanipulated essential oils are acceptable.

### LATIN NAMES

Perhaps the most valuable contribution of botany to the practicing aromatherapist is a knowledge of the system of naming plants using Latin binomials, as well as a familiarity with a number of botanical species, varieties, and chemotypes, ensuring the proper and safe use of essential oils. The essential oils of many plants look similar, and plants with many of the same components may even smell alike. Essential oils are often labeled with only a common name, such as Cedar.

This practice leads to much misunderstanding and misuse of essential oils. Cedar oil is from the leaf of *Thuja occidentalis* and is somewhat poisonous. Cedar oil from *Cedrus atlantica* is from the wood and is used by inhalation or application for the respiratory system. The properties of the oils depends greatly on which "Cedar" is used, and this is only apparent through use of the Latin binomial.

Similarly, essential oils from plants of the same genus may have components that vary according to species, variety, or chemical variety. For example, *Eucalyptus dives* has different percentages of chemical components, and therefore different uses from *Eucalyptus radiata*. Varieties of plants are plants of the same genus and species, but they may have some differing physiological characteristics.

## ESSENTIAL OILS AND THE HUMAN BODY

Aromatherapists must have an understanding of the human body and its interrelated systems. Essential oils and hydrosols are used through inhalation and application, with both forms of use affecting the person being treated in a number of ways.

Essential oils are volatile substances, which means that they evaporate easily, and their molecules are released into the air as a vapor. When this vapor of powerful chemical components is inhaled, the molecules are absorbed into the blood stream via the lungs and the nose. Upon inhalation, the vapor travels immediately to the lymbic system of the brain, which is responsible for the integration and expression of feelings, learning, memory, emotions, and physical drives.

### ABSORPTION OF ESSENTIAL OILS

Applied externally, essential oils are used to balance skin conditions, as well as to tend to the muscles and internal organs. They are most often applied diluted in a carrier substance, such as a vegetable oil, salve, or lotion. The essential oil is absorbed through the skin and carried to the muscle tissue, joints and organs. The essential oil molecules travel through the system to the kidneys, bladder, skin, and/or lungs for excretion. A familiarity with physiology provides the practitioner with the information necessary to choose essential oils and hydrosols specific to the condition presented.

*Right: a massage using aromatherapy oils can be relaxing and calming or stimulating and invigorating depending on the type of oil used.*

## THE AROMATHERAPIST AT WORK

A blend of essential oils in which the whole is greater than the sum of its parts is known as a synergy. Essential oils are not like prescriptions in which a particular pill is considered best for a specific malady. The skilled aromatherapist works with the client to select an individual oil or to develop a blend of oils that will suit their total profile. In this sense, the aromatherapist is an artist, as well as a scientist. The essential oils chosen work well together esthetically and are thought to address the condition presented while also confronting underlying causes.

When addressing muscle pain, for instance, an aromatherapist may create a blend of essential oils that is designed to relieve the tension of the muscle, but may also act upon the client mentally and emotionally to address the stress or mental pressure that may be the cause of the muscle tension.

## CARRIER OILS

These oils can be used singly or in conjunction with each other to dilute essential oils for making cosmetic preparations or aromatherapy massage oils. They include:
- Apricot kernel oil
- Avocado oil
- Grapeseed oil
- Jojoba
- Soya oil
- Sunflower oil
- Sweet almond oil
- Wheatgerm oil

The knowledge, awareness, and listening skills required to create synergies is quite complex. The creation of blends in which the balance of essential oils within the synergy is both therapeutic and esthetically pleasing is an art that is mastered only through study, continual practice and personal experience.

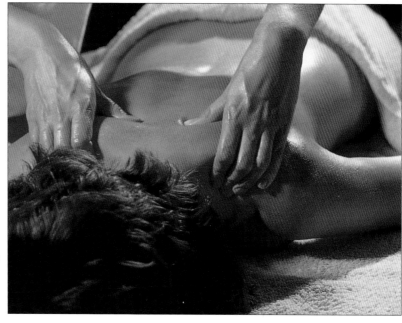

## A HOLISTIC PRACTICE

There are no legal standards of aromatherapy training, certification, or licensure in the United States as there are in Great Britain, although there are many schools and individuals offering aromatherapy training. American practitioners calling themselves aromatherapists are most often trained in some other form of therapy, e.g. they may be massage therapists, estheticians, or chiropractors, and have incorporated the use of essential oils into their practice. For this reason, diagnosis and treatment with a practitioner using essential oils will vary according to their primary licensing and with the extent of their aromatherapy training.

Aromatherapy combines well with other holistic practices, since it is based on botanicals and, when it is properly used by a trained professional, there should be no side effects. It has been combined successfully with the practice of psychotherapy, kinesiology, acupressure, various massage techniques, skin care, chiropractic, and other holistic approaches to health.

## SELF CARE WITH AROMATHERAPY

Not everyone who uses essential oils desires to become a practicing aromatherapist, incorporating the knowledge of chemistry, botany, physiology, and other training and practice into a professional healing art. It is possible to use essential oils and hydrosols for personal care to achieve maximum health. Essential oils can be used by application and inhalation for tending to colds and flu, stress, minor first-aid needs, women's care, emotional imbalances, muscle pain, beauty and body care and other needs. Essential oils are organic substances with antibiotic,

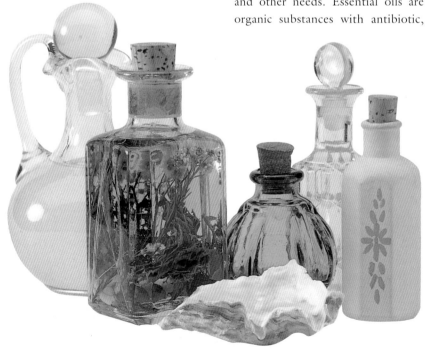

antibacterial and tonic properties which may help to prevent some illnesses that require more drastic medical approaches.

There are many uses for essential oils, and anyone wishing to use them for personal care would be wise to consult an authoritative reference book or the newsletters, quarterlies and journals produced independently and by aromatherapy organizations.

### USE OF ESSENTIAL OILS BY INHALATION

Inhalation of essential oils and hydrosols is thought to affect the mind, the emotions and the respiratory system. For personal use, essential oils can be inhaled from a handkerchief, or the aroma can be "diffused" throughout a room.

■ **Diffusors** are devices used to fill a room with essential oils to maximize the therapeutic benefits of inhalation. Some diffusors use heat as a means of evaporating the essential oils and spreading the tiny molecules throughout the room. Candle diffusors and ceramic rings placed on light bulbs are common forms of this type of diffusor.

■ **Other diffusors** are electric and consist of an electronically powered air pump and a glass vessel which holds the essential oil. Air is passed through a tube connected to the vessel holding the volatile oil which separates into tiny droplets small enough to be carried on currents of air and spread throughout a room.

■ **Hydrosols** are spritzed or sprayed into the air or on to the face and body and inhaled with a deep, relaxing breath.

## EMOTIONAL RESPONSES

When inhaled, micro-molecules of essential oils travel through the nasal passages to the limbic system of the brain which is the seat of memory and emotion. The inhalation of essential oils is thought to trigger memories and emotions within the limbic system, which in turn may stimulate a response within the entire system. For example, if the aroma of oranges is reminiscent of childhood summers, then inhalation of Orange essential oils may evoke feelings of carefree relaxation, refreshed playfulness, and pleasure. This emotional response, triggered by a mental association, can create a refreshed, rejuvenated response from the body. However, because of chemical composition, many essential oils produce a relaxed, stimulated, or soothed state, even if we have no memory associated with them.

## PHYSICAL EFFECTS

Another way in which chemical composition of essential oils affects the user by inhalation is physical. Eucalyptus essential oil, when inhaled through the mouth and nose, clears sinus passages and can aid in the treatment of chest colds and flus. Essential oils can be inhaled for many reasons: they are thought to reduce appetite for dietary considerations and weight loss; they may be used for respiratory ailments; they are thought to increase mental alertness and to help emotional conditions including depression, grief and anxiety; and they are used by some people as aphrodisiacs, or for

## USE OF HYDROSOLS

One drop of an essential oil can be more than is needed in a single treatment but the hydrosol can be used extensively, internally and externally, without any fear of overdosage. Hydrosols are a form of aromatherapy that can be used by children, babies, the sick or the infirm with no fear or worry of any skin irritation. Essential oils themselves are powerful forces for health but they are extremely concentrated and powerful. However, hydrosols are nearly free of irritating components and some are so gentle that they are used in the eyes as treatments for allergies or as antiseptics. These include hydrosols of Roman chamomile and myrtle (*Myrtus communis*).

Hydrosols are generally cooling and can be used as an anti-inflammatory compress for irritated or sensitive skin. There are some, such as Yarrow or Witch Hazel (called witch hazel extract), which are used as antiseptics. Others are considered mild toners, such as Lemon Verbena or Melissa water.

warming, soothing and other mental and emotional effects. Since inhaled essential oils travel throughout the body via the blood stream, their regular use can affect the harmony of the entire body.

## USE OF ESSENTIAL OILS BY APPLICATION

Essential oils are used by application in massage, bodycare products, aromatherapy perfumes, and in medicinal and first-aid preparations. Many practitioners believe that essential oils have the ability to permeate the skin and are then carried via the blood stream throughout the body to strengthen and heal internal systems. For this reason, essential oils are commonly used in baths, healing salves and lotions, compresses and massage oils. In such preparations, essential oils are used for their astringent, anti-bacterial, anti-biotic, or anti-inflammatory properties.

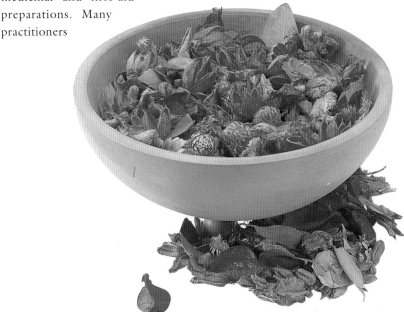

# USING ESSENTIAL OILS

## BATHING
Add 5-15 drops of essential oil to a tub of warm water. Swish the water with your hand to mix well. Soak yourself for 10-20 minutes.

## BODY LOTION OR OIL
Use $1/2$ to 1 teaspoon of essential oil per pint of unscented body lotion or botanical oil, such as sunflower, olive or vegetable oil.

## CANDLES
Light a candle and wait for the wax to begin melting. Add 1-2 drops of your chosen essential oil to the melting wax, being careful not to get inflammable oil on the burning wick.

## COTTON BALLS
Put 1-3 drops of essential oil on a cotton ball to diffuse the scent. Lavender oil on cotton promotes restful sleep.

## CULINARY
Use one drop of essential oil per four servings in salad dressings, sauces, desserts and beverages.

# ESSENTIAL OILS IN DAILY LIFE

Aromatherapy has myriad applications for health and wellbeing, and for adding to the sensual experiences of life. Whereas many healing modalities require some foul tasting, harsh smelling, or otherwise sensually unpleasant remedies, aromatherapy is a healing art that is a pleasure to incorporate into daily life, whether it is used to prevent ill health or to aid healing of an illness. Essential oils can be added to pot pourris, or spritzed around the home, car and office to spread pure, pleasurable aromas

They can also be added to cleaning agents to decrease harmful bacteria. Hydrosols are equally versatile and are used for bodycare, treating symptoms of menopause, stress relief, and in some culinary preparations.

## DIFFUSORS
These special products include the Lamp Ring Diffusor, Car Diffusor, Tabletop Diffusor, Glass Mister and Room Diffusor. Diffusors work with as little as 10 drops of oil, and at the highest setting 1 dram in 2 hours, or at the lowest setting 1 dram in 12 hours.

## DRAWER AND SHELF LINERS
Put several drops of an essential oil on some cotton and wipe down the liners with scent, or just add several drops directly to the liner. Avoid any contact with clothing or linen until the oil is dry, as some oils stain fabrics. Bay, Basil, Pine and Fir are good oils for kitchen cupboards.

## FACIAL WATERS
Add 6-8 drops of essential oil per fluid ounce of pure water. Lavender, Rose and Orange oils make wonderful facial waters.

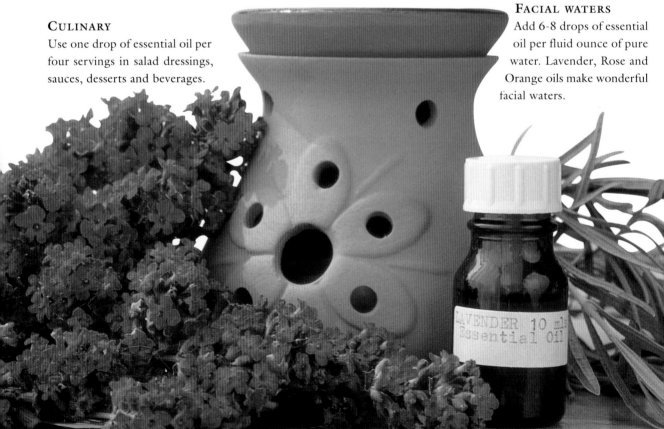

## THE ESSENTIAL OILS

**SCENTS AND THERAPEUTIC USES**

| ESSENTIAL OIL | SCENT | THERAPEUTIC USES |
|---|---|---|
| BENZOIN | Sweet, vanilla | Soothing, heals cracked skin, expectorant |
| BERGAMOT | Citrus, fresh | Calming, anti-depressant, healing, antiseptic, anti-viral |
| BLACK PEPPER | Spicy, peppery | Warming, stimulates blood flow |
| CEDARWOOD | Woody | Antiseptic, stimulating, toning |
| CHAMOMILE | Pungent | Calming, soothing, anti-inflammatory, antiseptic |
| CLARY SAGE | Herbaceous | Sedative, warming, anti-spasmodic, analgesic |
| CYPRESS | Sweet, spicy, balsamic | Anti-spasmodic, astringent |
| EUCALYPTUS | Woody, camphor | Anti-inflammatory, antiseptic, expectorant, anti-viral |
| FRANKINCENSE | Sweet, balsamic | Calming, anti-inflammatory, antiseptic, promotes skin healing |
| GERANIUM | Floral, sweet | Anti-bacterial, anti-depressant, anti-microbial, relaxing |
| GINGER | Spicy | Stimulating, warming |
| JASMINE | Floral, sweet | Cleansing, stimulating, anti-depressant |
| JUNIPER | Sweet, woody | Cleansing, calming, antiseptic, diuretic |
| LAVENDER | Floral, sweet | Calming, sedative, antiseptic, anti-spasmodic, analgesic |
| LEMON | Citrus, refreshing | Astringent, antiseptic, cleansing, refreshing |
| LEMON GRASS | Fresh, citrus | Antiseptic, sedative, digestive tonic |
| MANDARIN | Fruity, fresh | Refreshing, calming |
| MARJORAM | Sweet, camphor, herby | Calming, antiseptic, anti-spasmodic |
| MELISSA | Herby, citrus | Calming, refreshing, antiseptic, anti-viral, soothing |
| NEROLI | Floral, sweet | Sedative, calming |
| ORANGE | Citrus, fresh | Anti-spasmodic, uplifting, astringent |
| PATCHOULI | Woody, sweet | Anti-inflammatory, bactericidal |
| PEPPERMINT | Fresh, minty | Stimulating, decongestant, anti-spasmodic |
| PETITGRAIN | Citrus, floral | Calming, soothing |
| ROSE | Floral, intense | Anti-depressant, soothing, calming, antiseptic |
| ROSEMARY | Herby, fresh | Refreshing, invigorating, decongestant, anti-bacterial |
| SANDALWOOD | Woody, sweet | Calming, anti-inflammatory, soothing, antiseptic |
| SCOT'S PINE | Balsamic | Antiseptic, warming, stimulating |
| TEA TREE | Spicy, fresh | Anti-bacterial, anti-fungal, antiseptic |
| VETIVER | Woody, smoky | Calming, sedative, antiseptic |
| YLANG YLANG | Floral, exotic | Soothing, sedative |

## HERBAL SACHETS

Add several drops of an essential oil to moth-repelling dry herbs in muslin bags. Choose oil(s) compatible with the dry herbs used, particularly Cedar and Sage.

## HUMIDIFIERS

Add 6-8 drops of your chosen essential oil to water in a humidifier.

## HYDROSOLS

These are a product of distillation and can be added to any liquid or lotion in a ratio of 1 part hydrosol to 3 parts other. Use undiluted as a refreshing and healing spritz.

■ For hot flushes, or to cool the skin: use after cleansing the face as a toner, and after applying make-up to set it.

■ For diaper rash: use in the last rinse of hand-washables for a pleasant aroma.

## LAUNDRY RINSE

Add 2-3 drops of essential oil per quart of water. Use for hand-washables or add to the final machine rinse.

## LIGHT BULBS

Put several drops of Citronella oil on a cool outdoor light before illuminating to repel insects. Make sure that the essential oil does not drip

into the socket. Indoors, use a Lamp Ring Diffusor to release scents efficiently when the lights are turned on.

## MASSAGE

Use 5-15 drops of essential oil per ounce of base oil for aromatherapy massage.

## PERFUMERY

Most essential oils are too concentrated to apply to the skin undiluted. To make your own perfume: blend 1 dram of essential oil with 3 drams of ethyl alcohol or vodka. For a milder fragrance, make your eau de toilette with 15 drops of essential oil, 50 drops of ethyl alcohol or 60 percent vodka, and balance of formula 30-40 drops of distilled water. Age for two weeks before using. Shake well before each use.

## PET GROOMING

After bathing your pet, use 2 drops of Rosemary, Rose Geranium or Lavender in a pint of water as a conditioning rinse for pets. Between shampoos, soak the pet's brush in 2 drops of Lavender, Tea Tree or Cedarwood oil per pint of warm water. Shake out any excess and use

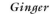

*Ginger*

to brush the coat with conditioning, flea-repelling scents.

## POT POURRI

Revive the faded bloom of your pot pourri with a few drops of essential oil. Stir to disperse the scents. Cover for two weeks before use.

## ROOM SPRAY

Use 4 drops per cup of warm (not hot) water. Use a new plant mister to diffuse into the air. Avoid contact with wooden furniture.

## SCENTED BOOKS AND PAPER

Use a few drops of repellent oils (Clove, Lavender, Rosemary) on absorbent papers to make scented bookmarks that also repel bugs. Scent stationery with a little oil to make your letters fragrantly memorable. Do not use on old, treasured books.

## WATER BOWLS

Use 1-9 drops of oil in a small bowl of warm water to scent a room. Put the water bowl on a radiator, allowing the heat to release the scents.

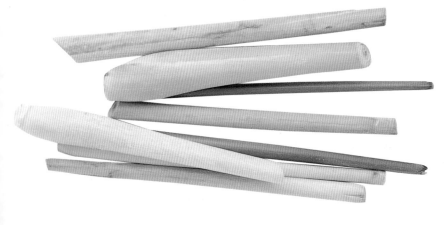

*Lemon-grass*

# THE ESSENTIAL OILS

| Common problems | Essential oils | Aromatherapy treatment |
| --- | --- | --- |
| ACNE | Bergamot, chamomile, geranium, lavender, lemon-grass | Facial massage or cold compress |
| BACKACHE | Chamomile, eucalyptus, lavender, melissa, rosemary | Aromatherapy massage |
| CATARRH & SINUSITIS | Eucalyptus, lavender, peppermint, rosemary | Gentle facial massage, inhalation |
| COLDS & COUGHS | Bergamot, cypress, eucalyptus, lavender, marjoram, peppermint, rosemary, sandalwood | Gentle neck massage, inhalation, adding oil to bathwater, air fresheners |
| CHEST INFECTIONS | Cypress, eucalyptus, lavender, marjoram, peppermint, sandalwood | Gentle chest massage, inhalation, adding oil to bathwater |
| CONSTIPATION | Black pepper, lemon-grass, marjoram, orange, rosemary | Gentle abdominal massage, adding oil to bathwater |
| DANDRUFF | Cypress, juniper, lavender, rosemary | Scalp massage and in shampoos |
| DEPRESSION | Clary sage, geranium, lavender, melissa, orange | Body and foot massage, adding oil to bathwater |
| ECZEMA | Cypress, geranium, lavender, sandalwood | Add oil to bath after patch test |
| HEADACHES | Chamomile, geranium, lavender, marjoram, peppermint, rose, rosemary | Massage shoulders, neck, scalp and face gently, cold compress |
| INSOMNIA | Lavender, marjoram, neroli | Gentle back massage, adding oil to bathwater or on pillow |
| MUSCULAR PAIN | Eucalyptus, juniper, lavender, marjoram, rosemary | Massage affected area, cold/warm compresses |
| NAUSEA | Lavender, orange, peppermint | Inhalation: 2-3 drops of oil in a handkerchief |
| SPRAINS AND STRAINS | Chamomile, cypress, juniper, lavender, rosemary | Gentle massage, cold compress |
| STRESS | Bergamot, geranium, jasmine, lavender, lemon-grass, neroli, orange | Body, neck, shoulders and facial massage, adding oil to bathwater |
| VARICOSE VEINS | Cypress, geranium | Gentle massage around veins, cold compress |

## GLOSSARY OF TERMS

■ **Aromatherapy:** healing with essential oils and hydrosols (from plants) through the sense of smell by inhalation and through application of these therapeutic volatile substances.

■ **Essential oil:** volatile materials contained within plant cells and derived by physical process (such as distillation) from the plant. Some essential oils are not in the living tissue but are found during destruction of the living tissue.

■ **Hydrosol:** the water from the distillation process which contains water-soluble parts of the plant material and micro-molecules of essential oil.

■ **Distillation:** process of vaporizing a substance by heat, condensing it by cold in a special vessel, and then re-collecting the liquid.

## AROMATHERAPY MASSAGE

Visiting an aromatherapist for a full body massage is a pampering, relaxing and calming experience. It can also be very therapeutic and can help to ease out sore muscles and a tired back. Depending on the aromatic oils used, a massage can be invigorating and energizing, dispelling tension and restoring wellbeing.

The patient should feel comfortable, warm and at ease throughout the massage. It is customary to undress but this need not be embarrassing as the patient is covered with plenty of towels and only the area of the body that is being worked on at any particular time is exposed.

The essential oil is mixed with a carrier oil; only a few drops of the former are used. The practitioner starts by pouring a little oil into the palm of one hand and warming it between the hands, before applying it to the patient's body.

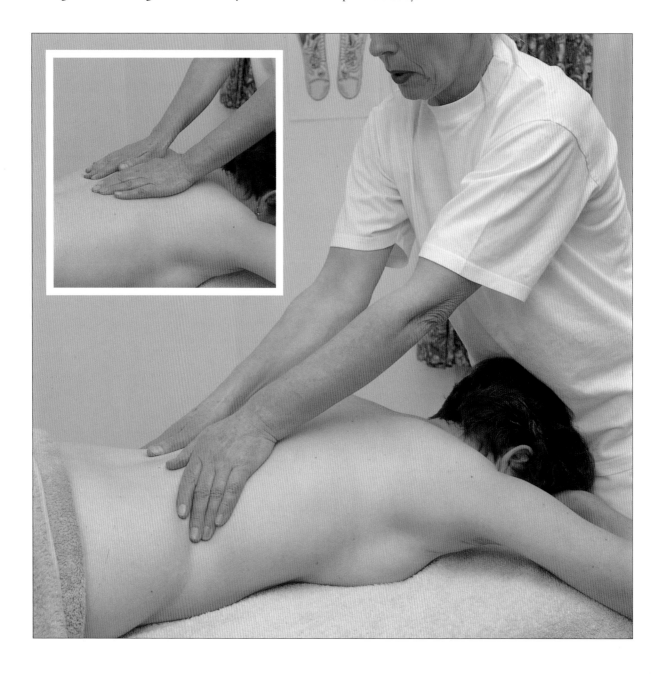

# AROMATHERAPY MASSAGE

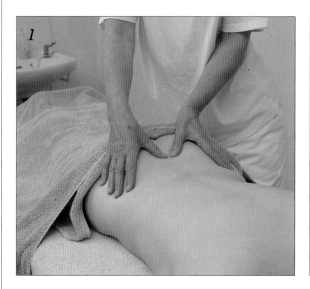

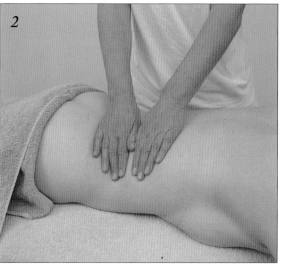

1 The aromatherapist slides her thumbs down either side of the patient's spine, working rhythmically and smoothly to gently stretch and relax the patient's back.

2 With the fingers on either side of the spine, the aromatherapist slides her hands over the side of the patient's body, stimulating the nerves and helping lymph drainage.

3 She then moves on to the neck area, working more deeply to ease out tense muscles and relax the whole area. The stroking movements are firm in order to dispel any tension in this area.

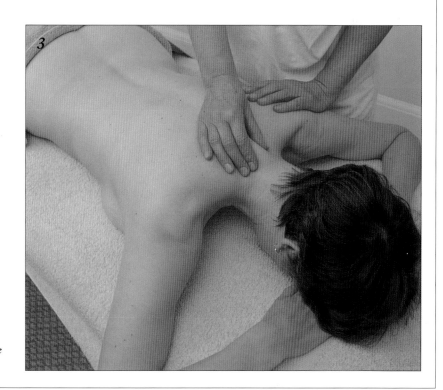

Opposite: the massage starts by stroking up and down the body to relax the patient.

# AROMATHERAPY MASSAGE

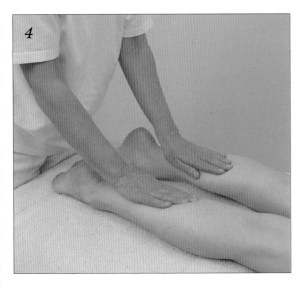

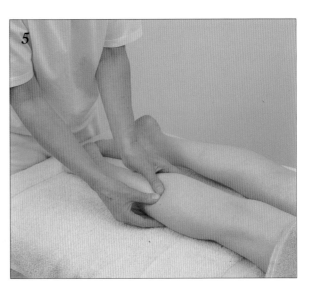

4 The legs are worked on next. The aromatherapist slides her hands up the calf muscles and behind the knees, stroking firmly and spreading the oil to stimulate the lymph system. The hands then glide back down again.

5 The thumbs then work more deeply on the sides of the lower legs, rhythmically massaging them in firm movements. Again, this helps to release tension and tightness in the muscles and relax the whole area.

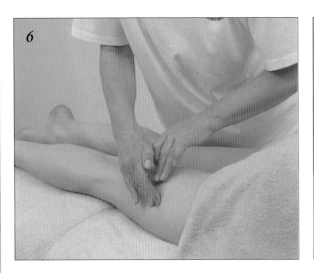

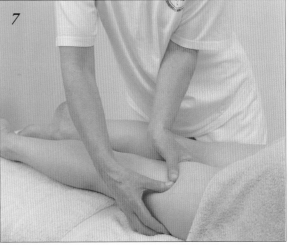

6 The aromatherapist moves her hands further up the legs to the backs of the thighs, her hands circling behind each other. This circular stroking technique is very smooth and helps create a steady rhythm.

7 She then works deeper on the thighs, using her thumbs to apply more penetrating pressure and working on any taut muscles to relax and unknot them. This firm thumb technique applies circular pressure.

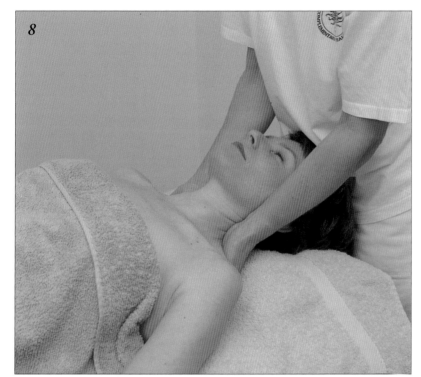

**8**

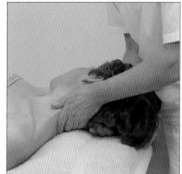

8 At this point in the massage session, the patient is asked to turn over on to her back and the aromatherapist works on the base of her neck, using firm but penetrating circles on the back of the neck and side of the spine.

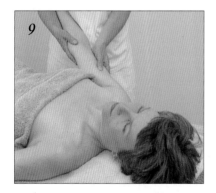

**9**

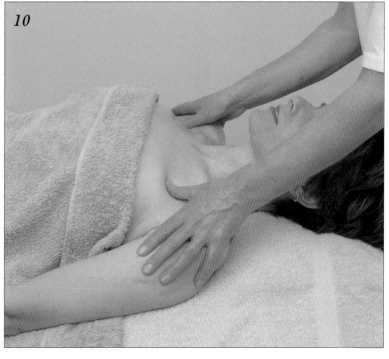

**10**

9 The upper arms are stroked and massaged gently in relaxing, draining movements.

10 The hands move up the arms to the shoulders, then across the shoulders and upper chest where the lymph returns into the veins.

# AROMATHERAPY MASSAGE

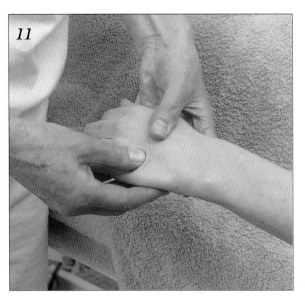

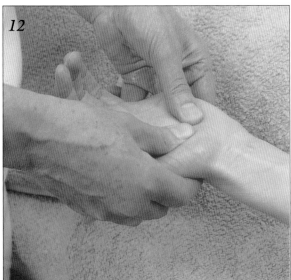

*11 and 12 The patient's hands are stroked on both sides. The palms are stretched out and massaged gently, then the hands are turned over and the wrists and backs of the hands are stroked.*

*13 To help with sinus drainage and the release of tension, the aromatherapist presses firmly with her fingers on either side of the base of the nose.*

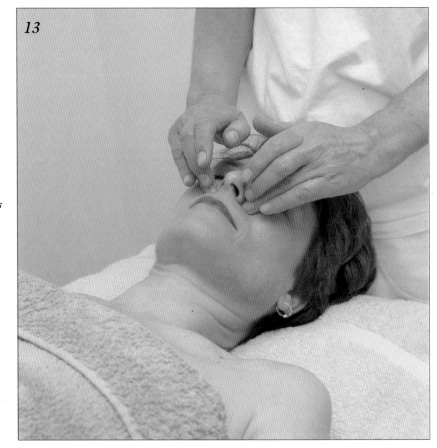

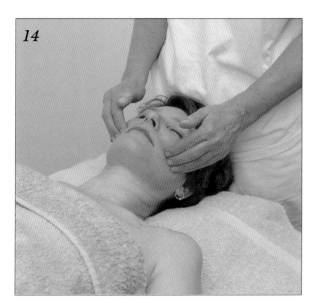

14 All the fingers are used to slide down the sides of the face. Only gentle pressure is used. When massaging the face, patients who wear contact lenses should remove them.

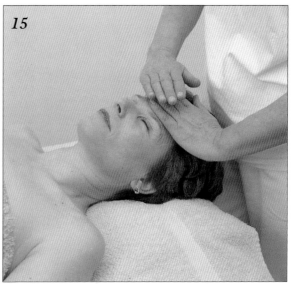

15 The fingers and palms stroke the forehead rhythmically, with the whole palm moving backwards and forwards across the forehead without any release. This form of massage can be helpful in relieving headaches.

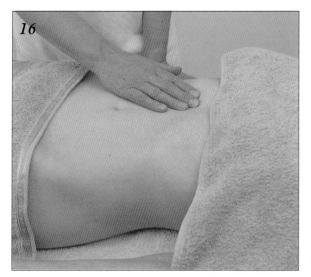

16 The abdomen is stroked in clockwise circular movements with one hand always staying in touch. This is a rhythmic circular stroke with one hand following the other and the arms crossing each other.

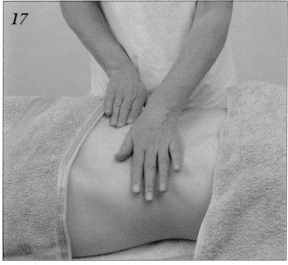

17 The solar plexus is stroked gently in an anti-clockwise direction. This is an emotional area where many people hold tension—the hands slide down over the side of the body to drain it.

# REFLEXOLOGY

## CHAPTER TWENTY FOUR

*R*eflexology is the treatment modality that deals with the principle that there are reflex areas in the feet and hands which correspond to all of the glands, organs and parts of the body. Reflexology employs a unique method of using the thumb and fingers to apply specific pressures to these reflex points to achieve numerous therapeutic benefits.

The reflexologist works each reflex, thereby triggering a release of stress and tension in the corresponding area or body zone, as well as an overall relaxation response. The release of tension unblocks nerve impulses and improves the blood supply to all parts of the body. Because reflexology works from the inside, it also has a balancing effect on each gland, organ and body region. Clients typically express relief from tension and pain, greater feelings of wellbeing and increased energy.

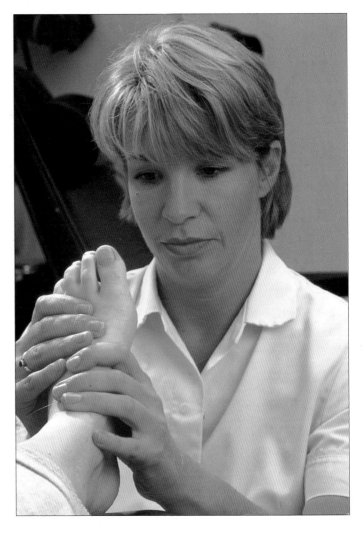

The reason for this is still being debated, but it may be shown eventually that foot reflexology removes blockages in the body's energy flow. It may also help to normalize blood and lymphatic flow to various regions of the body, promoting oxygenation of tissues and removal of waste. There are 7,200 nerve endings in each foot and this may help explain why we feel so much better when our feet are treated. Nerve endings in the feet have extensive interconnections through the spinal cord and brain with all areas of the body, making the feet the ideal site from which to release tension and enhance our health.

## ORIGINS OF REFLEXOLOGY

Popular belief holds that some form of reflexology has been practiced by many cultures through the ages. Reflexology is thought to have roots in the ancient art of Oriental Pressure Therapy or acupuncture, which are based on the theory that energy pathways exist throughout the body, and that blockages of those pathways lead to energy loss, discomfort or illness.

The earliest documentation of reflexology practiced by an ancient culture was found at Saqqara, in a wall painting in the tomb of an Egyptian physician (Ankhmahor, the highest official after the pharoah), dating back to the early sixth dynasty (approximately 2330B.C.). The

prominence of the inscriptions and drawings in what is known as the Physician's Tomb indicates that reflexology was a major therapeutic tool of the ancient Egyptians.

Zone therapy, considered the precursor to reflexology as we know it today, was practiced as early as the fourteenth century. Neurological studies conducted by Sir Henry Head of London in the late 1800s provide a scientific basis for reflexology. He is credited with identifying the hypersensitivity of zones on the skin connected neurologically to diseased organs. These were termed "Head's Zones" or "zones of hyperalgesia."

The work of Russian scientists and psychologists in the nineteenth century, including Ivan Pavlov's theory of conditioned reflexes, provided

the groundwork for the later studies of reflexology from both the physiological and psychological perspectives. Today, in Russia, reflex therapy is used to complement traditional medicine in treating a variety of problems.

At the beginning of this century, a German version of reflexology called "reflex massage" was being used in the treatment of disease. In 1912, Dr. Alfons Cornelius published the manuscript *Druckpunkte* (or "Pressure Points, The Origin and Significance"), describing the therapeutic benefits of pressure-point massage to "reflex zones."

*Below: it is not uncommon to practice reflexology outside in the streets of Bangkok in Thailand.*

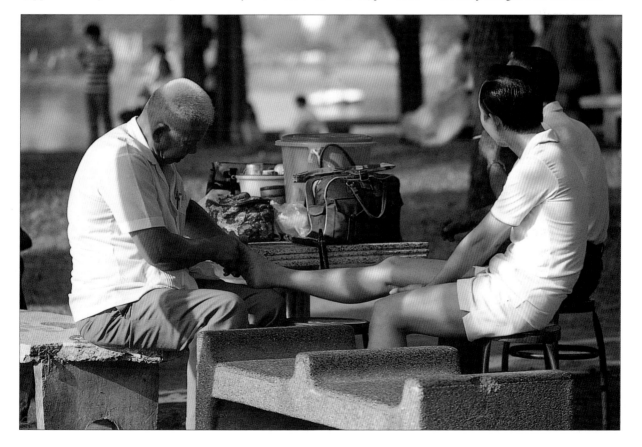

## MODERN REFLEXOLOGY

This traces its origins most directly to the work of the Connecticut-born physician, William Fitzgerald. After graduating from the University of Vermont School of Medicine in 1895, he practiced in Vienna and London where his study of pressure point therapy led to the development of his theory of zone therapy. On returning to the U.S., he continued his research into zone therapy while head of the Ear, Nose and Throat Clinic at St. Francis Hospital in Hartford, Connecticut.

He found that pressure applied to the fingers acted as an analgesic to various parts of the face, ear, nose, shoulder, arm and hand. Using only this pressure technique with elastic bands or small clamps, he was able to perform minor surgical operations. Dr. Fitzgerald divided the body into 10 longitudinal zones, running the length of the body from head to toe. He proposed that the parts of the body within each zone were linked by an energy flow, and so could affect one another.

In 1917, Dr. Fitzgerald and his colleague Dr. Edwin Bowers published *Zone Therapy, or Relieving*

*Pain At Home*, in which they described their success at relieving pain using various devices on the hands and fingers. However, with the advent of modern anesthesia, interest in zone therapy waned. Although it made no great impact on the medical world, and did not particularly emphasize the reflex zones of the feet, it did lay the groundwork for the work that followed.

Dr. Fitzgerald was later hailed as "the discoverer of zone therapy" in an article titled *Mystery of Zone Therapy Explained*, describing a dinner party attended by him and a well-known concert singer. The upper registers of

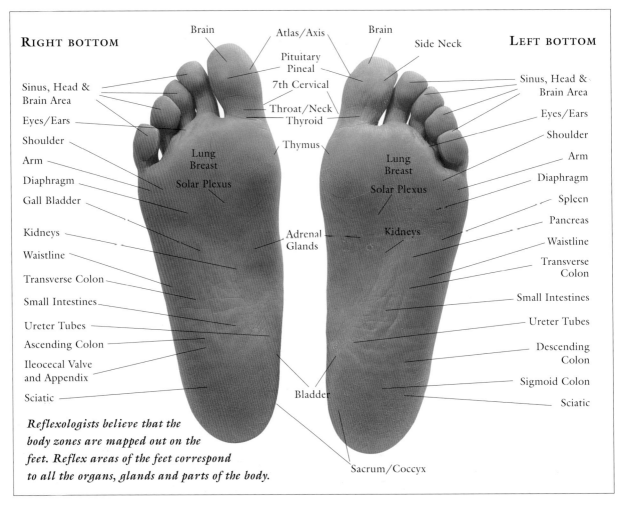

*Reflexologists believe that the body zones are mapped out on the feet. Reflex areas of the feet correspond to all the organs, glands and parts of the body.*

her voice had gone flat, and treatment by throat specialists had been unsuccessful. Dr. Fitzgerald examined her fingers and toes and, on discovering a callous on her right great toe, applied pressure to the corresponding part in the same zone. Not only did the pain in the toe disappear but also the singer was able to surpass her previous vocal capacity.

Dr. Joseph Shelby Riley used Zone Therapy in his practice for many years, refining Fitzgerald's techniques and also adding his own discoveries, including the first detailed diagrams and drawings of the reflex points located in the feet.

## THE ORIGINAL INGHAM METHOD

Reflexology in its current form was developed by the late Eunice Ingham [1889-1974], a physiotherapist in Dr. Riley's office, who separated foot reflexology from zone therapy in general, and made the greatest contribution to the development of modern reflexology.

She theorized that the highly sensitive feet would be even more responsive gateways to various parts of the body than the hands, the primary focus of Dr. Riley's work. Encouraged by him, she began developing her theory of foot reflexology in the early 1930s. Correlating sensitive spots on the feet with various body parts, she charted the feet anatomically and found that by probing with her fingers and thumbs she achieved the best results in terms of identifying tender areas on the feet

*Right: reflexology should be a relaxed and enjoyable experience for both the patient and therapist.*

and achieving a therapeutic effect.

Eunice Ingham traveled around the United States, practicing and teaching her Original Ingham Method of reflexology to thousands of people, both in and out of the medical profession. She is considered the pioneer and developer of reflexology as it is known in the world today.

Her nephew, Dwight Byers, continued her work. As a child, he had been a "guinea pig" for his aunt's research when she worked on his feet to relieve his hay fever and asthma. He founded the International Institute of Reflexology (IIR), which conducts seminars around the world, and now has regional directors in 13 countries, including four in Great Britain. The Original Ingham Method is universally acknowledged as one of the foremost systems of

reflexology, producing the most highly trained practitioners and instructors.

## REFLEXOLOGY TODAY

Reflexology has been widely practiced in England since the mid-1960s and throughout Europe since 1970, but only in recent years has it achieved wide acceptance in the United States. It has grown steadily, as those helped by it learned reflexology to help their family and friends. During the past 10 years, reflexology has evolved from a quietly practiced healing modality to one of the fastest growing forms of alternative therapy, and it is now widely practiced around the world. Its use is common in many European hospitals, and it is the most popular form of alternative treatment in Denmark.

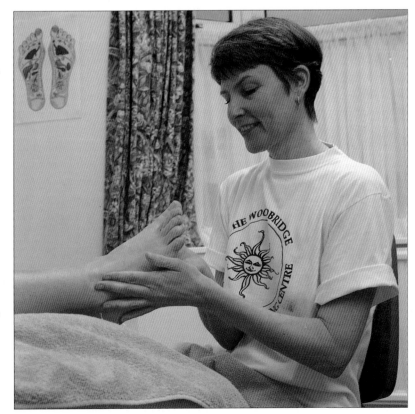

# HOW REFLEXOLOGY WORKS

The original concept of heavy-finger pressure breaking up the "grains of sand" at the tender spots under the skin has given way to much lighter treatments. The discomfort and bruising which were occasionally a feature of the original techniques was found to be counter productive and stress creating as well as causing excessive strain on the practitioner's fingers. The hands provide a similar pattern to the feet and can be used to treat the various organs. This is most helpful for self-treatment.

During the 1980s in England, a number of reflexologists found that treatment using feather-light pressure was successful. This method also allowed practitioners to induce relaxation more easily and to observe the patient's response to the various areas' of sensitivity. This approach has been widely used by the British teachers Christine Jones and Pat Morrell, who has also developed methods of diagnosis using the appearance of the areas of distress whilst not actually touching the flesh.

Whilst reflexologists who are not medical doctors may not comment on specific named diseases unless qualified, they are expected to be able to express their own specialist interpretation of the sensitivity as charted in the feet or hands. Thus reflexology diagnosis will often point to potential areas of illness which require referral to other specialists.

Reflexology can be given successfully by anyone who has completed a course and has been assessed by an external examiner. However, the levels of competence may vary from therapists who treat simple relaxation and stress control within a beauty salon to practitioners who are able to treat illness. These variations of skills are often associated with particular insurance cover which may limit their use. Practitioners may also find that when they offer healing, the patient may remark on additional sensations of peace and calm. The act of healing should be understood by practitioners since it can have a substantial added value.

**Conditions that benefit from reflexology**
Recent trials in the UK suggest that when reflexology is given to post-operative patients, the healing process is accelerated. Morrell reflexology has been used on patients receiving hip and knee replacement surgery and the results have been so interesting that further research is planned.

## A HEALTHY MODALITY

Reflexology is a holistic healing modality which attempts to address the entire body, as well as individual conditions, through the application of pressure to specific reflex points on the feet and hands. By systematically working various reflexes, using an inchworm-like motion of the thumb and fingers, the reflexologist claims to relieve stress and tension. With medical reports indicating that at least 75 percent of all medical ills are stress-related, reflexology can have a major impact on health and wellbeing. Reflexology helps to relax the effects of stress and tension on the body's musculature, nervous system and blood supply, laying the foundation for all other healing to take place. People are often surprised to feel energized as well as relaxed following a treatment.

By looking for tenderness in the feet or hands, or areas which feel like tiny peas or grains of sand under the skin, the reflexologist is able to identify congested zones of the body and attempts to improve the blood supply and promote the unblocking of nerve impulses to those areas, enhancing the body's ability to heal itself. Because every gland, organ and part of the body is represented by reflexes in the feet and hands, reflexologists believe that these same indicators help to identify areas that are out of balance and working at less than optimum levels. Reflexology seems to help restore the body's dynamic state of homeostasis or balance.

While reflexologists do not diagnose, prescribe or treat for specific problems, these clues give them a clearer picture of what's going on. A highly trained reflexologist may also be able to identify problem areas just by looking at the foot for discolorations, calluses or swollen areas.

## UNDERSTANDING REFLEXOLOGY

A good way to understand reflexology is to visualize the human body superimposed on the feet (see page 224). Reflexologists see the foot as a mini-map of the body to guide them in their work, and so begin treatment by working the entire foot before focusing on specific areas. Note the correlation between reflexes, zones, and body parts on the charts. Each foot represents one half of the body, and the five zones on that side of the body.

■ The toes represent the head, neck and sinuses.

■ Each toe represents a zone, but the big toes each encompass all five zones. The reflex for the pituitary, or master gland, is found in the center of the big toe, and the base of the big toe represents the neck.

■ The other toes represent the sinuses and specific areas of the head.

■ The ball of the foot represents the thoracic area, which encompasses the lungs, heart, chest, upper back, and shoulders, etc.

■ The area just below the metatarsal or ball of each foot represents the diaphragm or solar plexus, the highly important area which has neural connections to many body parts.

■ The arch represents the abdominal area, including the liver and gall bladder on the right foot, the stomach and spleen on the left foot, and the kidneys, adrenal glands, and pancreas on both feet.

■ The heel represents the pelvic area, including the intestines, colon and sciatic nerve.

■ The top of the ankle represents the lymphatic system.

■ The points between the ankle bone and heel on each side of the foot represent the reproductive areas.

■ The length of the inside edge of the foot represents the 26 vertebrae which comprise the spine, as well as the 31 pairs of nerves connected to the vertebrae, leading to every body area.

■ The outer sides of the foot represent the knee, hip and lower back regions.

Drawing on the principles of zone therapy, the reflexologist believes that an organ or gland or muscle group found in a specific zone will have its reflex in the corresponding zone of the foot, and that an abnormality in any part of the zone may affect anything within that zone.

A well-trained reflexologist will believe that one cannot address the complex condition of diabetes, for instance, by pressing the button that says "pancreas." Such a reflexologist understands the functionality and anatomical interrelationships of each physiological system in order to provide maximum benefit, and so is doing much more than pressing spots on the foot.

## PRACTICAL APPLICATIONS

Although reflexology is not a substitute for seeing a medical doctor, it can be of benefit to virtually every physiological system: the skeletal, nervous, muscular, cardiovascular, circulatory, lymphatic, respiratory, digestive, urinary, endocrine and reproductive systems, as well as the sense organs. It is often the preferred modality to reduce pain, especially with regard to chronic pain or terminal illness.

Some traditional research into reflexology has already confirmed its healing powers. For example, in 1993, Beijing Medical University

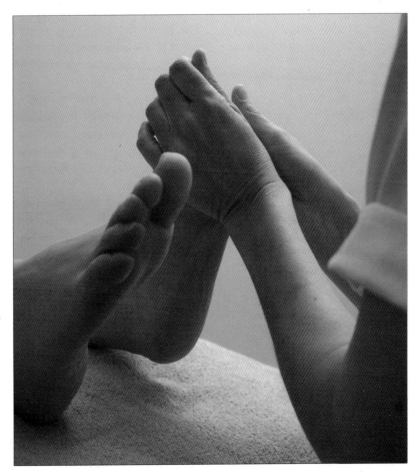

reported on a study conducted on 32 diabetics showing that foot reflexology is an effective treatment for Type II diabetes mellitus. There are over 10,000 case histories documented by doctors in China to verify the efficacy of reflexology in treating ailments ranging from colds and flu to heart problems.

In 1992, in Denmark, a study was carried out with postal employees requiring them to have reflexology treatments at least twice a month. At the end of the year, absenteeism was reduced by 13.3 percent.

Although few formal American studies have been conducted on the effects of reflexology, one study conducted at the Burbank-based American Academy of Reflexology reported by the *American Obstetrics and Gynecology Journal* showed a nearly 50 percent reduction in premenstrual syndrome (PMS) symptoms in a group of women who received reflexology treatments.

Case histories abound describing the numerous benefits of reflexology. A skilled reflexologist can even provide first aid in certain situations. Working the pituitary reflex in the middle of the big toe could help to resuscitate a fainting victim. Working the sigmoid flexure on the heel of the left foot could benefit a heart-attack victim whose attack was triggered by excessive gas buildup from the colon. Surgery patients may report reduced postoperative healing times when receiving reflexology treatments before and after surgery.

While a systems approach to reflexology yields the best overall results, a reflexologist will focus primarily on the specific areas required to achieve desired results.

■ Working the toes and the base of the toes where they join the feet may help alleviate headaches, stress, sinus congestion, eye strain, a stiff neck and pain from the temporomandibular joint (T.M.J.).

■ Stimulation of the wide band across the ball of each foot may produce relief from asthma, shortness of breath and some allergies.

■ Reflexing the entire inside edge of the foot, from the middle of each big toe to the base of the heel may help alleviate back pain and spinal problems, as well as related neurological problems.

■ Stimulating the diaphragm reflexes along with the kidney reflexes on both feet may improve circulation and normalize blood pressure.

■ Reflexing the zone on the inside edge near the top of the heel of each foot may help alleviate urinary infections and incontinence.

Professional reflexologists achieve the highest levels of success when working an entire physiological system and its associated systems. For example, on finding sensitivity in the digestive reflexes, a reflexologist might inquire about constipation. On confirming that suspicion and working the digestive system along with associated systems, the client is likely to find relief from constipation. Reflexes worked would include the intestines, the colon, especially the sigmoid flexure at the base of the colon, the lower spine (which is responsible for the nerve supply to the intestines), as well as in the diaphragm, pancreas, gall bladder and liver (which aid digestion), adrenals (for soft muscle tone), and the iliocecal valve (which regulates mucous).

### REFLEX AND REFERRAL AREAS

The body's reflex areas are not limited to the feet and hands; they are simply the easiest to access. The foot's resemblance to body structure and sensitivity to touch makes it an ideal site from which to perform reflexology. But, in fact, direct pressure applied to any point along the zone will affect the entire zone.

## VISITING A THERAPIST

It is wise to ask about the methods of reflexology being used and the methods of course examination and course accreditation used. Patients should confirm that the practitioners are insured and work within an accepted Code of Practice, etc.

The initial session should last

## REFLEXOLOGY AND YOUR LIFESTYLE

Reflexology is perhaps the simplest of all healing modalities to fit into your lifestyle. It is a do-anywhere, anytime, no paraphernalia kind of therapy. Because reflexology is widely practiced around the world, scheduling treatments is not usually difficult. Increasingly, working people will schedule a lunchtime massage or reflexology treatment, sometimes even in their own offices. And it is relatively easy to learn a few basic reflexology techniques with which to help oneself or one's family

from 45 to 60 minutes. Subsequent sessions typically last from 30 to 45 minutes. If the hands are included, add an additional 15 to 20 minutes. Weekly sessions are helpful to maintain health; two to three weekly sessions usually are needed to remediate a problem. Costs vary from area to area.

The reflexologist starts by asking about client concerns or problems. The session usually begins with a few relaxation movements. The majority of the session involves the inchworm-like "walking" of thumbs and fingers over every area of the foot. Movements should be smooth and deeper than massage. Particular attention is given to problem areas. It is important for the client to communicate about any tender areas covered, and the reflexologist should be sensitive to client expressions of discomfort. Sensitivity will decrease as the congestion in the area diminishes. If there is considerable pain or serious illness, sessions should be briefer, lighter, and more frequent.

## SELF-HELP TECHNIQUES

With a basic understanding of the principles of reflexology, you can help yourself with treatment in the home. It is always wise to consult a professional practitioner who will give you a full diagnosis and suggest treatment patterns before attempting to help yourself. Since each patient is different, you will need to be assured that you are giving your body the support that it needs. You will also need to know that your problem has been correctly assessed and this can best be confirmed by a professional.

Study the chart on page 224 and then work on areas you know need help. You can learn to be sensitive to tender areas that appear on your hands and feet and work them out regularly. The use of foot rollers, or even the edge of a coffee table, can help you to spot areas that need work. Going barefoot on the beach— or even in the forest—is a pleasurable way to stimulate the reflex zones of the feet.

Reflexology involves highly effective relaxation techniques, which are difficult to perform on yourself but are simple to perform on others, and very specific movements of the thumbs and fingers, which can be used on yourself or others. The following sampler of techniques will get you started.

## BASIC REFLEXOLOGY TECHNIQUES

**The basic thumb technique**
This can best be demonstrated by placing your hand palm down on a table. You will notice the natural position of your hand on the table and particularly the angle of the thumb where it meets the table. This is the working area of the thumb. The inside (medial) edge of the thumb makes contact with the table. The secret of using the thumb technique successfully is to walk it over the reflex zone by slightly bending and unbending the first joint of the thumb and creeping forward with a steady, even pressure. It is important to leverage this movement with the slight, even pressure of the other four fingers in opposition to the thumb on the other side of the foot.

**The finger technique**
This is basically the same as the thumb technique in that you use the inside edge of the finger just as you use the inside edge of the thumb, in conjunction with the bending of the first joint of that finger.

**The thumb, hook-in, back-up technique**
This is used when pinpoint accuracy is needed in a reflex zone.

Again, the technique is to bend the first joint of the thumb and exert pressure with the inside corner of the thumb. Once you have placed the thumb on a reflex point on the foot, you push in and pull back across the point with the thumb, without sliding, but keeping it in contact and only moving the underlying tissue.

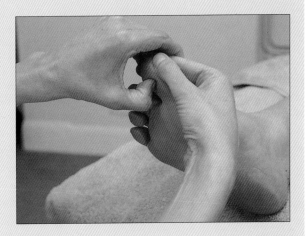

# REFLEXOLOGY RELAXING TECHNIQUES

### THE BACK AND FORTH TECHNIQUE

This is accomplished by placing the palms of your hands, one on the inside and one on the outside edge of the metatarsal padding, and then moving your hands rapidly back and forth, with fingers relaxed.

### THE ANKLE LOOSENING TECHNIQUE

This is done by placing the heel of your hands in the back of the ankle bones on either side of the foot, resting the palms gently on the ankle bones, and moving your hands rapidly forward and back. The foot will shake from side to side.

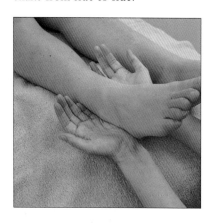

### THE SPINAL TWIST

This is done by placing both hands firmly around the foot, fingers on the inside top of the foot, index fingers touching, the webbing of the thumbs on the spinal reflex area, and thumbs on the bottom of the foot. Keep the hand closest to the heel stationary while the other hand rotates slowly and smoothly back and forth. After several rotations, move the two hands together gradually up toward the toes and continue the rotation, keeping

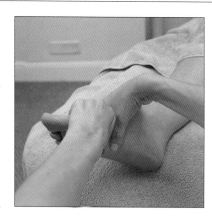

the hand toward the heel stationary at all times. Inch upward until the hand toward the toes is over the big toe. Twist the foot evenly in both directions.

### THE DIAPHRAGM-TENSION RELAXER TECHNIQUE

This works the whole diaphragm reflex area, starting at the inside edge of the foot below the metatarsals. Place your working thumb on the reflex at a slight angle up under the metatarsals. With the holding hand, grasp the toes, lift slightly, and pull the foot toward you. This pulls the foot onto the thumb. Your thumb should then take one small step toward the outside and repeat the process. Continue until you reach the outside edge.

### THE DIAPHRAGM-DEEP BREATHING TECHNIQUE

This is done by placing the ball of your thumbs in the center of the diaphragm/solar plexus reflex on both feet at the same time, allowing the fingers to comfortably lay on the top of the foot. Then ask your subject to take a deep breath and hold it each time you press on this reflex.

### INTERACTION BETWEEN REFLEXOLOGY AND MASSAGE THERAPY

Massage therapy and reflexology are being combined across the United States and Europe with dramatic results. Therapists trained in both modalities are in agreement over their synergistic power.

■ Massage is the systematic manipulation of the soft tissues of the body.

■ Reflexology is the application of specific pressures to reflex points in the feet and hands.

■ Massage treatments benefit the muscles or connective tissue which are the direct recipients of the manipulation.

■ Reflexology benefits the contact treatment sites (feet or hands) only incidentally.

The primary benefits of reflexology are thought to result from the generalized relaxation of the entire body, as well as from the balancing effect on specific organs, glands, zones or body regions.

Reflexology, when it precedes massage therapy, seems to bring about a state of internal and external relaxation which enables the therapist doing deep muscle massage to achieve far greater results with less effort than if the client had begun the massage with a tense body.

With reflexology, clients can feel the benefits of the treatment quickly, with particularly dramatic results when treating such conditions as stress, tension, neck and shoulder pain, lower back, leg and knee pain, menstrual discomfort, or bowel irregularity.

## SELECTING A PROGRAM

In selecting a program, seek the recommendation of reflexologists and therapists who have been practicing successfully; research the background of the program and instructors you are considering, and find out how long they've been practicing and teaching. Evaluate the training program, the certification process, and instructor qualifications. How credible and accurate are the training materials, books, and charts? Does the program teach students how to work physiological systems or merely how to "push buttons" for related parts of the body? How stringent are the standards of certification? What are the criteria? Does it involve both written and practical tests? How are instructors trained and qualified?

The length of the program is another major indicator of credibility. Reflexologists agree that the magnitude of knowledge and experience required for competence calls for a program that incorporates approximately 200 hours of combined classroom, practical experience and home study. A minimum of one year of experience is essential for basic certification

## REFLEXOLOGY SESSION

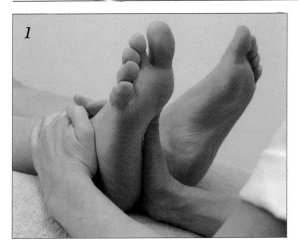

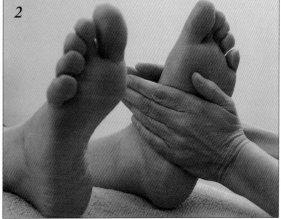

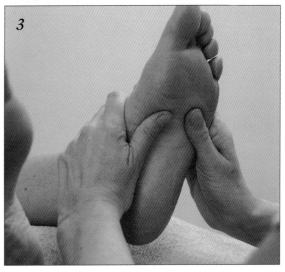

*1 Most reflexology sessions start with the practitioner warming up the feet with some soothing movements over the top of the feet and the soles to help the patient to relax.*

*2 Often the reflexologist will then move on to the "prayer" movement in which the hands are placed around the foot as if clasped in prayer and then moved up and down and around the foot.*

*3 The hands move in a circular movement with the fingers circling, gently pressing in with the thumbs.*

# REFLEXOLOGY SESSION

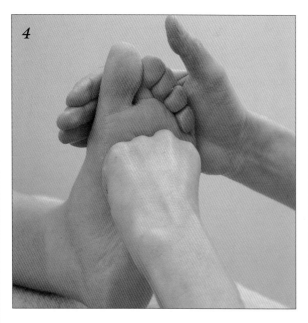

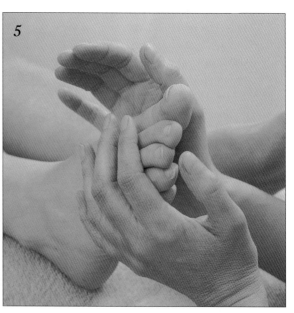

4 *The reflexologist uses her fist to climb up the foot from the heel to the toes, pressing in with the knuckles and then sliding back down the foot.*

5 *The reflexologist continues to use her hands to open the chest and lung area, releasing tension and relaxing the foot with gentle stroking movements.*

6 *Using the thumb and hook technique, the practitioner works the pituitary reflex area to stimulate the pituitary gland and the endocrine system which is connected with the control of hormone levels. This is quite a deep movement.*

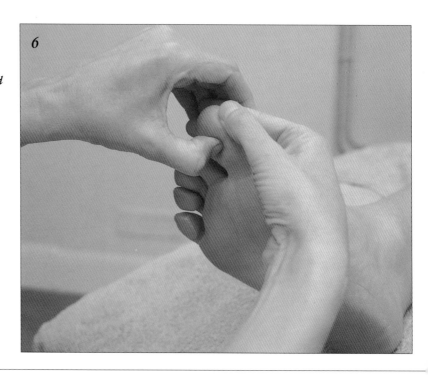

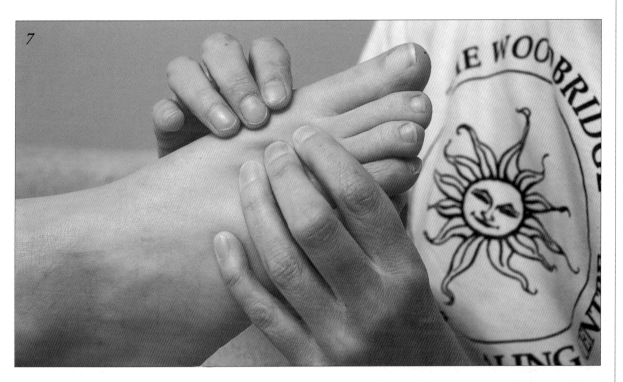

7 This is the metatarsal movement which works to mobilize the feet and reduce tension in the joints. The movement involves sliding the metatarsals slightly to achieve the right effect.

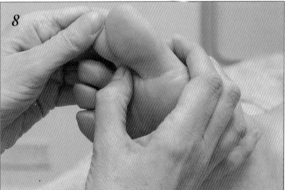

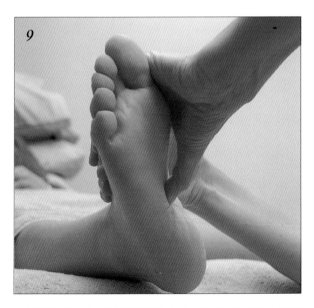

8 The spinal twist works to release the spine and encourage the release of tension in the back. The thumb works on the specific point of the foot while the hands gently twist the spinal area.

9 The big toe is worked on to concentrate on the occipital point. This is particularly good for relieving headaches, migraines and tension.

## REFLEXOLOGY SESSION

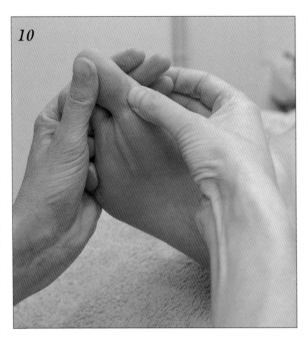

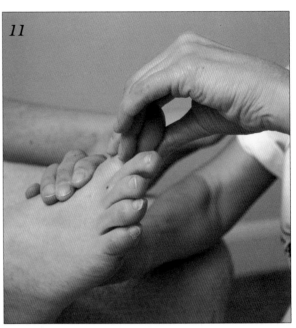

10 Working on the big toe affects the whole of the head and brain area. The thumb "walks" over the pad of the big toe and works up the side.

11 The treatment of the big toe continues with a finger roll technique to promote a beneficial effect in the head and brain areas, and to relieve tension.

12 The practitioner moves on to the base of the toe, which represents the base of the neck. This is an important area for relieving headaches, and reducing stress and tension.

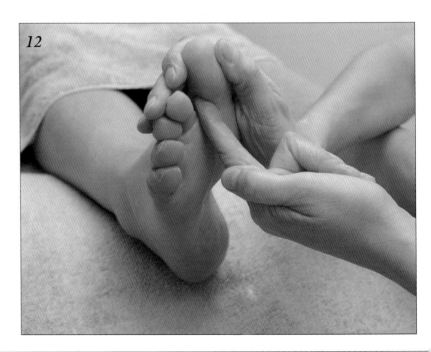

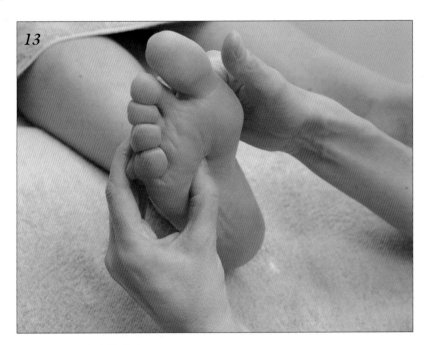

13 This movement works on the solar plexus to find and treat any areas of tenderness, which could be an indication of respiratory problems. Problems in this area are a good indicator of stress, and relieving them helps promote more even, steady breathing. Treating this area of the foot works the diaphragm at the same time.

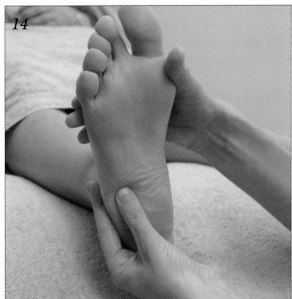

14 This photograph shows the thumb walking technique up the side of the foot in order to work on the ascending colon and promote its healthy functioning.

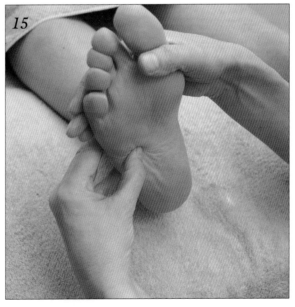

15 This movement, which is designed to work on the kidneys, involves one hand over the top of the foot and the thumb of the second hand working up the middle of the foot. This helps stimulate kidney function and improves elimination of toxins.

# REFLEXOLOGY SESSION

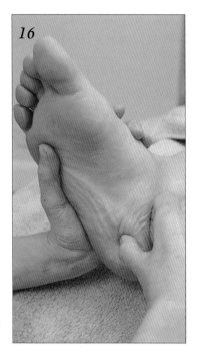

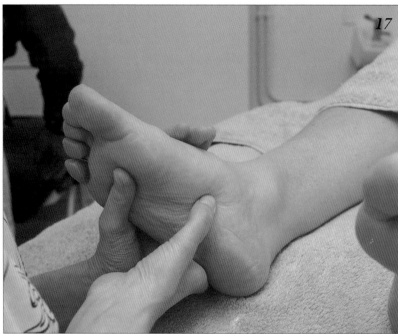

16 The heel represents the pelvis, buttock muscles and the area of the sciatic nerve which is located at the base of the heel. Working across the base of the heel greatly helps any sciatic nerve problems.

17 The reflexologist continues to work around the heel, concentrating on the pelvis, buttock muscles and sciatic nerve, and using thumb pressure to relieve problems in the pelvic area.

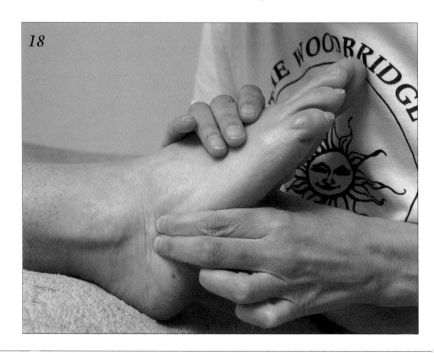

18 This photograph shows finger walking around the heel, again concentrating on the hip and pelvic areas.

*19 The pads of the small toes are worked on to relieve congestion in the sinuses which is often very effective. In some patients, it can have almost instantaneous results, relieving the symptoms of catarrh, colds and sinus headaches.*

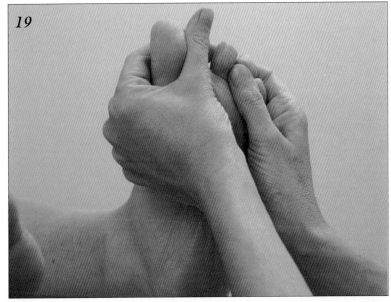

*20 This is a continuation of the treatment on the pads of the small toes, working on the sinus area to clear, relieve and reduce any congestion. The session then finishes with some relaxing ankle circling.*

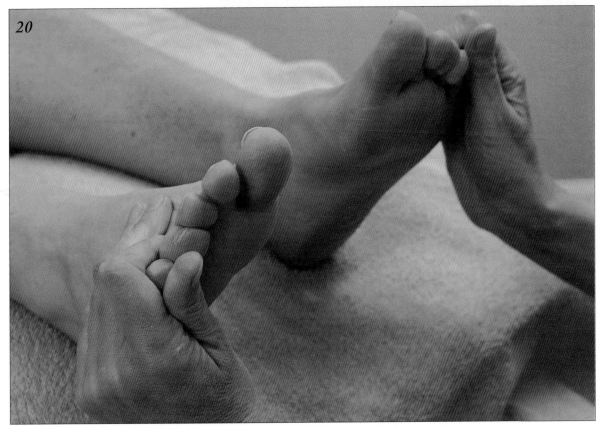

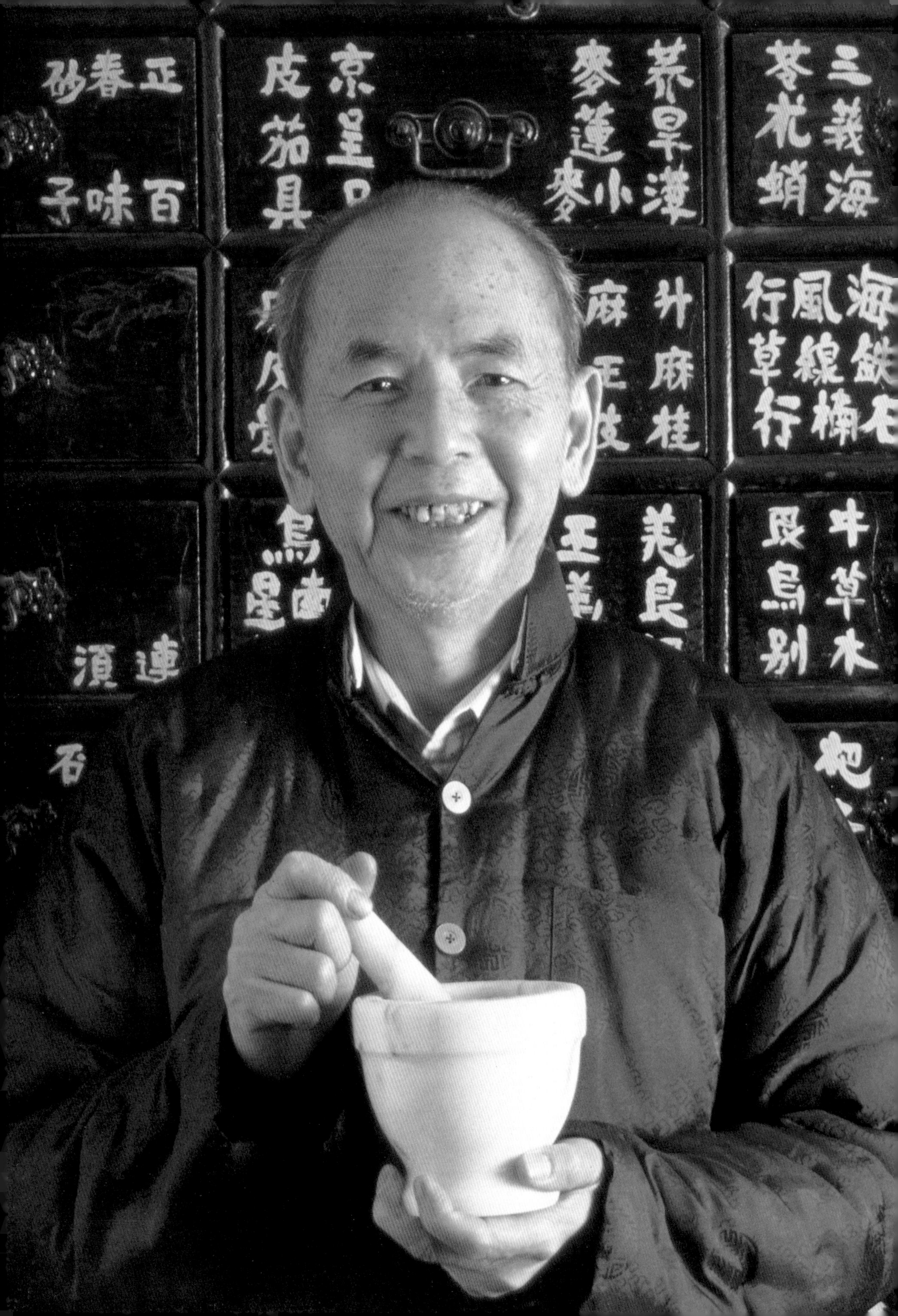

# EASTERN THERAPIES

## PART SEVEN

*All of the therapies featured in this section originated in China, with the exception of Shiatsu which developed in Japan. Chinese medicine is a complete medical system, dating back over 2,000 years. Like other forms of holistic medicine, it emphasizes the interaction between the individual's body, mind and spirit, and his relationship with the environment. Traditional Chinese medicine aims to encourage good health and wellbeing and prevent dis-ease, as well as being a means of diagnosing and treating illness. This is unlike orthodox Western medicine which tends to focus on specific isolated areas of disease.*

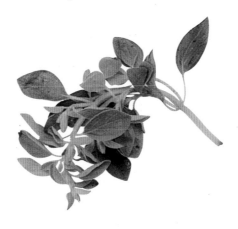

# ACUPUNCTURE

## CHAPTER THIRTY

*C*hinese medicine has been a long-kept secret behind the Great Wall. The purpose of this chapter is to lead the reader into a fascinating voyage through the intricacies and marvels of a medical system which is as prevalent and effective today as it has been through the last 3,000 years.

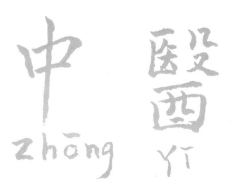

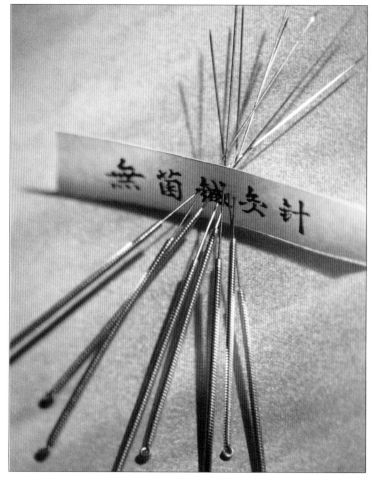

*The word acupuncture originates from the Latin words* acu, *which means needle, and* punctura, *which translates into puncture, a term first proposed by the Dutch physician William Ten Rhyne in the seventeenth century. Acupuncture is a method to treat disease and maintain health by inserting very fine needles into precise points, called Acupuncture Points, located along energy channels running on the surface and traversing the body, called Meridians. In China, the scientific name for acupuncture translates into "Methods of Needles and Moxa." The layman calls it* Cha Zen, *which means "to stick a needle," which is often also the Westerner's understanding of acupuncture.*

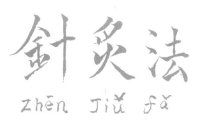

# THE HISTORICAL PERSPECTIVE

Acupuncture originated in China where it was practiced as far back as 1200B.C. and as a result, Chinese

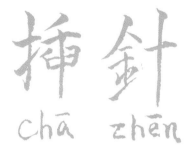

chā zhēn

medicine is considered to be the most widely used system of medicine in our history; more so than all other systems of medicine combined.

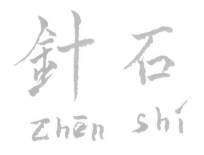

zhēn shí

The *Nei Jing* or the *Internal Classic* (or Cannon) *of Medicine,* also called *The Yellow Emperor's Classic of Internal Medicine,* is the oldest medical book in China, and it is estimated to have been written by numerous medical authors around 475 to 221 B.C. In this ancient text, nine differ-

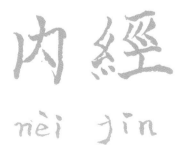

nèi jīn

ent types of needles are mentioned as being used for acupuncture treatments, each one with a precise length and width and a different tip. These were used for various conditions, from rheumatic diseases to pediatrics.

Interestingly enough, over 2,000 years later in an archeological discovery in 1968, nine acupuncture needles (four gold and five silver) were actually found in the tombs of Liu Cheng and his wife in the Hopei province of China. This confirmed the existence of what was known only through the ancient texts.

## HOW WAS THE SYSTEM OF POINTS AND MERIDIANS DISCOVERED?

Everybody would like an answer to this question. It is really puzzling how Chinese doctors in ancient times were able to organize such a complex system of points and channels 3,000 years ago without any of today's technology. Some scholars of Chinese civilization propose that the acupuncture points were discovered through the observation of injured or sick people, who by rubbing certain areas of the body would obtain pain relief and even cures for their ailments.

## ACUPUNCTURE NEEDLES

The earliest needles date back to the Paleolithic Age, when they were crafted out of stone. During the Neolithic times, needles were made out of bone, later of bamboo, gold, silver and copper, and, today, most commonly of stainless steel with a copper handle.

Others postulate that warriors were the first to report "miraculous cures" of various conditions in arrow-shooting survivors. A few others yet suggest that the acupuncture points and the meridians were "visualized" by Taoist priests during their meditation practices.

## THE KOREAN HAND ACUPUNCTURE SYSTEM

In modern times, there is a living example of how an acupuncture system was discovered. This is the Korean Hand Acupuncture System, or Koryo System, which was discovered by Dr. Tae-Woo Yoo.

Already a seasoned acupuncturist in Korea, Dr. Yoo woke up one night and felt an intense pain on one side of the back of his skull. At the same time he noticed that there was a sore spot on the side of his middle finger. As he rubbed it, the headache resolved almost immediately. He thought that there must be a corresponding point between his head and the small spot on his middle finger. And since he was a very curious and methodical scientist, Dr. Yoo spent the next several years dedicated to the discovery of a new microsystem, in which every acupuncture point on the body had an exact correspondence on the hand.

This system allows an acupuncturist to treat any condition that he would usually treat on body points directly on the hand, with equal effectiveness as with body acupuncture. Such an option might be quite desirable and practical when one needs to be treated outdoors or in a public place, or if one has a fear of larger needles. Korean acupuncture needles are very tiny and are barely felt.

## BODY-HAND CORRESPONDENCES IN KORYO ACUPUNTURE

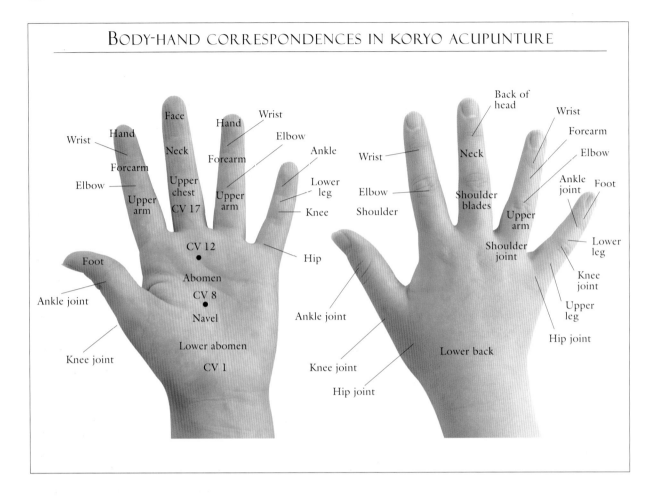

# PHILOSOPHY

## WESTERN MEDICINE

All science has a philosophical base, upon which its theories are founded, and which provides the scientific thought with a reasoning model so that one can move from an initial observation to a final conclusion of "scientific truth."

Western medicine is based on the Cartesian philosophy of René Descartes (1596-1650), who published his *Discourse on Method* in 1637. Descartes was actually interpreted by his contemporaries as being linear, meaning that his emphasis was on cause and effect, yet, after a careful review of his discourse, one might

disagree with his contemporaries. Nevertheless, to this day he is still known as the promoter of our present linear, analytical form of reasoning, a philosophy that has led to a scientific thinking of dissecting everything to its smallest visible part—the cell, the molecule and the atom—in an attempt to understand how it all works, what keeps us healthy and what makes us sick.

"If we can't see it, then it is not there," or "perhaps it is just a product of our imagination," or something like what clinical researchers call "placebos." This is the mind-set of today's Western practitioners and researchers, and therefore any exceptions to such an understanding are

labeled as "spontaneous healing," or an "unexplained phenomenon."

## CHINESE MEDICINE

The philosophical base for Chinese medicine and one of its major divisions, acupuncture, is at the opposite end of the spectrum.

## YIN AND YANG

All things in the world carry within themselves two qualities which are in opposition, yet which are also in constant transformation into each other. Therefore, they form an interdependent and continuous, rhythmic movement which aims at achieving a balance between the two.

The ancient Chinese called the

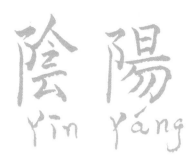

陰 陽
Yin Yáng

quiet, cold, dark quality of all things yin, and its active, warm, bright counterpart, Yang, and chose "water" to represent Yin, and "fire" to represent Yang.

This theory was conceptualized from observations of nature. The concept of day would not exist without its opposite concept of night. Neither would cold be perceived as such, were it not compared to heat. Or light with dark, or low with high, or wet with dry.

Chinese medicine is based on Taoist philosophy, which is founded on the principles of Yin and Yang. Within this context, people, their organs, meridians, and diseases are all viewed within their Yin/Yang perspective. As a result,

▪ Health is at its most basic level when it is in proper balance between Yin and Yang energy.
▪ Disease is a break in such order.
▪ Treatment is aimed at restituting the normal movement between the two opposites.

## TREATING PATIENTS AS A "WHOLE"

In Chinese medical thought, nothing is seen in a vacuum or in isolation, nor are human beings arbitrarily divided into parts or viewed within specialties, as in Western medicine. Rather, man is seen as a creature of Nature and, as such, is subject to its laws. Each human being is appreciated as a complete and individual microcosmos. Patients are treated as a "whole," with the understanding that all symptoms and signs within one person interrelate and influence each other. Finding the original driving force behind the cascade of manifestations for each syndrome, is the real challenge for the physician.

"If one disregards the location of an illness entirely and employs drugs to attack (contrary to what would be correct) a place that is absolutely free of illness, this is what the *Nei Jing* calls 'punishing the innocent'." (From the *I-hsueh Yuan Liu Lun* of 1757 by Hsu Pa-ch'un, 1693-1771.)

## DIFFERENCES BETWEEN WESTERN AND CHINESE MEDICINE

All that a patient comes with, even what is thought of as totally inconsequent during a Western medical evaluation, is of great importance to a practitioner of Chinese medicine.

The common saying, "some person's garbage is another person's treasure" is quite applicable to the difference in observations between a Western-trained and an Eastern-trained physician.

What a biomedical doctor may toss out of the medical interview and exam as "clinically non-significant, redundant or negligible information," is really the "golden nugget," the most valuable information for the practitioner of Chinese medicine, who pays careful attention to the patient's personal history after it has been narrated, rather than have the story fit into a set number of questions which are pertinent for his diagnostic formulation.

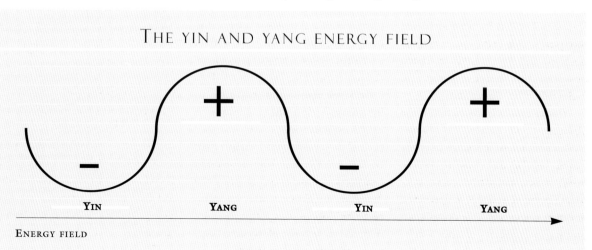

## THE YIN AND YANG ENERGY FIELD

YIN        YANG        YIN        YANG

ENERGY FIELD

Although many theories have been postulated to explain how acupuncture works, none by itself is complex enough to support the multiple beneficial effects this form of treatment has on human beings as well as on animals. In addition, understanding how it works very much depends on where one stands historically, geographically, ethnically and academically. It also depends on one's science background and mode of thinking, and especially on one's ability to accept cultural and epistemlogical differences. Epistemology is the philosophy of knowledge; it is the way in which one thinks through a set of concepts from an initial observation until one reaches a conclusion.

Understanding how it works also depends on what sort of evidence one needs for accepting or rejecting a theory as valid. For example, for those with a background in Mathematics and Physics, the theory of the needle acting as a metal conductor may be the most acceptable.

## THE THEORY OF THE NEEDLE ACTING AS A METAL CONDUCTOR

It is known that acupuncture points are areas where there is an increased electrical activity and lowered resistance of the skin; and it has been observed that nerve endings are much denser at these points.

▪ When a needle is inserted into the body, the tip of the needle is submitted to a higher temperature than the handle due to the warmth of the body tissues, and therefore an electrical potential gradient is generated between the tip and the handle. In Physics, this property of a metal conductor is known as the Thermo-

# HOW THE THERAPY WORKS AND ITS PRACTICAL APPLICATIONS

electric Effect of Thomson-Kelvin. The electrical gradient that results, transforms the tip into a positive electrode and the handle into a negative one. This is known in Physics as the Seebeck Effect.

▪ The copper spiral that surrounds the handle of the needle generates an electromagnetic field as it comes in contact with the stainless steel, and, therefore acts as a bimetalic battery.

▪ If one uses a 0.3 mm thick ($^1/_8$ in.), 8 cm (3 in.) long stainless steel needle with a spiral copper handle, and introduces it into an acupuncture point, a small current of 2 to 3 microamperes can be measured along the length of the instrument. Because the tip of the needle has a positive polarity, it will attract negative ions from the tissues surrounding it, until an equilibrium is reached. If the needle is left in a neutral position, this process takes between 10 and 15 minutes, and such a technique is called dispersion in acupuncture practice.

▪ If, instead, the handle of the needle is stimulated by heat, the polarity of the tip will change to negative, and positive ions are attracted from the surrounding medium. This process of equilibrium takes 60 to 90 minutes and the technique is called tonification.

▪ It is then easy to understand that, by strategically inserting needles in tonification and dispersion along the meridian lines, one is able to influence the flow of ions along the lines in predictable ways, based on a diagnostic and therapeutic design.

## THE NEURO-TRANSMITTER THEORY

For those who are trained in Neurophysiology, Molecular Biology, and Biochemistry, the neuro-transmitter theory may be more satisfactory. A simplified explanation of such theory is as follows:

▪ Signals from a pain in the shoulder are transmitted to a nerve cell (posterior neuron) in the spinal cord. From there it is conducted through pain pathways (spinothalmic tract) to the hypothalamus, and then from there to the brain, which recognizes the localization of the pain.

▪ Through the introduction of a needle into an acupuncture point, (in this case LI4 or *He Gu*), the stimulation of the spinal cord nerve cell is inhibited, and the release of beta-endorphins at the hypophysis and

## THE CONCEPT OF CHI

The Chinese are actually more concerned with the concept of Chi than with the scientific explanations that Western physicians find it necessary to elucidate the mechanism of action of acupuncture.

Chi, or Qi, is a concept for which there is no parallel in the English or European languages. Chi is translated by some as "energy," "essence of life," "living force," or "vital energy." It is Chi that gives life to all living matter and it is Chi which circulates along the Meridians. Its flow and distribution depend on the balance of Yin and Yang.

the hypothalamus, is thus activated.

In addition, other neuro-transmitters such as serotonin, substance P, norepinephrine, dopamine and ACTH are also released, and are thought to have an important role in pain control, in mechanisms mediated through acupuncture.

Several other observations have been made during acupuncture treatments, such as increased gamma and beta globulins and increased activity in cells fighting inflammation, such as lymphocytes and phagocytes, an increase in skin temperature due to vasodilatation and improved blood flow, and finally improvement of blood sugar levels during treatment, both from an excessive high or excessive low level, as well as a decrease in cholesterol and triglycerides.

Many of these theories are interesting but they miss the "wholeness" that is the mainstream of Chinese diagnosis and therapeutics. The comprehensiveness in which a patient is perceived suggests that its mechanism of action may be much more complex and multifactorial than is understood to this day.

### UNDERSTANDING THE ROOTS AS WELL AS THE SYMPTOMS

A physician trained in Chinese medicine must have the skills not only to recognize the symptoms of disease, e.g. cough, fever, headaches, constipation, or "branches" of the illness, but he or she must also understand its "roots," or at what level the balancing mechanism has been originally injured. Within this reasoning, some types of asthmatic conditions require that the "kidney energy" must also be balanced before the lung can be properly affected, due to the very

close energetic relationship between the two organ "energies."

So while Western medicine would aim at treating the symptom or "branch," the bronchospasm, Chinese medicine would be more concerned with the "roots" or origin of the disease, and at regulating the kidney function, for example, so that further balancing of the related energies may lead to reversal of the condition.

Too much mental activity can weaken the spleen Yin, for instance, leading to loose stools and ankle swelling, among other symptoms. That explains why treating diarrhea with anti-diarrheals, or water retention and swelling just with diuretics, may not be as effective in the long run as paying attention to the "root" of the "spleen energy deficiency," which, once treated with acupuncture, herbs and a change in some habits and lifestyle, might have a totally curative effect.

We can find some parallels with the Yin and Yang theory in today's

Quantum Theory of Physics, as well as in Einstein's Theory of Relativity, Yin being just the negative polarity and Yang the positive polarity of the waves of the universal energy field.

## VISITING AN ACUPUNCTURIST

The office visit experience to an acupuncturist may vary greatly depending on who one sees. Acupuncture is a highly operator-dependent intervention. The more skilled and educated the therapist is, the more accurate the diagnosis will be and the more effective the treatment. The proportion of Eastern and Western medical training the acupuncturist has, number of years in practice, ability to master multiple, simultaneous bits of information, the sharpness of the intuitive edge, the listening and observational talents, all are factors that will ultimately affect the outcome of the intervention by a particular practitioner. A competent

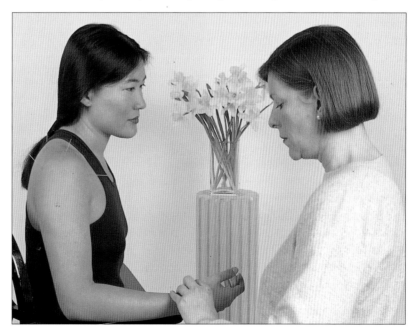

# THE MERIDIAN SYSTEM

The layout of the Meridian system, as shown here, has been thought of as "energy channels, like rivers flowing through the body," or "like electromagnetic (EM) fields surrounding and traversing the body, just as the EM fields behave as they embrace the Earth and all living systems."

There are 12 principal Meridians on the surface of the body of which six are Yin and six are Yang, Yin usually being on the front of the body, and Yang on the back. There are also two Meridians running through the center of the body, the Conception vessel on the front and the Governing vessel on the back. In addition, there are multiple other deeper Meridians which are used for more complex illnesses, and which use points from several of these superficial Meridians and communicate between each other.

Originally 365 points were described along the Meridians on each side of the body, but more than 1,000 points can be counted now, if one includes the extrameridian points. In addition, multiple new points have been added to the microsystems of the scalp, ear and hand among others. The ear alone has over 200 points described on it. The scope of this chapter does not permit a more extensive discussion on this topic, which can be found in more detail in technical and medical books on Chinese Medicine.

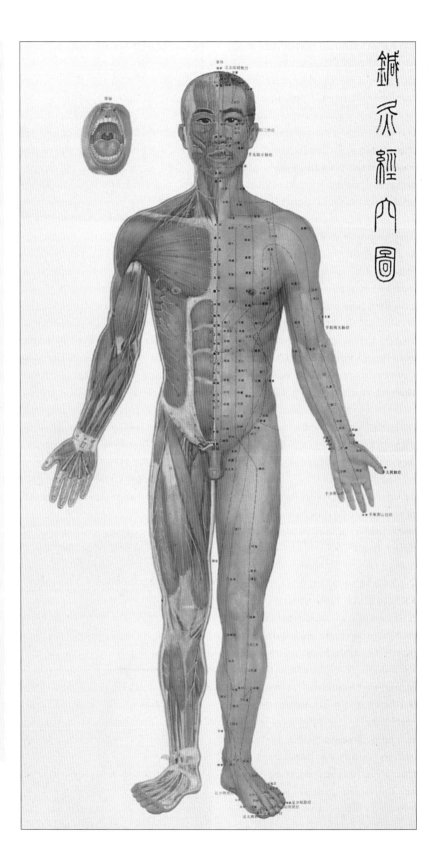

*Very fine needles (average size of between 1.5 and 7.5 cm and a diameter of 0.26 to 0.46 mm) are inserted into various points, depending on the condition being treated.*

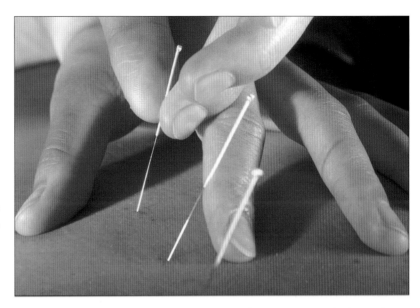

therapist will be able to arrive at a comprehensive diagnosis, delineate a practical treatment plan and submit the patient to the least number of sessions, obtaining the most desirable results with a minimum number of needles and a minimum period of time.

The famous sixteenth-century Chinese physician Yang noted: "It is obvious that there are channel pulses. Those who use them are the true doctors (*Liang Yi*). Those who ignore them are clumsy workers (*Zu Gong*)."

## PATIENT'S HISTORY AND EXAMINATION

At the time that a patient is first seen, a history is usually taken and, depending on the physician's expertise, a purely Chinese medical examination or a combination of an Eastern and Western approach is in order. This may consist of the standard medical evaluation with the addition of the following:

▧ Inspection of the tongue.

▧ Palpation of the pulse for rate and rhyth. A second palpation, which would consist of evaluating the pulse in six positions on each wrist, representing the function of all 12 Meridians.

▧ The ears may be examined inside with an otoscope as it is done in most traditional offices, and the auricle may also be probed for "active points" for later treatment.

▧ The abdomen will be palpated for organs as it is done in the traditional way, but may also be searched for tender points and zones which are clues within the Chinese diagnostic system.

▧ Palpation of Meridians is often done prior to needle insertion.

▧ Testing of Meridian circulation can also be done by heating the tips of the toes and fingers with an incense-like stick or, for the technologically inclined, with electrical devices designed for that purpose.

## THE TREATMENT

When the needle is inserted, a slight ache, dull pain, tingling or an electrical sensation is felt for a few seconds, which acupuncturists call the "De Chi" sensation, and which means that the Chi has been accessed, this being important feedback for proper point location. Once the needles are in place, no further discomfort should be experienced. On the contrary, an occasional pleasant, tingling or warm feeling may be experienced moving along the Meridian lines, which is just a mani-

festation of energetic (the body's electrical function) activity passing through these channels.

The needles are usually left in place for between 15 and 30 minutes, depending on the condition being treated. Removal of the needles causes no discomfort, and only rarely minor bleeding may occur at points where a number of small blood vessels tend to converge.

In addition to inserting the needles, the practitioner has to decide

## TYPES OF NEEDLE

Many practitioners, especially in the United States, now use disposable needles to avoid any risks of spreading the hepatitis and HIV viruses. Acupuncturists using reusable needles may resort to gold or silver, depending on the material the treatment calls for. Disposable needles are usually made of stainless steel and often have a copper wire spiraled around the handle.

which of these will remain in a neutral position, or be manipulated for dispersion, and which of them will be manipulated to obtain a tonification effect. The needle can be manually rotated clockwise or heated with a moxa stick when tonifying, or it can be rotated counterclockwise or its handle cooled with an alcohol swab, when dispersing. Both procedures can also be done by electrically stimulating the needle at various frequencies and intensities; tonification can be obtained at low frequencies and dispersions at higher ones.

## ACUPUNCTURE TREATMENTS

Often patients wonder why their back pain is not treated only with needles placed on their back, but even with some placed on their hands, legs and ankles. This is because acupuncture treatments are designed like "electrical circuits," and the real "switch" may actually be at the opposite end of the injury. Local treatments are of little value and are not an indication of therapeutic sophistication.

## MOXIBUSTION

This is a procedure in which the herb, *Artemisia vulgaris* is used in various forms as a source of heat, applied to points or needles. This herb was once called "the mother of herbs" and was cherished throughout Europe and Asia. The Chinese name for it is *Ai*, and its common name is mugwort. It is a perennial plant which grows three to four inches high with dark green leaves and yellowish-brown flowers. It has been used in earlier times to flavor beer, to stimulate the appetite, as a diuretic, to treat intestinal worms and as an insect repellent.

Its "wool," which is the finely ground dried herb, is used in the form of cones, applied directly or indirectly to the skin, as sticks which are formed by the rolled-up leaves of the plant. Sometimes small jackets are crafted to fit around the needles.

Moxibustion is usually used for "deficiency" and chronic conditions, and it is generally contraindicated in the presence of high fever or on certain points or parts of the body. It can be used with or without needles and for some severe long-standing conditions, patients can be taught to use it at home.

### LENGTH OF TREATMENT

It is reasonable to expect a cycle of no more than six to twelve sessions as an average length of treatment for most common conditions, by which time significant changes should have become evident. If this has not happened by then, the treatment plan should be reevaluated and the appropriateness of using acupuncture for that condition reassessed.

Some patients may require a few more treatments, others may have reached 100 percent resolution within just a few treatments. Months or years of treatment are not usually indicated for common ailments, but "maintenance" treatments at monthly, bi-monthly or quarterly intervals are useful for long-standing, chronic illnesses, once they resolve.

### REACTIONS TO TREATMENT

During the acupuncture session, and sometimes 24 to 48 hours after the treatment, a patient may experience slight mood changes as well as a reaction in their body functions, such as frequency and flow of urination, change in bowel movements and sleep patterns. Symptoms may at times worsen slightly during this period. This is a sign that the area treated is going through an increased energetic activity and therefore it

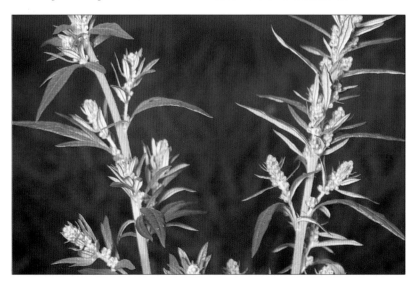

*The common mugwort is used in the ancient technique of moxibustion.*

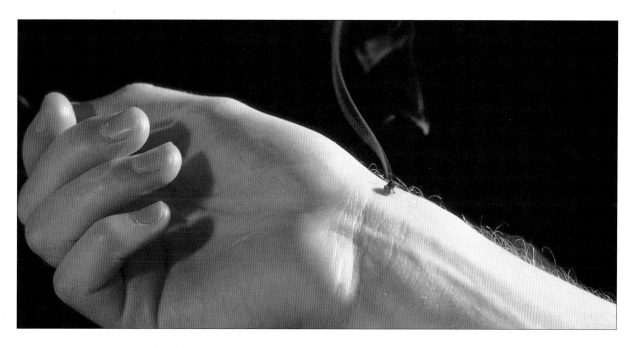

*In moxibustion, the moxa "wool," the finely ground mugwort, is burned on top of an acupuncture needle.*

is moving towards change.

The symptom response to treatment varies widely. German practitioners have classified patients' responses to acupuncture into early, mid and late responders, but a reliable mechanism to predict the time of response has not yet been developed. Some patients respond immediately, "like a miracle"; one treatment is all they need to resolve a neck pain, an old headache or to stop smoking. Other patients have a very slow initial response, which increases with each visit. A third group yet may not experience any change at all until well into their fourth or fifth visit, often becoming impatient and at times not returning, believing that "acupuncture just doesn't work for them."

What could have happened in reality, had they persevered with their treatment, is that after the fourth or fifth session they would have suddenly experienced a 50 percent improvement, which would be a major change from their baseline condition. This is due to acupuncture's "cumulative effect," which occurs from visit to visit, but as we shall see, this does not follow a straight line but rather a ragged one.

## THE GOAL OF TREATMENT

For most conditions that qualify for acupuncture therapy, the goal of treatment should be a 100 percent resolution. If a patient stops at a 30 percent or 50 percent improvement level, for example, all accomplishments so far may be lost over time because the cumulative effect has not yet "kicked in." On the other hand, this cumulative phenomenon may also explain those cases when, after achieving an 80 percent to 90 percent resolution, a patient had to stop for various reasons and then the remaining 20 percent to 10 percent extra effect still occurs over several weeks without any further acupuncture intervention.

This is not an unusual observation in an acupuncture practice. Once the 100 percent resolution goal is achieved, recurrences are very unlikely, but in some more complex cases, such as rheumatoid arthritis or psoriasis, a maintenance program of several treatments a year is in order. These maintenance sessions are usually limited in number, and give both the patient and practitioner an opportunity to observe how strongly the results are holding, providing the necessary information that the physician needs in planning to dismiss the patient from treatment.

## OTHER FORMS OF CHINESE MEDICINE

### CHINESE HERBAL FORMULAS
In addition to acupuncture and moxibustion above, practitioners may also

## REACTION TO TREATMENT

The graph shows that a 40 percent improvement, for example, may bounce back to 30 percent before it moves on to a 50 percent level. This is due to the resilience of the body, as it adjusts to new stages. Therefore it is very important for patients not to become discouraged and discontinue treatment before maximum benefit could have been achieved. Each person has an inherent and individual capacity for healing.

However, the pace of such is highly variable and dependent upon multiple, often incalculable personal factors.

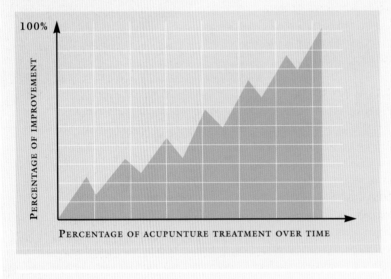

prescribe Chinese herbal formulas, either raw to be prepared as a decoction, or in a pill form to be swallowed with water.

Cupping is used by practitioners for some conditions, such as colds, bronchitis and long-standing arthritis or other rheumatic diseases. Cupping is the stimulation of the points by applying a glass, bamboo or ceramic cup or small jar on a point, after a partial vacuum has been obtained inside the container with a flame. Sometimes a needle is inserted and then a cup applied over it. A small bruise will result. Do not worry as this is necessary for the desirable therapeutic effect.

### DIETARY CHANGES AND EXERCISE

Most practitioners will also prescribe dietary changes based on Yin and Yang principles, as well as recommending T'ai Chi or external movement therapy, a gentle form of the most powerful of martial arts, and Chi Kung, or internal breathing exercises, which is often prescribed and taught to patients as another form of directing the flow of the Meridians for various dysfunctions. Tui-na may be ordered, which is a very effective form of therapeutic massage in which the acupuncture points are massaged rather than just general muscle groups. Massage prescriptions for Tui-na include a set number of points for each condition and also precise massage techniques for each of these points.

## CONDITIONS FOR WHICH ACUPUNCTURE CAN BE USED

Chinese medicine, especially its divisions of acupuncture, moxibustion and herbology, has been a self-contained system of medicine for at least 3,000 documented years and most likely for one or two thousand years beyond that. Therefore, Chinese medicine was designed to treat all diseases known to man in the different eras of civilization into which it was born.

Yet in the Western world it is a system that has been mostly associated with pain control. Contrary to our Western understanding of pain management, acupuncture is not the equivalent of an aspirin or another narcotic; it resolves pain not only through a direct action on pain but also through a normalization of dysfunctions that led to the pain symptom in the first place.

In some way one could say that pain resolution is a "by product" or "fringe benefit" from receiving acupuncture treatments. If the patient's condition is treatable with acupuncture, then an appropriate designed "circuit" for that particular patient will normalize all functions and, therefore, pain should no longer have a place in the organism once it is functioning again.

A list of treatable conditions will vary from practitioner to practitioner. Some conditions for which acupuncture and other forms of Chinese medicine are commonly and effectively used are as follows:

### ▦ ORTHOPEDIC PROBLEMS,

These include tennis elbow and other tendinitis, and many degenerative (arthritic) and post-traumatic (sport and other injuries) joint disorders.

### ▦ RESPIRATORY AND EAR, NOSE AND THROAT DISORDERS

These include bronchitis, recurrent respiratory infections, allergic rhinitis, toothaches, ringing of the ears, functional vertigo (like Meniere's disease) and TMJ (temporo-mandibular joint dysfunction).

### ▦ ALLERGY PROBLEMS

These include certain eczemas as well as seasonal allergies, manifesting as itchy eyes, runny noses and sinus headaches.

### ▦ DIGESTIVE DISORDERS

These include constipation, diarrhea, spastic colon, colitis, excessive acidity and gastritis.

## NOTE

A general rule of thumb is that acupuncture works best for conditions that are functional and reversible and it works least with more established diseases or degenerative processes, such as cysts, tumors, kidney or heart failure or diabetes. One may want to remember that acupuncture can heal what is disturbed; it cannot heal what is destroyed.

### ▦ URINARY AND GENITAL PROBLEMS

These include recurrent cystitis, vaginitis and urethritis, menstrual irregularities, as well as painful intercourse and a lack of sexual desire or enjoyment.

### ▦ NEUROLOGICAL DISORDERS

These include most types of headaches, post-herpetic neuralgia, Bell's palsy, post-stroke paralysis, torticollis, sciatica, tremors and facial tics.

### ▦ NEURO-PSYCHIATRIC PROBLEMS

These include anxiety, tension, depression and insomnia.

### ▦ SOME RARE, YET OTHERWISE DIFFICULT TO TREAT, CONDITIONS

These include certain types of hair loss, non-organic infertility problems, psoriasis, and stress urinary incontinence, and various forms of post-operative pain, often resolve with acupuncture when it is delivered by expert hands.

## INTERACTIONS WITH OTHER THERAPIES

In general, there is no contraindication to using acupuncture with most other therapies, although there are some exceptions.

▦ High doses of sedatives, narcotics, steroids or anti-depressants may interfere with the release of endorphins and therefore with at least one of the well known mechanisms of the action of acupuncture. This could make the acupuncture intervention less effective, slower or

## TREATABLE CONDITIONS

In the author's practice, the top 15 conditions that have been treated very successfully with acupuncture throughout the years are as follows:

- Migraine headaches
- Allergic sinusitis
- Fibromyalgia
- Cervical Spine Syndromes (neck pain)
- Lumbar Spine Syndromes (low back pain)
- Trigeminal Neuralgia
- Premenstrual Syndrome (PMS), especially Dysmenorrhea or premenstrual and menstrual cramps
- Peripheral Neuropathy
- Plantar Fascitis (painful feet)
- Frozen shoulder
- Forms of arthritis
- Asthma
- Irritable Bowel Syndrome
- Addiction and Substance Abuse (Alcohol, Tobacco, Drugs)
- Chronic Pelvic Pain (functional)

The conditions enumerated above are not listed in order of effectiveness. Results of treatment do not depend on the condition, but on the associated dysfunctions the patient with the condition may have, although time of onset of the illness, as well as intensity or severity of the illness may be factors influencing faster or better outcomes.

in some cases not effective at all.

▦ Massage, chiropractic, physical therapy and other physical modalities, if performed within six to eight hours of an acupuncture treatment, could disturb the energetic changes produced by the needles and, to a

certain extent, inactivate its therapeutic impact.

■ Patients are also advised not to
engage in sexual activities, strenuous
exercise or consume a large or heavy
meal within four to six hours after
their treatments. Some practitioners
advise six to eight hours abstinence,
but after being asked, "How long
before, you know, doctor, did you say
I have to wait?" they may decide to
become more lenient on this issue.

■ With respect to nutritional therapy
it is advisable that during acupuncture treatment, patients do not "try
yet another diet." It is a time for
rebalancing, and the body, in its own
wisdom, will ask for a variety of foods
and taste preferences in its attempt to
return to order. It is more natural to
follow dietary advise based on
Yin/Yang principles, and to use food
as a therapeutic intervention based
on the same philosophy as the treatment of pain.

Combining acupuncture and
moxibustion with Chinese herbs is
often quite appropriate and very
helpful. Sometimes homeopathy can
be used in conjunction with acupuncture as well as native American herbs
from different countries, as long as
they are used within a well thought
through system, and by an expert
practitioner.

A number of naturopathic
approaches can also be used. Among
these are aromatherapy, hydrotherapy, reflexology, rolfing, shiatsu, yoga,
therapeutic touch, Alexander technique, hypnotherapy, autogenics,
biofeedback and meditation.

Western homeopathic medicine
can be used in addition and does not
usually interfere with acupuncture
treatments.

# HOW ACUPUNCTURE CAN FIT INTO YOUR LIFESTYLE

Acupuncture is a simple intervention
that can easily fit into various
lifestyles which patients may have. If
time permits and your practitioner so
proposes, you may choose to go for
treatment two to three times per
week to obtain faster results. If you
travel frequently, you may be able to
skip a week, but probably should
avoid prolonging intervals between
treatments for more than two to
three weeks, at least during the first
six to eight treatments

■ **The "Chinese Clock"**
Ideally, some conditions are best
treated at different times of the day,
depending on the peaks of meridian
circulation which follow a pattern
called "Chinese Clock." But in a
busy urban life, such purism in therapeutics may not be possible for either
the doctor or the patient.

If work is very stressful, it might
be better to schedule acupuncture
treatments in the afternoon, and go
home from there for a small nap, or
during your lunch time if it is long
enough.

For the "morning person," a
morning session may be more effective than a later one in the afternoon.
If a patient is very hungry or very
tired, it is best to postpone acupuncture treatments. Some offices, which
are more patient-centered, may have
tea, juices and crackers available to
solve this problem.

## ACUPUNCTURE AND MENSTRUATION
It is not advisable to do acupuncture
at least during the first two days of
a woman's menstrual period—
although this is done quite often
because the question rarely gets
asked. During the time that a
woman happens to be on her cycle,
the acupuncture may have an effect
that could be desirable for some
women and undesirable for others;
it could either shorten the period
or stop it all together. Although
this might not seem like a major

## PHYSIOLOGICAL REACTIONS

Some patients have a very severe physiological reaction to the insertion of
needles, such as sweating, a small drop
in their blood pressure, feeling of nausea and dizziness, which, although not
in any way dangerous, it is best to
avoid. On occasions, such reactions are
called "needle shock" and are seen
during patients' first treatments but
usually not during subsequent ones. A
skilled practitioner can handle this with
ease. Koryo Hand Acupuncture can be
done with pellets, which are little metal

pointed buttons, as well as with magnets, so that needles are not always
necessary.

Auricular or ear acupuncture can be
done with a laser beam or simply with
a low-intensity electrical device without a needle insertion. Results are
similar to those obtained with needle
insertion. Patients who prefer these
approaches must seek a practitioner
who is skilled in such techniques,
which are called microsystems of
acupuncture.

this might not seem like a major problem, such effect may be followed by changes in the cycle and subsequent irregularities.

## SELF-HELP PRACTICAL MEASURES

Rest, exercise, good natural nutritional food (without any additives, pesticides and hormones) as well as listening to your body are the most important measures an acupuncture patient might take. A positive attitude helps, but it is not a requirement for the effectiveness of acupuncture. Acupuncture works in dogs, cats, horses and a variety of other domestic animals and, as we know, animals do not have a belief system. So placebo is not a good argument when it comes to veterinary acupuncture.

Other more specific measures may be prescribed by your doctor, such as moxibustion at home, acupressure at certain points, rubbing in certain ointments or taking prescribed herbs.

Following the plan as outlined by your practitioner is the most important measure a patient can take for self-help. Lifestyle changes are as important in Chinese medicine as they are in Western medicine. Certain exercises may be beneficial, whereas others may not. Heat and cold are used differently in Chinese medicine than they are in Western medicine and it is important not to use any of these without proper advice from your practitioner.

The use of magnets may also be helpful between visits and should be specifically prescribed and applied to points as instructed by your physician.

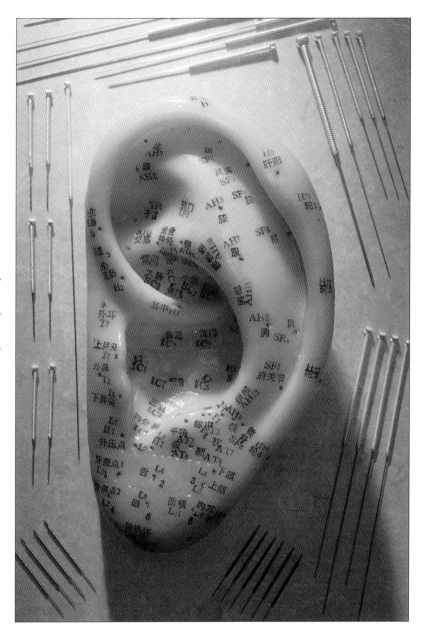

*As seen here, the entire body is represented on the ear and, although the representation that has been included is a very schematic simplified map, it should be known that over 200 points corresponding to the body have been identified on this rather small surface, and in close proximity to each other.*

Finally the most important aspect of self-help is probably to read about what is happening to you as you are doing now. In order that you may continue to educate yourself there is a selected bibliography at the back of this book, which will extend your knowledge of acupuncture. Consult

# ACUPRESSURE

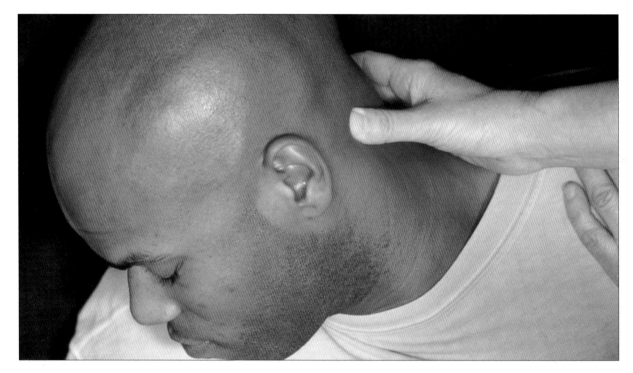

## CHAPTER TWENTY SIX

*A*cupressure is as old as instinct itself—the natural response to hold a place on your body that is aching, wounded, or tense. The impulse that makes you double over and press your stomach in response to abdominal cramps is an example of the instinctive practice of acupressure. Everyone at some time or another has used their hand spontaneously to hold tense or painful places on the body. It may well be the most ancient form of physical therapy.

More than 5,000 years ago, the Chinese discovered that pressing certain points on the body relieved pain where it occurred and also benefited other parts of the body more remote from the pain and the pressure point. Gradually, they found other locations that not only alleviated pain but also influenced the functioning of certain internal organs.

In the early Chinese dynasties, when stones and arrows were the only implements of war, many soldiers wounded on the battlefield reported that symptoms of disease that had plagued them for years had suddenly vanished. Naturally, such strange occurrences baffled the physicians who could find no logical relationship between the trauma and the ensuing recovery of health. After years of meticulous observation, ancient Chinese physicians developed ways of curing certain illnesses by striking or piercing specific points on the surface of the body.

# A NATURAL, HANDS-ON HEALING ART

As with the Chinese soldiers, people through the ages have found the most effective ways to help themselves by trial and error. The art and science of acupressure was practiced by the contributions of people whose awareness was so highly developed that they could feel where the bodies of people in pain were constricted and sense which trigger points would alleviate the problem. The Chinese have practiced self-acupressure for over 5,000 years as a way of keeping themselves well and happy.

You, too, can learn how to complement the care you receive from your doctor. You can help your body relieve itself of common ailments by pressing the proper spots. In the course of trying out these points, you may even find others that work better for you. More recently, high-tech equipment has scientifically revealed that these points actually have a higher electrical conductivity on the surface of the skin.

In traditional Chinese medicine, methods range from the most natural to the most intrusive. The most down-to-earth, natural healing methods, such as breathing exercises, dietary therapy, acupressure and herbalism, were used as a people's form of hands-on, organic healing. If more treatment was needed, acupuncture and chiropractic were used, being more complex and manipulative, followed by drugs and surgery, which use the most drastic interventions in last-resort medicine.

## BALANCING SYSTEMS OF THE BODY

Many ailments can be the result of too much stress challenging the body's balancing systems beyond their limits. The resulting tension and internal stress inhibit the body's ability to cope effectively with the disrupting condition. In order to relax muscular tension and balance the vital forces of the body, acupressure uses a system of points, which tend to collect muscular tension, and meridians, the pathways along which healing energy flows from point to point.

Acupressure considers symptoms to be an expression of the condition of the person as a whole. Thus, acupressure sessions focus not only on relieving pain and discomfort, but also on responding to these tensions and toxicities in the body before they develop into illnesses. Thus, acupressure works before the toxin constrictions have caused damage to the internal organs.

## THE BODY'S WARNING SIGNALS

From an acupressure point of view, tension is a stagnation of the bodily flows: the nerves, meridians, lymphatic ducts and blood vessel. Lack of exercise, poor diet, alcohol and drugs all contribute significantly to this stagnation. Emotional repression, neurotic habits, as well as the common stresses of day-to-day living, cause blockages within the body. These physical tensions or blocked emotions (whether conscious or not) lock the homeostatic mechanism of the body, restricting proper functioning. Instead of taking aspirin to repress such a signal by cutting off the body's natural alarm system, acupressure releases the tight, constricted muscles to correct the imbalance and its cause. There are a number of possible causes of headaches. These can include emotional stress; chronic shoulder and neck tension, which can partially block the circulation of the blood to the head; meridian imbalances; cervical misalignment,

---

## ACUPRESSURE AND ACUPUNCTURE

Acupuncture and acupressure use the same points. The fundamental distinction lies in the needles used in acupuncture and the gentle but firm pressure of hands (and feet in some techniques) used in acupressure. Although the older of the two techniques, acupressure tended to be overlooked. However, using the power and sensitivity of the human hand, acupressure continues to be more effective in relieving tension-related ailments in self-treatment and in preventive health care.

Many of the health problems in our society—from bad backs to arthritis—are the result of living unnaturally. Stress, tension, lack of exercise, poor eating habits, and poor posture contribute to the epidemic of degenerative diseases in our culture. Acupressure is one way to help your body fight back and balance itself in the face of the pressures of modern life.

which creates strain on head/ neck muscles and pinched nerves; intestinal congestion; and dietary imbalances, such as the contracting effect of salt, the expanding effect of sugar, the toxicity of most meats. In extreme cases, headaches can signify more serious conditions, such as earaches, toothaches, rheumatism and even internal hemorrhaging.

The practise of acupressure has developed primarily through a combination of instinct and hands-on experience. Its principles and healing techniques have also been influenced by individuals who could feel or see trigger points and meridian pathways. Some healers integrated breathing meditations and *mudras* (hand positions), while

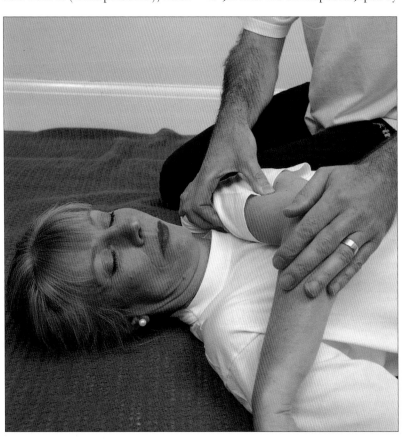

others added herbal remedies and massage. This exciting evolution of acupressure continues today among contemporary practitioners who incorporate traditional principles while discovering new point formulas and bodywork styles of their own.

## A VARIETY OF APPROACHES

The ancient points are common to all types of acupressure. Each type has distinctive characteristics that incorporate unique ways of touching and interacting with clients. The following descriptions focus on the primary styles or methods in an acupressure practice.

■ Jin Shin was developed in Japan by

Jiro Murai, who rediscovered the ancient "ki flow" (bioenergy) in his own body and mapped out a powerful healing system of points. Combinations of acupressure points are held with the fingers for a minute or more, usually with the client lying on his back.

■ Shiatsu (literally "finger pressure") is also Japanese in origin. This well-known method uses firm rhythmic pressure on the points for three to ten seconds (with the thumbs in the Namakoshi style) following a sequence of points which are designed to awaken the meridians.

■ Zen Shiatsu incorporates the creative use of the whole body along with stretches and leverage to awaken the healing channels of the body.

■ Barefoot Shiatsu uses the foot, allowing the practitioner the added advantage of leaning weight into the recipient.

## HOW ACUPRESSURE WORKS

Acupressure points (also called potent points) are places on the skin that are especially sensitive to bio-electrical impulses in the body and conduct those impulses readily. Traditionally, Asian cultures conceived of the points as junctures of special pathways that carried the human energy that the Chinese call *chi* and the Japanese call *ki*. Western scientists have also mapped out and proven the existence of this system of

*Left: acupressure is a natural healing art which focuses on relieving pain, balancing the body's vital forces and relaxing muscular tension.*

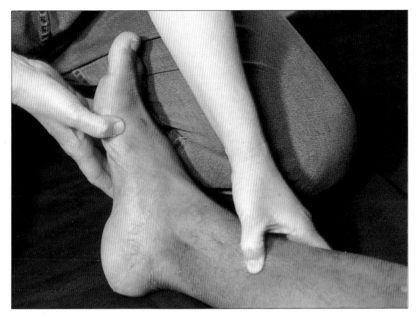

*Left: practitioners of acupressure believe that there are acupressure points all over the body which can be stimulated by applying varying degrees of pressure.*

tension yields to the finger pressure, enabling the fibers to elongate and relax, blood to flow freely, and toxins to be released and eliminated. Increased circulation also brings more oxygen and other nutrients to affected areas. This increases the body's resistance to illness and promotes a longer, healthier, more vital life. When the blood and bioelectrical energy circulate properly, we have a greater sense of harmony, health, and wellbeing.

## WAYS TO USE ACUPRESSURE

Acupressure's potent points can be used to enhance many aspects of life. In addition to managing stress, you can use acupressure to relieve and prevent sports injuries. Sports massage has been widely used by athletes

body points by using sensitive electrical devices.

Stimulating these points with pressure, needles, or heat triggers the release of endorphins, which are the neurochemicals that relieve pain. As a result, pain is blocked and the flow of blood and oxygen to the affected area is increased. This causes the muscles to relax and promotes healing.

Because acupressure inhibits the pain signals sent to the brain through a mild, fairly painless stimulation, it has been described as closing the "gates" of the pain-signaling system, preventing painful sensations from passing through the spinal cord to the brain

Besides relieving pain, acupressure can help rebalance the body by dissolving tensions and stresses that keep it from functioning smoothly and that inhibit the immune system. Acupressure enables the body to adapt to environmental changes and resist illness. Tension tends to concentrate around acupressure points. When a muscle is chronically tense or

in spasm, the muscle fibers contract due to the secretion of lactic acid caused by fatigue, trauma, stress, chemical imbalances, or poor circulation. For instance, when you are under a great deal of stress you may find you have difficulty breathing. Certain acupressure points relieve chest tension and thus enable you to breathe deeply.

As a point is pressed, the muscle

## SELF-HELP TECHNIQUES

Two techniques designed specifically for self-application are Acu-Yoga and Do-In (or self-acupressure massage). Acu-Yoga uses whole body postures along with deep breathing, finger pressure, meditations and stretches. Do-In also incorporates body awareness, stretching and breathing, but focuses on vigorous techniques that stimulate the points and meridians.

Whether used to relieve pain and muscular discomfort or to prevent

illness, acupressure techniques are intended to correct imbalances, working toward the regulation and harmony of all systems of the body. Since acupressure requires no special tools, and many people respond to the touch of hands-on contact more than they trust needles, the growing appeal of the ancient Chinese healing arts has led to increased interest in acupressure as a means toward optimum wellness.

# THE MERIDIANS

The Meridians are pathways that connect the acupressure points to each other as well as to the internal organs. Just as blood vessels carry the blood that nourishes the body physically, the Meridians are distinct channels that circulate electrical energy throughout the body. They are thought to be part of a master communications system of universal life energy, connecting the organs with all sensory, physiological, and emotional aspects of the body. This physical network of energy also contains key points that we can use to deepen our spiritual awareness as we heal ourselves.

Because the stimulation of one point can send a healing message to other parts of the body, each acupressure point can benefit a variety of complaints and symptoms. Therefore, you will find a particular acupressure point used for a variety of problems. The highly effective acupressure point in the webbing between our thumb and index finger, for instance, is not only beneficial for relieving arthritic pain in the hand, but also benefits the colon and relieves problems in the facial area and the head, including headaches, toothaches, and sinus problems. Tonic points improve your condition and maintain general health. They strengthen the overall body system and fortify various internal organs and vital systems of the body.

before and after Olympic events. Acupressure complements sports medicine treatments by using points and massage techniques to improve muscle tone and circulation and relieve neuromuscular problems.

The Chinese have also used acupressure as a beauty treatment for thousands of years. You can use potent points to improve skin condition and tone and relax the facial muscles, which can lessen the appearance of wrinkles without drugs.

Although acupressure is not a substitute for medical care, it may be an appropriate complementary treatment. It may, for instance, speed the healing of a broken bone once it has been set, or aid a cancer patient by helping to alleviate some of the associated pain and anxiety of the disease.

Similarly, acupressure can be an effective adjunct to chiropractic treatment. By relaxing and toning the back muscles, acupressure makes the spinal adjustments easier and more effective, and the results last longer. In fact, the two therapies were originally practiced together in ancient China.

Psychotherapy patients can derive benefits from acupressure by using it to heighten body awareness and deal with stress. When powerful emotions are free and unresolved, the body stores the resulting tension in the muscles. Acupressure can help restore emotional balance by releasing the accumulated tension caused by repressed feelings.

## ACUPRESSURE POINTS

An acupresssure point actually has two identities and ways of working. When you stimulate a point in the same area where you feel any pain or tension, it's called a "local point." That same point can also relieve pain in a part of the body that is distant from the point, in which case it is called a "trigger point." This triggering mechanism works through a human electrical channel called a Meridian.

### HOW TO FIND A POINT
Acupressure Point Names and Reference Numbers
You locate an acupressure point by referring to anatomical landmarks. Some acupressure points lie underneath major muscle groups. While points located near a bone structure usually lie in an indentation, muscular points lie within a muscular cord, band, or knot of tension. To stimulate the point, press directly on the cord or into the hollow.

As acupressure evolved, each of the 365 points was named poetically, originally with a Chinese character. The imagery of its name offers insight into either a point's benefits or location. For instance, the name Hidden Clarity refers to the mental benefit of the points: it clears the mind. Shoulder's Corner refers to that point's location. The Three Mile Point earned its name because it gives a person an extra three miles of energy. Runners and hikers have used this famous point to increase stamina and endurance.

Some of the names of the acupressure points also serve as a powerful meditation tool. By pressing a point and silently repeating its name while you visualize its benefit and breathe deeply, you can realize the full potential power that each point offers. As you hold the Sea of Vitality points in your lower back, breathe deeply and visualize each breath replenishing your deep reser-

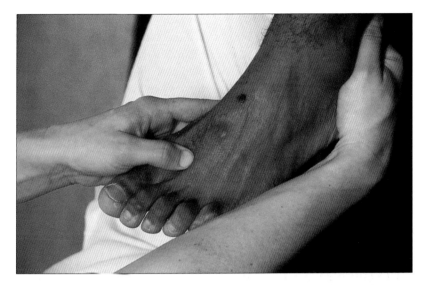

*Left: there are 365 acupressure points located on the body, each of which is poetically named. They are connected by the Meridians.*

voir of vitality. Use the power of your mind to strengthen and help heal your lower back.

You can create affirmations with the names of the points—powerful action statements that amplify a point's benefits. For example, hold the Letting Go points on the upper, outer chest with your fingertips. Breathe deeply. Imagine yourself

## THE HEALING BENEFITS

The healing benefits of acupressure involve both the relaxation of the body and its positive effects on the mind. As any tension is released, you not only feel good physically, but you also feel better emotionally and mentally. When your body relaxes, your mind relaxes as well, creating another state of consciousness. The expanded awareness leads to mental clarity and to a healthier physical and emotional healing, dissolving the division between the mind and body.

letting go of tension, frustration, and stress. As you hold and breathe into these points, repeat to yourself that you are now letting go of all the negativity and irritability.

In addition to its name, each point was assigned an identification number to track its placement along the body. Point location numbers, such as ST 3 or GB 21, are a standard referencing system used by professional acupressurists and acupuncturists.

### ARTHRITIS AND NONARTICULAR RHEUMATISM

It is believed that acupressure can relieve both muscle aches and arthritic pain, increase the mobility of your joints, strengthen them, and prevent further joint deterioration.

With some types of rheumatoid arthritis, it does take longer to increase joint mobility and reduce pain. Most people with arthritis will need to practice these self-acupressure techniques two to three times a day for six months and continue once a day for prevention and health maintenance.

Acupressure may be especially effective for relieving nonarticular (non-joint-related) rheumatism. This soft-tissue condition, also referred to as myofibrosis or fibrositis, has symptoms similar to rheumatoid arthritis, such as morning stiffness, muscle tenderness, debilitating fatigue, and often depression.

Medical doctors have found that patients who suffer from fibrositis, a disorder involving musculoskeletal pain and aching, especially in the morning, numbness, disturbed sleep, and fatigue, have tender areas that researchers have termed "tender points." These tender points on the body correspond to acupressure points used in traditional Chinese medicine. If you have arthritis, you can easily locate many of these points simply by pressing the areas where the pain concentrates. When you find the area, instead of massaging, rubbing, or kneading, simply hold it firmly for a few minutes. If it is extremely sensitive, then gradually decrease the pressure until you find a balance between pain and pleasure.

Acupressure can also be extremely effective in reducing the inflammation that accompanies arthritis. The potent points presented in this chapter are selected from 12 anti-inflammatory points. If they are stimulated on a regular, daily basis, they increase circulation, which in turn reduces inflammation and at the same time increases joint mobility.

## POTENT POINTS FOR RELIEVING ARTHRITIS

### JOINING THE VALLEY (HHOKU) (LI 4)

**Caution:** This point is forbidden for pregnant women until labor because its stimulation can cause premature contractions in the uterus.

**Location:** In the webbing between the thumb and index finger at the highest spot of the muscle when the thumb and index finger are brought close together.

**Benefits:** Relieves pain and inflammation in the hand, wrist, elbow, shoulder, and neck.

### OUTER GATE (TW 5)

**Location:** Two and one-half finger widths above the wrist crease on the outer forearm midway between the two bones of the arm.

**Benefits:** Relieves rheumatism, tendonitis, wrist pain, and shoulder pain.

### THREE MILE POINT (ST 36)

**Location:** Four finger widths below the kneecap, one finger width to the outside of the leg.

**Benefits:** Strengthens the body, benefits the joints, and relieves the fatigue that often results from the drain of dealing with arthritic pain.

### CROOKED POND (LI 11)

**Location:** On the upper edge of the elbow crease.

**Benefits:** Relieves arthritic pain, especially in the elbow and shoulder.

### GATES OF CONSCIOUSNESS (GB 20)

**Location:** Below the base of the skull, in the hollow between the two large, vertical neck muscles, two to three inches apart depending on the size of the head.

**Benefits:** Relieves arthritis, as well as the following common complaints that often accompany arthritic pain: headaches, insomnia, stiff neck, neck pain, fatigue and general irritability.

■ You do not have to use all of these points. Using just one or two of them whenever you have a free hand can be effective.

## BACKACHE AND SCIATICA

Back problems are one of the most common ailments in our society. Four out of five people have had severe back pain at least once in their lives. The majority of sciatica and lower-back problems are related to stress, poor posture, accidents, or weak abdominal muscles. Back muscle or ligament strains are possible causes as well, so it is extremely important to keep your spine and back muscles strong and flexible. Acupressure may be highly effective in relieving the muscular tension associated with lower-back pain and sciatica.

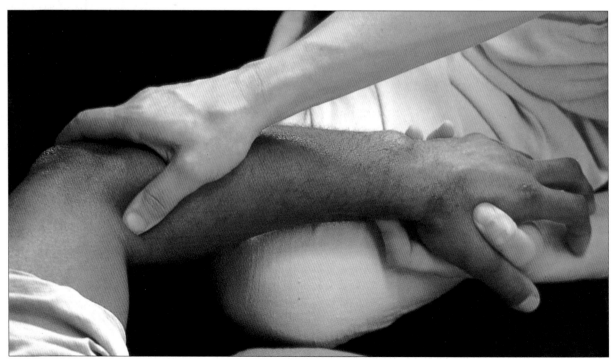

# POTENT POINT EXERCISES

Sit yourself down comfortably for the following routine.

**Step 1**

Press into LI 4: To press this anti-inflammatory point on your left hand, place your right thumb into the webbing between the thumb and index finger to gradually direct pressure underneath the bone that attaches to your index finger. Press for a couple of minutes while breathing deeply, then switch hands and work on your right hand.

**Step 2**

Press TW 5: To find this point, place the knuckles of your left hand on top of your right forearm two-and-one-half finger widths from the wrist crease. Use your knuckles to apply firm pressure on this joint as you breathe deeply for one minute. Switch hands and work on your left arm.

**Step 3**

Press LI 11: Bend your right arm in front of you with your palm facing down. To find this point, place the fingertips of your left hand on top of the right arm where the elbow crease ends. Press into the elbow joint firmly with your left fingers as you breathe deeply for one minute. Then switch sides and work on your left elbow.

**Step 4**

Firmly press GB 20: Place both of your thumbs underneath the base of your skull, two to three inches apart, into two hollow areas. Apply pressure gradually, as you slowly tilt your head back. Firmly press up and underneath the skull for one minute.

When your hip hurts or your lower back aches, your body automatically compensates for this weakness by taking pressure off that area and shifting it to another. This, unfortunately, shifts an extra burden to another area of your back, compounding the problem.

The effectiveness of acupressure can be enhanced by a healthy diet and the proper use of heat. According to traditional Chinese medicine, eating too much salt; drinking too much liquid; eating excessively cold foods as well as catching cold; and an excess of jarring exercise, fear, or paranoia can cause problems in the lower back area. Regularly practicing gentle back care exercises can help to prevent back problems.

Using a heating pad, hot water bottle, or hot bath (if there is no inflammation) can also be helpful because heat provides temporary relief from stiffness and pain. But when you use heat in conjunction with acupressure on a muscular problem, the relief from tension and pain often lasts longer.

**Caution:** Do not press on disintegrating discs or on fractured or broken bones. For severe lower-back or sciatic pain, you must always first consult a medical or osteopathic doctor, chiropractor, or physical therapist.

## POTENT POINTS FOR RELIEVING LOWER BACK ACHES

The following potent points stimulate the lower back to strengthen and heal it. The point behind the knee (B 54) is a special trigger point for alleviating lower-back pain. The Sea of Vitality points (B 23 and B47) in the lower back, and the Sea of Energy point (CV 6) in the lower abdomen help relieve back pain and especially benefit the kidneys and the urore-productive system. The Womb and Vitals point (B 48) in the buttocks is an effective lower-back and sciatic pain point. You can use any of these points separately or together in sequence for a more complete routine for relieving both sciatica and lower-back aches.

### SEA OF VITALITY (B 23 AND B 47)

**Caution:** If you have a weak back, the Sea of Vitality points may be quite tender. In this case a few minutes of light, stationary touch instead of deep pressure can be very healing. See your doctor first if you have any questions or need medical advice.

**Location:** In the lower back (between the second and third lumbar vertebrae) two to four finger widths away from the spine at waist level.

**Benefits:** Relieves lower-back aches, sciatica, and the fatigue that often results from the pain.

### WOMB AND VITALS (B 48)

**Location:** One to two finger widths outside the sacrum (the large bony area at the base of the spine) and midway between the top of the hipbone (iliac crest) and the base of the buttock.

**Benefits:** Relieves lower-back aches, sciatica, pelvic tension, hip pain, and tension.

# SHIATSU

## CHAPTER TWENTY SEVEN

*Shiatsu is a Japanese word made up of two written characters meaning "finger" (shi) and "pressure" (atsu). It describes a form of manipulative therapy, licenced by the Japanese government, which focuses on the use of static pressure applied to specific points and pathways all over the body. These points, called* tsubo *in Japanese, are also used in acupuncture and are sometimes called "acupoints" in English. The pathways along which most of the points are located are known as "channels" or "meridians." These form a comprehensive bodily system fundamental to the theory and practise of all oriental healing arts, involving the flow of bio-energy (Ki in Japanese or Chi in Chinese). Shiatsu therapy works to restore normal flow of this vital life energy to create optimum balance and health in the mind and body.*

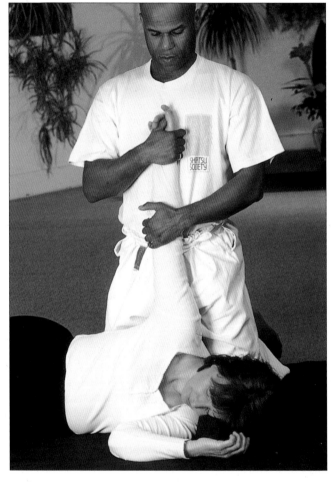

*Shiatsu is often called "acupressure," and stimulation of the points with pressure is one of the main, though not the only, technique used. In practice, pressure is applied to wide areas as well as precise points all over the body, using not only the fingers and thumbs but also the palms, elbows, knees and even the feet. Pressure may vary from light to quite firm and may be sustained or may involve rubbing, kneading and "brushing," much like massage. At times, very light "holding" techniques may be used almost like palm healing. In addition to meridian and point pressure, gentle stretch and manipulation techniques are used which work on the soft tissue and joints. Shiatsu then incorporates a variety of approaches, drawn from different traditions, both ancient and modern, all of which share a common element—touch. Shiatsu, therefore, is first and foremost a "hands-on" therapy.*

# HISTORY AND ORIGINS

The origins of Shiatsu lie in the natural response to injury, pain or discomfort—to rub the affected area feels comforting and often relieves the pain. From this automatic response to dis-ease in the body there evolved, through trial and error, a systematic approach to the relief of certain ailments by concentrating on certain key areas and points which were observed to trigger specific repeatable results. Originally this was done in an intuitive manner; but, over time, theories developed which attempted to explain such phenomena. These theories became the basis of a healthcare system which has remained in practical use for several thousand years in the East, and to which Shiatsu belongs.

In the earliest recorded Chinese medical text, *The Yellow Emperor's Classic of Internal Medicine*, written over 2,000 years ago, the origins and development of different medical disciplines was attributed to the different regions of China; the geography, diet and lifestyle varied enormously between these regions, and so did disease patterns. Thus acupuncture, massage and herbal medicine evolved side by side to treat the range of diseases encountered.

The traditional massage of ancient China was known as "Anmo" and found its way to Japan in the eighth century to be adopted and adapted by the Japanese, who called it "Anma." In Japan, Anma therapy gradually became a profession associated with blind people and enjoyed an excellent reputation for several centuries. However, as Western medical influences began to predominate by the nineteenth century, it began to be looked down upon as folklore and almost suffered extinction during the Meiji era. Not until recently, as part of a general revival of Far Eastern traditional medical systems, has Anma therapy begun to re-emerge as a popular and effective form of healthcare.

The term "Shiatsu" itself is relatively new and refers specifically to the pressure techniques employed in the original Anma or Do-In-Ankyo system, which also involved a comprehensive range of exercise, diet, meditation, massage and manipulation. The recent incorporation of elements of physiotherapy reflects the integration of Eastern and Western approaches in modern Japan where Shiatsu is now gradually regaining stature.

In Western countries, Shiatsu is really coming into its own as a respected therapy and is being enjoyed by thousands in Europe and North America for the prevention and treatment of many common ailments. It is enjoying a particular upsurge in popularity in Britain where there is a National Society with a register of qualified practitioners and accredited schools.

Shiatsu is readily available as private treatment in multi-disciplinary complementary health clinics or at home, but there are many examples of Shiatsu being used in hospital settings and of family doctors referring patients directly to practitioners. The role of Shiatsu within the healthcare system, public and private, is therefore in the process of developing rapidly in response to a genuine demand for this type of safe, effective therapy.

# PHILOSOPHY AND OBJECTIVES

Oriental Medicine, although it embraces the logic and empiricism of a science, has its roots in philosophy and cosmology. In observing natural phenomena, the earliest philosophers attempted to describe the laws that determine life and its processes. Universal theories evolved that employed symbolic language and concepts in an attempt to express the particular through the general. For example, the terms Yin and Yang, literally meaning the "shadow" and the "light," derived their symbolic meaning from nature (the moon and the sun respectively). These terms could then be used to symbolize many other natural phenomena with similar characteristics, such as cold, night and winter in the case of Yin, and heat, day and summer in the case of Yang.

Similarly, the naturally occurring elements of fire, water, wood, metal and earth were each used to symbolize a quality of energy and movement that corresponded to their organic state. For example, the energy of fire was seen as expansive and dynamic and therefore came to symbolize heat, summer, the color red and the day, whereas the energy of water was associated with a downward, contracting movement symbolic of cold, winter, the color black and the night. Thus fire was considered Yang compared to water which was Yin.

The use of such symbols lay in their descriptive universality. The theories of Yin and Yang and the Five Elements were used, not only to define the external physical environment, but also to interpret the life process itself. In clinical medicine, for example, a patient with a red face, fever and daytime sweats was characterized as having a Yang disease, while chills, pallor (with black circles under the eyes) and night sweating belonged to Yin. In physiology, because the heart was seen as extremely dynamic and is responsible for circulation and warmth, it was

## THE MERIDIAN SYSTEM

The principle on which the mechanism of "external" treatments like Shiatsu rest is the existence of a physiological system unique to Oriental medicine—the channel or meridian system. Oriental healing and martial arts have always believed that all energy circulates and vitalizes the whole person via these specific pathways. The written character for "meridian" suggests a criss-cross network of interconnected channels which link the skin, flesh, muscle, bone and vital organs into a unified whole. The character for the energy that flows in the meridians literally means "breath" or "gas" and suggests something vital which characterizes movement and change within the body, symbolic of all physiological processes.

associated with the element of fire, while the kidney, with its connection to fluid metabolism and moisturizing (cooling) was connected with water.

The theory and practice of the healing arts were therefore guided in every aspect by these basic philosophies which explains the highly symbolic language of Traditional Chinese Medicine (TCM) today.

### BALANCING YIN AND YANG

In TCM, health and disease are seen as manifestations of the delicate balance between Yin and Yang, between the subtle energy movements within the organism. A plant needs light (Yang) and also water (Yin), a human being food (Yin) and oxygen (Yang). The diagnosis of disease rests on the accurate assessment of which part of

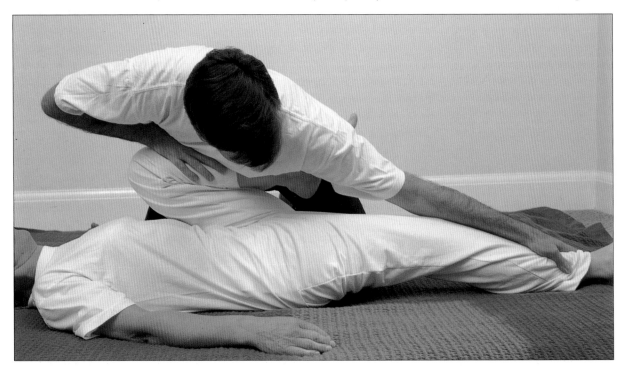

the energetic whole is out of balance. The treatment principle and method then follows automatically. For example, a patient with cold hands and feet can be characterized in TCM terms as suffering from heart (associated with fire and the warming function) Yang (dynamic circulatory function) deficiency. Treatment is aimed at supplementing the Yin of the kidney. Treatment methods vary according to the condition. For example, treating the Yin (vital body substances) is usually done from the inside with herbs, while treating the Yang (vital body functions) is mostly achieved from the outside by either acupuncture, moxibustion (a form of heat treatment) and by various manipulative therapies including Shiatsu.

## DIAGNOSING ENERGY IMBALANCE

In martial arts, learning to sense and direct the flow of energy through the meridians is the key to harnessing the power needed in combat. In medicine, the practitioner learns to detect deficiencies and blockages of this energy and directs treatment at restoring its normal flow. In Shiatsu this is done through careful and continuous palpation of each of the meridians both before, during and after treatment.

"Diagnosis" involves characterizing the nature of the energy imbalance in terms of the affected meridian(s) and successful treatment implies a palpable change in the movement and balance of the energy flow. The meridians are named according to the vital organ each connects with so that a Shiatsu diagnosis might be "heart deficiency,"

## DEVELOPING INTUITION AND SENSITIVITY

In Shiatsu, the "form" consists of a series of interconnected movements to enable the giver to apply correct leaning pressure to the different parts of the receiver's body. It requires a level of precision and skill which seems almost mechanical at first, but which, like the Zen example, encourage concentration and quieten the mind to allow the direct experience of giving and receiving the pressure to be felt. Through the "form" the giver develops a level of body awareness and sensitivity which far outweighs their ability to understand what it is that is actually felt or done in Shiatsu. Curiously, perhaps, it is through the discipline of strict technical application that intuition, one of the key elements of Shiatsu, can be developed. The practice of the "form" can become a liberating rather than a limiting experience.

which may not refer to a physical heart problem as such; rather to the fact that the energy of its meridian is hypofunctioning.

Treatment is then aimed at restoring normal energy flow in that channel by balancing the total meridian system. The practitioner does not transmit energy into the patient; he uses the patient's own energy and simply guides the re-balancing process.

## PRACTICAL APPLICATION

Shiatsu involved the application of static pressure to the body and is governed by the basic laws of physics. Gravity is the main ally, not muscular strength and the most important principle, universally applied to all techniques in Shiatsu, is that of natural, leaning pressure. Only the body weight is used, without pushing, pressing or squeezing, like a crawling baby whose body is supported without effort by its arms and legs.

This may sound easy, and it certainly requires no effort, but in practice it often involves rediscover-

ing the kind of unconscious, automatic and highly integrated way in which we first began using our bodies as babies. The basics of Shiatsu therefore involve as much how to apply pressure as to where. This involves the careful positioning of the body so as to lean or "rest" on the receiver, from any angle, in any position, comfortably and without effort.

### THE "FORM"

Initially, then, the practice of Shiatsu involves perfecting the art of moving into precisely the correct position to apply natural leaning pressure to any given area of the body. Such movements assume a rhythm and flow of their own, in which precision and grace, discipline and spontaneity combine in a dance-like sequence. This is often referred to as the "form." All martial arts practitioners are familiar with the concept and practice of a particular "form" of movement associated with their chosen discipline, be it Karate, Judo, T'ai Chi or any other. In fact, this notion of form extends to the study and practice of all oriental art and sciences, from calligraphy to flower arranging, from the tea ceremony to paper folding.

Indeed, a broader understanding of oriental culture in general reveals many subtle levels at which this concept of "form" operates. The way one looks, behaves and even thinks are all greatly influenced by how these factors may appear to others. Conformity is considered a virtue and contributes to the collective "form" of society and ultimately to its peace and harmony. To act out of self-interest shows a disregard for the group and goes against the common good.

In the field of medicine, to threaten such harmony (in this case symbolized by the accepted laws of nature) would be literally to endan-ger your health. Many of the medical classics emphasized the need to live in harmony with such laws, which governed all aspects of life including exercise, rest, diet, emotions and relationships as well as climate, season and geography.

Thus a concern for the "form" of things is paramount, though this is not to say that such a concern is for things simply to look good; it has a purpose which is both subtle and powerful. It aims to liberate the mind and allow the body to experience things directly. For example, in Zen meditation there is a form of sitting and walking while focusing on the breath, and maintaining a certain posture for a certain length of time.

The ultimate purpose may be to attain a spiritual goal (enlightenment), but the form is essentially practical. The more you concentrate on sitting, walking and breathing the less your mind tries to work out the purpose of it all. Only when the mind is quiet can the value of the experience of meditation be fully appreciated. What may at first seem empty ritual actually provides the focus for developing concentration, awareness and, ultimately, peace of mind.

## TECHNIQUES OF APPLYING PRESSURE

There are specific principles which govern the practice of Shiatsu and the actual techniques of applying the pressure. These include vertical pressure which is perpendicular to the surface being worked on; steady pressure which is sustained and flowing;

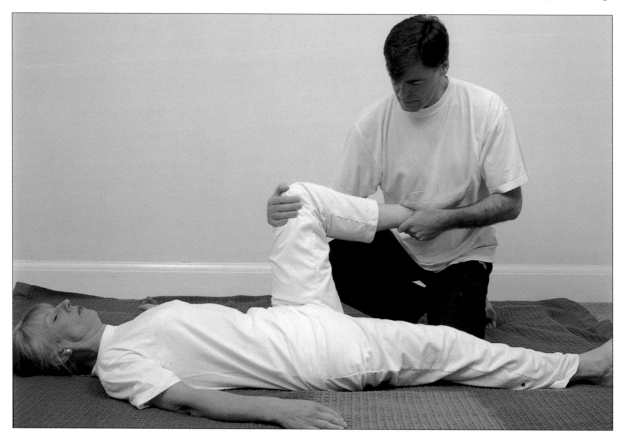

supporting pressure which allows the giver to rest their weight comfortably on the receiver without effort or strain; and equal pressure which maintains a uniform weight distribution causing minimum disturbance to the receiver. Pressure is applied variously with the thumbs, fingers, palms, elbows, knees and feet all over the body in four different positions—prone (on the belly), supine (on the back), side and sitting.

# VISITING A PRACTITIONER

## WHAT TO EXPECT
Shiatsu is always given on floor level, usually on the kind of Japanese cotton mattress known as a "futon." Any foam mattress or blanket that is fairly firm and not springy will do—a sprung mattress is no good. The receiver must be supported properly as pressure is applied which is why a bed is not suitable. The floor is preferable to a treatment couch, as the giver can move around the receiver much more easily and can lean their body weight over the top of them without effort. If a pillow is used it should be firm and small; an ordinary bed pillow is not usually appropriate.

The giver and receiver of Shiatsu should both wear loose, comfortable natural-fiber (cotton) clothing—a thin tracksuit is fine.

When giving Shiatsu to areas of exposed skin, such as the hands, feet, face and neck, a thin cotton hand towel or cloth is often used. Unlike in other massage forms, there is generally no direct contact with the bare skin in Shiatsu, since there is neither anything applied to it (e.g. oils) nor is there any need to slide along it.

The thin layer of cotton between the giver and receiver allows the giver to move easily from one position to the next without stretching or pinching the skin, and avoids any unpleasant contact if the giver or receiver has cold, sweaty or clammy skin.

## CONDITIONS
Conditions, such as room temperature, light, sound etc., are designed to make the receiver feel comfortable in every respect, but not so much so that they switch off to their surroundings and to the giver. The ideal state to be in when receiving Shiatsu is somewhere between being awake and asleep, in a state of complete relaxation as in meditation. This level of deep relaxation allows the receiver to be more receptive to the effects of the treatment.

## TIME OF DAY
Shiatsu can be given at any time of the day, though according to the theory of energy circulation and season there is always an ideal time for each individual. Evening is naturally an ideal time to receive Shiatsu for relaxation

before going to bed though it can be very invigorating in the morning before starting the day also. Shiatsu is not advised, however, when over-tired, on a full stomach or under the influence of drugs or alcohol.

## A SHIATSU SESSION
It is usually best to rest for about 15 minutes following the treatment and to allow the mind and body to "come to" slowly again as Shiatsu can produce a sleepy, euphoric feeling. Each session usually lasts about an hour, rarely more as the effects can often be counter-productive. It seems that the body has its own kind of attention span like the mind, which varies from person to person. In some cases 30 minutes will be enough. It is perfectly healthy to receive up to two or even three Shiatsu treatments a week, though in practice one is usual. Treatments for specific problems, such as a stiff neck, require a series of treatments lasting weeks and perhaps even months to make a lasting difference, though the first time a person receives Shiatsu is often the most dramatic.

# BASIC GUIDELINES

The basic guidelines as to when and where not to receive Shiatsu are similar to those of any treatment which affects the flow of energy, blood and body fluids through the system. These include times of high fever, especially when accompanied by local infection or inflammation or by infectious disease of any sort, cancer, heart disease, and areas where there may be cuts, bruises, scar tissue, injury or swelling. However, since Shiatsu techniques vary from the very dynamic to the soft and gentle, it could still be possible to use the supportive quality of some of the holding techniques in most of these situations. In fact, Shiatsu has been used effectively to complement other approaches in the treatment of various forms of cancer, heart disease, HIV and AIDS.

**A two-way process**

Shiatsu is a two-way process and relies to some extent on the responsiveness of the receiver as well as the giver. When receiving treatment the receiver will often be expected to participate actively in the treatment by using their breath to relax the whole body and in between sessions by following a series of exercises designed to enhance the therapeutic effect. Essentially, Shiatsu works best when it is able to impact the various factors which affect overall health and this naturally extends beyond the treatment time itself. In turn, this requires a certain level of commitment on the part of the person receiving the treatment.

## THE BENEFITS OF SHIATSU

The main principle of treatment relied upon in Shiatsu is that of the body's own innate ability to balance and heal itself. The method by which this is achieved relies on the proper stimulation of the body's energy system which includes the meridians and points. In practice, when correct pressure is applied, a positive effect is always achieved. That is to say the receiver's homeostatic or self-regulating abilities are activated and the system will begin to balance itself naturally. A "Kyo" type person who is basically weaker will respond more slowly to this process than a "Jitsu" type who is basically stronger. The job of the Shiatsu practitioner is to assess these strengths and weaknesses in terms of the person's illness and in their ability to respond to it and to redistribute

## EVALUATING SHIATSU

In trying to describe the benefits of Shiatsu, it is difficult to list specific results in terms of the systems of the body as we understand them from a Western perspective. The fact is that Shiatsu does not lend itself well to this approach, and, unlike Western massage which has been adopted for its specific remedial effects in cases of tension, injury and so on, Shiatsu must be evaluated in terms of the system to which it belongs.

Attempts have been made to equate the oriental concept of the energy system with, for example, the nervous system, but these correspondences are imprecise and ultimately invalid. Naturally, since Shiatsu works on the body it affects the nervous, circulatory, respiratory and musculo-skeletal systems. However, through its stimulation of the hormone system it can also affect the digestive and reproductive systems. In fact, the more specific one attempts to be in describing the effects of Shiatsu, the more general and wide reaching seems to be the picture.

It is enough to say that Shiatsu can and does help with a variety of ailments, particularly chronic, persistent ones, helping to reduce stress, aid the digestive system, relieve pain, improve mental, physical and sexual functioning, help musculo-skeletal problems and promote overall health. Apart from bringing relief to symptoms, it gradually corrects longterm postural and behavioral imbalances leading to improved body/mind awareness and a general sense of wellbeing and peace of mind. It is the ultimate purpose of Shiatsu to regulate the energetic system linking mind, body and spirit, to create a more whole and complete experience of ourselves.

their available energy resources to restore harmony to the system using the meridians.

Stimulation of the meridians and points frees up blocked energy and draws it toward areas of weakness. According to one of the laws of Yin and Yang an extreme of one can transform to its opposite. So in areas of blockage (Jitsu) where there may be Yang phenomena such as tightness, heat and pain which feels uncomfortable to the touch, firmer, quicker pressure (also Yang) is used to disperse the blockage—Yang meets Yang and turns to Yin producing release and relaxation. Conversely, in areas of weakness (Kyo) where there may be more Yin phenomena, such as emptiness, cold and aches, which welcome touch, softer, lingering pressure (more Yin) may be used to draw energy to the area—Yin meets Yin and turns to Yang, producing an invigorating, revitalizing effect.

These are basically the two main approaches to giving Shiatsu: the one more dynamic and releasing, and the other more gentle and nourishing. The elements of stretch and manipulation obviously relate to the former, whilst the latter include the more static pressure techniques. However, within any one technique you can bring both Yin and Yang elements into play, and most Shiatsu is in reality a natural combination of these.

## SHIATSU THERAPY

Shiatsu is not a therapy that lends itself to self-help and which you can do yourself at home. However, the following guide helps to explain what happens in Shiatsu and shows that it is a two-way process between the giver and the receiver, working on moving energy from one part of the body to another.

## SHIATSU TECHNIQUES

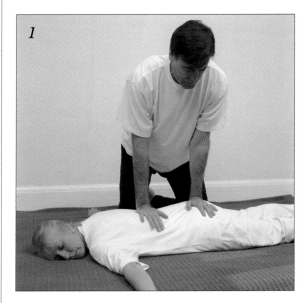

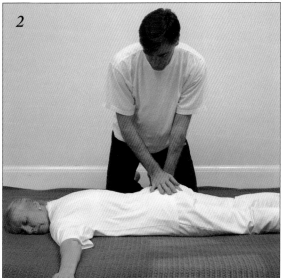

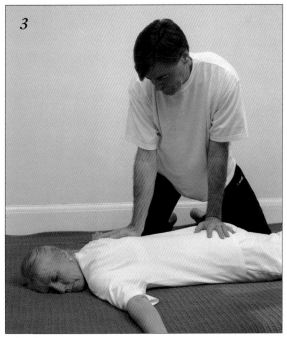

*1 The Shiatsu practitioner may start by gentle rocking up and down the body to encourage a degree of relaxation in the patient.*

*2 Pressure is applied to the sacrum, with the practitioner using his body weight. He then applies pressure along the spine, working up along the Governor Vessel, the important channel that runs up the spine.*

*3 He stretches out the spine, including the meridians that run along it, the muscles, tendons and ligaments. This, too, helps to encourage a state of relaxation in the patient.*

# SHIATSU TECHNIQUES

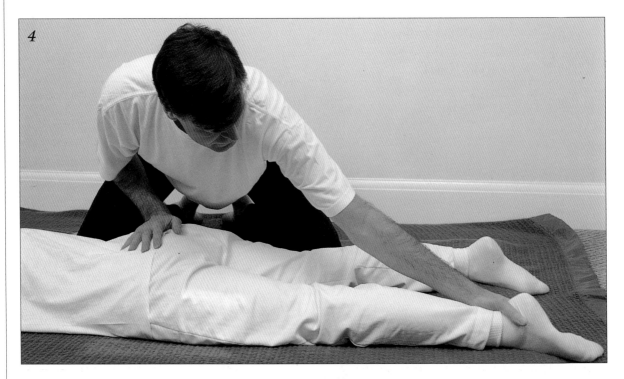

4 The Shiatsu practitioner then stretches out the feet and legs. In so doing, he stretches the hamstrings, the calf muscles and the meridians.

5 He stretches out the whole of the lower torso by pulling.

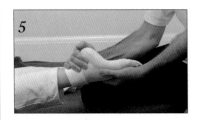

6 The legs and feet are bent back and held while pressure is applied to the lower back.

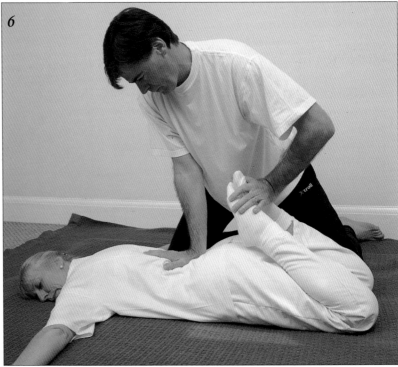

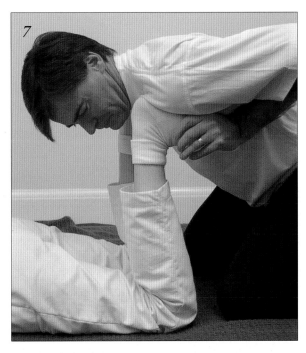

7 The gall bladder meridians run down the side of the body and the legs. The Shiatsu practitioner works on the legs gently.

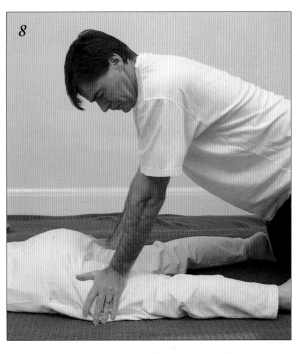

8 The backs of the legs and the muscles in the hips and thighs are stretched out, and pressure is applied along the meridians.

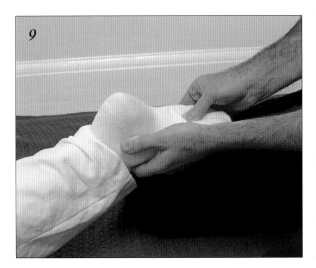

9 There are some important acupuncture points on the bottom of each foot and these can be pressed to revitalize the patient's whole body.

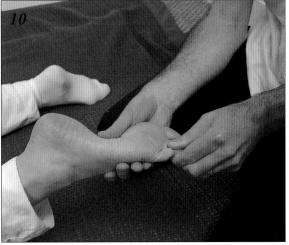

10 The ends of the meridians finish in the toes, so the Shiatsu practitioner ends this part of the session by tweaking the toes of the patient.

# SHIATSU TECHNIQUES

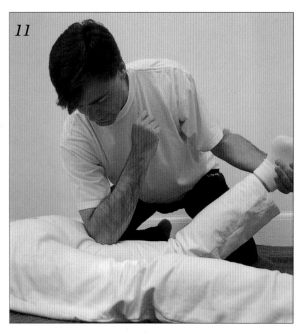

11 The Shiatsu practitioner applies the kidney crunch, lifting the patient's leg up. This is sometimes beneficial for people who have lower back problems.

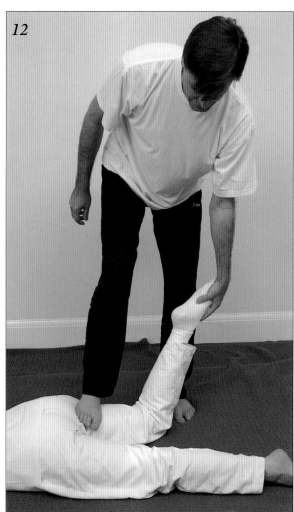

12 The treading technique applies deeper pressure to the meridians. It can be done either with a foot or an elbow. Shiatsu can bring relief by putting pressure on the trigger points.

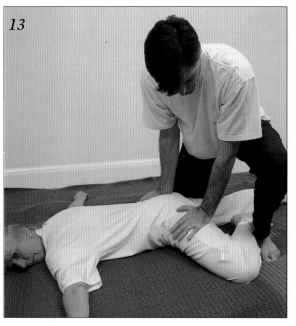

13 The practitioner works on the leg meridians, twisting with one leg across the other and working on the gall bladder meridian.

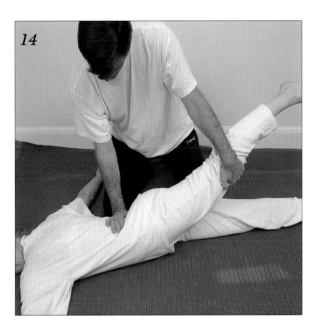

14 For treating the meridians on the legs, one hand is placed on the "hara" while fingertip pressure moves along the direction of the meridian.

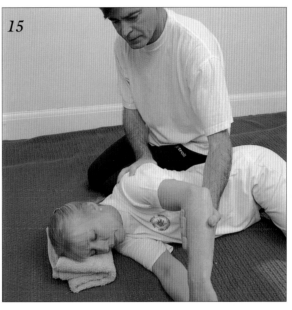

15 With the patient in the "recovery" position, the arm and shoulder are circled in a relaxed position and then at full stretch.

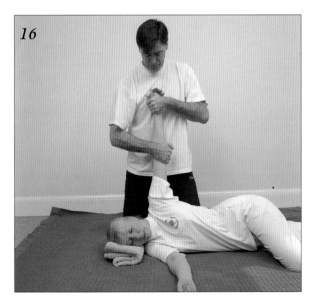

16 The Shiatsu practitioner works on the patient's hands and arms, again stretching out the meridians at full stretch.

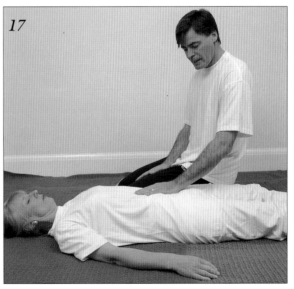

17 He also works on the "hara" area (the stomach), starting with the palm of the hand pressing down on the hara, gently but firmly.

## SHIATSU TECHNIQUES

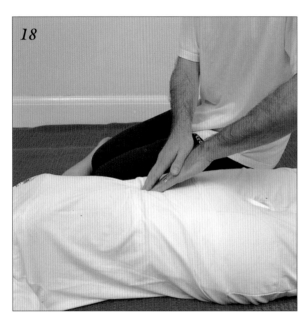

18 The Shiatsu practitioner continues to work on the "hara," pressing down on the stomach with the fingertips of both hands.

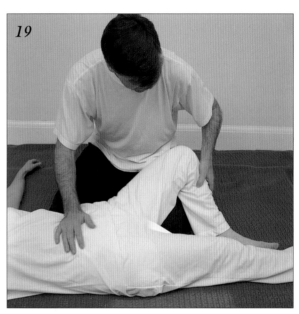

19 With the palm of one hand still resting on the "hara," he moves on further down the body to the legs, stretching them out gently.

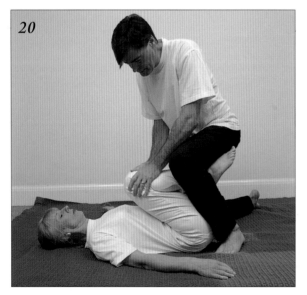

20 The patient's legs are bent at the knees and pushed back into the body, the practitioner pressing down with his body weight.

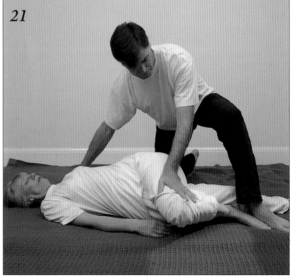

21 The patient's leg is bent across her other leg to the side and the hips turned as the practitioner presses down on the upper leg.

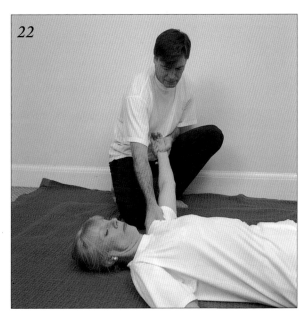

22 The practitioner works on the arms to pull them, stretching them out to the sides and pressing down firmly on the shoulder.

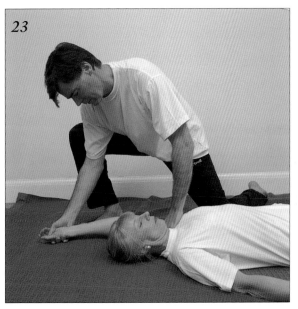

23 With pressure still being applied to the shoulder, the patient's arm is pulled back at full stretch behind the head.

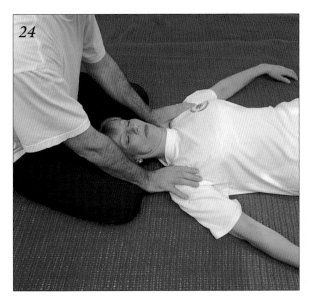

24 The Shiatsu practitioner then moves on to the patient's shoulders, pressing down and applying pressure.

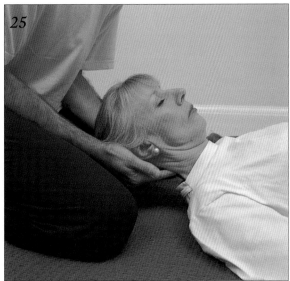

25 The session ends with the practitoner working on the neck, supporting the patient's head and pulling back gently.

# T'AI CHI CH'UAN

## CHAPTER TWENTY EIGHT

*T*he Chinese martial arts, from their inception, were always valued for improving fitness, health and longevity as well as for their usefulness as self-defense systems. This has been particularly true for a special kind of Chinese martial art called T'ai Chi Ch'uan (Tajiquan), which originated several hundred years ago and which has become one of the most popular forms of exercise in the world.

It is estimated that more than 10 million people practice some kind of T'ai Chi Ch'uan daily in China and that over one million practice in Japan. During the past 30 years, it has grown more and more outside of Asia, and is now widely practiced in Australia, the United States, Canada and Europe. It is recognized readily by millions of people who have seen its exponents in parks or on television, practicing the graceful, slow, liquid movements that look like a ballet underwater.

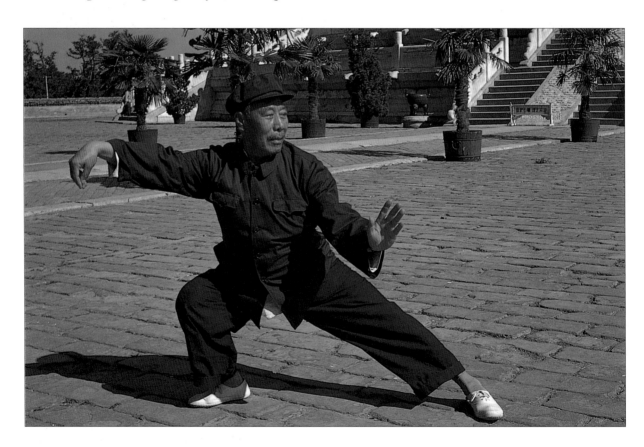

# THE HEALTH BENEFITS

## PHYSICAL BENEFITS

There have been many claims for the health benefits of T'ai Chi Ch'uan, which has some of the qualities of Hatha Yoga, but is performed while standing. Some of the more obvious benefits that can be derived from this are greater flexibility, improved circulation, better balance and, equally important, the intangible benefit of achieving a greatly enhanced sense of wellbeing.

Studies both inside and outside of China have shown that old people who practiced T'ai Chi enjoyed better health than other people of the same age in terms of cardiovascular function, breathing function, bone condition and metabolism. A growing number of medical and healthcare professionals are becoming aware of the benefits of T'ai Chi Ch'uan and are recommending it to their patients and even taking classes themselves. However, for many healthcare providers, T'ai Chi is still virgin territory. Many scientists in physiology, biochemistry, immunology and endocrinology have made studies in recent years of the health benefits that can be experienced from practicing T'ai Chi Ch'uan, and they found, among other things, that practitioners have lower than average blood pressure and blood viscosity.

Research studies also indicate that while T'ai Chi promotes an even circulation of blood, the metabolism remains normal, and acid and alkali are basically balanced. It also seems to help maintain a high level of oxygen, which improves the metabolism of oxygen and the storage of energy.

The slow movements allow for

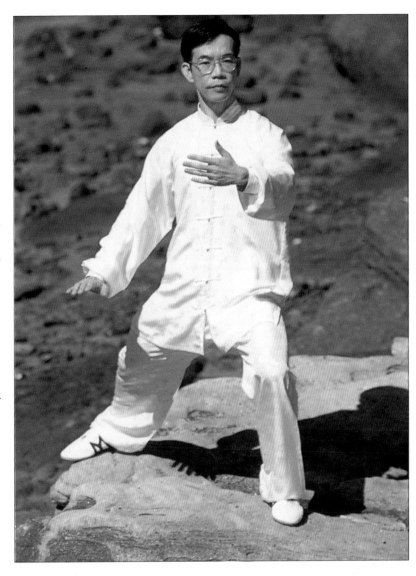

training the muscle fiber of the bones and elasticity of the smooth muscle of the vascular wall, improving the stability of the vascular motor nerve and the circulation of the blood.

## PROMOTING RELAXATION

Some studies have also indicated that T'ai Chi can be helpful in achieving a state of relaxation of the whole body which helps to quiet the mind and promote relaxation. Some forms of T'ai Chi, which are practiced more

vigorously, also help to strengthen the cardiovascular system.

One study in China observed a group of 120 persons, aged between 50 and 80 years, and who had practiced T'ai Chi Ch'uan for many years. They found that after practice 92.3 percent of the group became noticably more cheerful and optimistic. Another study examined a group of patients in a sanitorium who were given treatment that combined T'ai Chi Ch'uan with medicine and

# THE GUIDING PRINCIPLES

Some of the guiding principles of T'ai Chi Ch'uan are listed as follows:

■ **Relaxation**
This involves being loose and also providing extension in the arms, legs and torso to loosen the joints. It is also required to achieve proper alignment of the arms, legs, hips, back and shoulders.

■ **To sink**
This refers to letting the intrinsic energy, or Qi, go to the dantian, or lower abdomen, so that it can accumulate energy and be the power behind all movements. Advanced practitioners have drumlike abdomens and attribute their skill and good health to their success in letting the energy sink to the dantian.

■ **Coordination**
All the movements in T'ai Chi should be coordinated properly so that the whole body is connected and each movement involves bringing energy up through the legs, hips, back and shoulders, and out through the arms and hands.

■ **No external or awkward strength is used**
External strength is segmented and not connected with the rest of the body. It is not as effective or efficient as the unitary, coordinated energy of the entire body which is the ideal of T'ai Chi.

■ **The movements must be slow and continuous**
In T'ai Chi, all movements should be slow and continuous, without stopping. The speed of the movement can vary with the styles of the individual. Although some movements may appear to pause, this is not the case.

■ **The cultivation of a calm mind and clear spirit**
This process starts from the very beginning of T'ai Chi practice and continues, helping to support that practice over the years. If properly developed, a calm mind and clear spirit support all the activities of the practitioner.

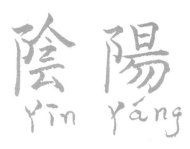

China, tries to harmonize various parts of the body, the emotions, mind and spirit, while at the same time becoming more aware of the various states of inner conflict, such as tension and relaxation, that exist in the body and mind.

The arena for this practice is what is called the "form," or solo practice, but it can also include weapons exercises, two-person self-defense routines and even contact sparring. It can also involve standing in certain postures from a few minutes to an hour to foster tranquillity, inner strength and rootedness.

## INTERNAL STRENGTH

All methods are intended to cultivate what is referred to as an internal strength, an inner strength based on Qi (chi), a Chinese concept referring to the intrinsic energy that courses through the body along pathways called meridians. Points along these pathways are acupuncture points, which are treated by acupuncturists to alleviate disease and are used by some T'ai Chi practitioners as points of focus to direct the internal energy which can make a T'ai Chi practitioner very strong. In fact, the longer a person practices, the stronger he or she may get if he is practicing correctly. Persons of 70, 80 or 90 years old, men or women, may be very strong from their practice and tend to

physiotherapy. The results indicated an improved rate of recovery for 80 percent of the group, as compared with 34.6 percent when the patients were treated with medicine only.

## PHILOSOPHY OF T'AI CHI

Although there are five major styles of T'ai Chi Ch'uan, all are based on certain root principles and characteristics and draw deeply on China's rich cultural history. The name itself, which means "Supreme Ultimate

Fist," is taken for the concept and philosophy of T'ai Chi, which is symbolized in the Yin and Yang symbol. This represents polar opposites that are brought into dynamic harmony and balance. However, the philosophy of Yin and Yang can be taken to mean the great diversity of the phenomenal world being brought into harmony and balance even as all the same elements of diversity are constantly sinking into conflict.

As part of the practice of T'ai Chi Ch'uan, the serious practitioner, or player, as they are referred to in

show fewer signs of aging. And since the exercise is done slowly, smoothly and with relaxation, it can still be practiced at an advanced age. There are practitioners in China who are over 90 years old, and one famous master lived to be over 100 years old.

## ORIGINS OF T'AI CHI

According to the T'ai Chi Ch'uan mythology, it was conceived in the Sung dynasty, in the thirteenth and fourteenth centuries by a Taoist known as Chang San-Feng, who had studied martial arts at the Shaolin Temple as well as various spiritual disciplines, such as Buddhism and Taosim. While at a retreat at Wadang Mountain, he was said to have looked out of a window

*Right: T'ai Chi Ch'uan may involve slow, continuous graceful movements or standing in a particular posture for anything from a few minutes to an hour. It increases flexibility and promotes relaxation.*

### OVERALL LIFE IMPROVEMENT

Perhaps one of the most important aspects of T'ai Chi Ch'uan is that when people study and practice it over a long period of time, it is usually one of many activities in which the individual participates to improve his or her health and life. In this way, T'ai Chi can be used to complement and support healthy diet, other exercises, meditation, or spiritual practice.

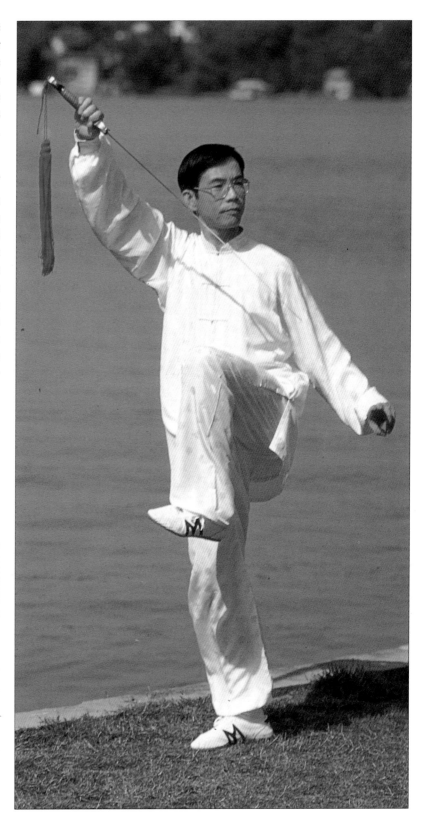

and to have observed the interplay between a magpie and a snake as they fought. The swooping attacks of the bird and the elusive movements of the snake inspired him to create a martial art based on the interplay of Yin and Yang, as opposed to the practice of using strength to overcome an opponent.

T'ai Chi Ch'uan is also attributed to Chen Wang-ting, who lived in seventeenth-century China. He drew on his extensive martial art experience to create five routines in the Chen family village. This form of T'ai Chi Ch'uan came to be known as the Chen style. It was later learned in the nineteenth century by a man named Yang Lu-ch'uan, who became famous for his martial skill. He modified T'ai Chi so that more people could learn the form, and the Yang style has subsequently become the most popular form of T'ai Chi Ch'uan in China and throughout the world.

Later major styles were also developed from the Yang style, and there were also Wu and Sun styles, which were named after other important practitioners. There are a number of other styles too, but they have not become as popular. T'ai Chi Ch'uan was later embraced as a health discipline by the Communists when they siezed power in China in 1949, and it was promoted, with modifications, to reduce the self-defense aspects. Today, shortened, modified forms of T'ai Chi Ch'uan are still practiced throughout China, but the traditional forms also thrive.

## A LONG LEARNING PROCESS

Be aware that learning T'ai Chi Ch'uan is not necessarily easy. Although it looks simple when you watch an experienced player practice the art, it does take time to learn the movements and to be relaxed and coordinated in them. Depending upon your mind-set, the effort required is part of the fun. Even when you have learned one or more T'ai Chi forms, the learning process can continue as long as you practice, if that is your bent; masters with decades of experience continue to learn in internal, if not external, ways.

## PRACTICE REGULARLY

When you have selected a place to learn, make practice a part of your regular routine, preferably at a particular time of the day, so that you don't have to find special time each day to do it. If you have to make a decision each day, then the chances are that some other activity may crowd it out. You can derive benefits by practicing T'ai Chi occasionally, but the benefit and enjoyment you will get are directly related to the amount of time and effort you apply. You should regard your study as a long-time practice in which small gains which are accumulated regularly over a period of time are more important than momentous breakthroughs. It is always a good idea to supplement your practice with readings about the principles and philosophy of T'ai Chi Ch'uan and to include as part of your development the exploration of other alternative health methods.

*Below: T'ai Chi Ch'uan is so popular in China that 10 million people still practice it daily.*

## FINDING A TEACHER

■ To find a teacher, it is best to contact a local martial arts school and ask if they know of a reputable teacher. It may also be useful to check with local colleges and universities, municipal recreation departments and health spas.

■ Determining the quality of the teacher is very subjective and depends in large part on the chemistry between the student and teacher. Foremost, you should be satisfied with the character of the teacher and the method of teaching used.

■ Then you should try to determine if the practice conforms to generally accepted T'ai Chi principles, such as being relaxed, coordinated, calm, fluid and balanced.

■ For some people, it helps to talk to the instructor, but some instructors are best teaching rather then talking about their teaching.

■ You can go along and observe a class or sign up for a short period only, such as a month. It is sensible to avoid long-term commitments or contracts until you have had a realistic experience with a teacher.

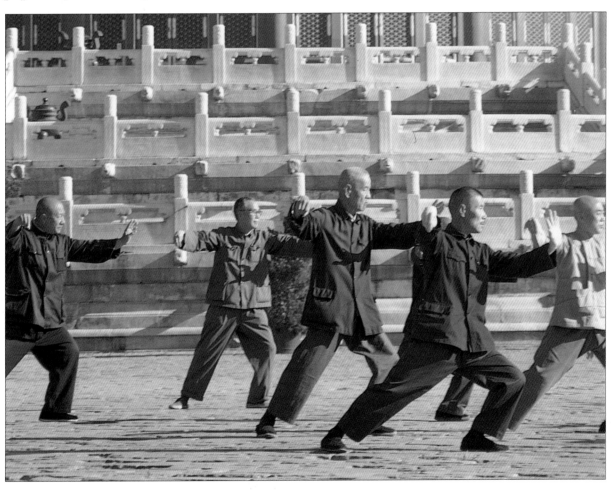

# CHINESE HERBAL MEDICINE

## CHAPTER TWENTY NINE

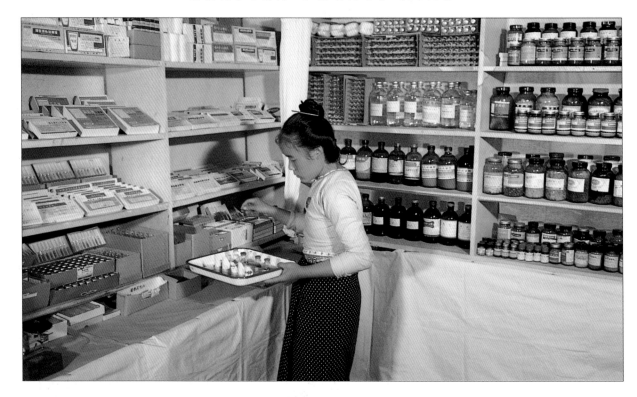

*C*hinese Herbal Medicine has been used for nearly the last 4,000 years; the earliest written record dates from 2000B.C. Obviously through the passing of the years some of the ideas have radically altered. Initially the Chinese considered that the main cause of disease was due to displeasure of ancestors. However, from about 1000B.C. it was attributed to attacks by demons. Then herbs were used in conjunction with spells, incantations and rituals to exorcize them.

In ancient China, large prosperous households retained their own Herbalist. The Herbalist was paid when the household was healthy and not when they were unwell. Thus Herbalists were concerned with preserving health, as opposed to purely treating disease.

# TRADITIONAL CHINESE MEDICINE

As it is practiced today, Traditional Chinese Medicine dates from the "Warring States" era (476-221B.C.) It was during this period that all of the main foundations were laid:

◼ Yin and Yang
◼ The Five Elements
◼ Energetics and Flavors
◼ Qi and Blood.
◼ The Eight Principles (This term was coined in the seventeenth century. but the main aspects were discussed at this time.)

## ◼ ZANG FU

Traditional Chinese Medicine is a theoretical understanding of how the body works, how we are born, live, get sick, subsequently get well again and finally die. The way that it is used is either through Herbs, Diet, Acupuncture or Qi Gong.

# THE THEORIES OF TRADITIONAL CHINESE MEDICINE

### 1 YIN-YANG

The Yin-Yang symbol is becoming increasingly well known throughout the Western world. It symbolizes opposites.

| Yin | Yang |
| --- | --- |
| Shady side of the valley | Sunny side of the valley |
| Night | Day |
| Cold | Hot |
| Female | Male |
| Rest | Activity |

Not only are Yin and Yang opposite to each other, but also one cannot exist without the other. For

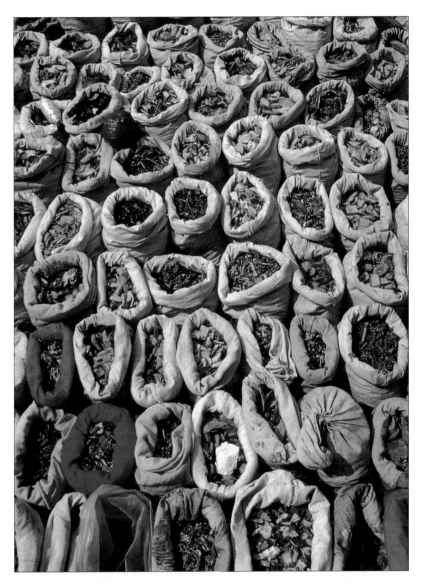

instance, if we did not have Night we would not have a point of reference to be able to have the opposite—Day.

In health Yin and Yang are balanced. When we become diseased this balance is lost, but Yin and Yang adjust their relative levels to each other, even in disease. If there is excess Yang, Yin correspondingly goes down. Finally, Yin can turn into Yang, or Yang into Yin as Summer turns into Winter.

Chinese thought has always been

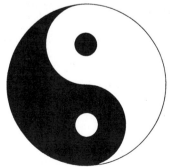

fluid, and this is expressed by there being no absolutes. Therefore in the symbol, in the Yang (white) side there is a dot of Yin (black), and in the Yin (black) side there is a dot of Yang (white). Yin was not associated with evil, and Yang was not associated with good.

## 2 THE FIVE ELEMENTS

The Chinese recognized Five Elements: Wood, Fire, Earth, Metal and Water. These Elements represent many different ideas, some of which are listed in the table (right).

As you can see, "Wood" not only relates to Spring but also to the Liver, and it has a taste, which is "sour." (Herbs and foods are also categorized into tastes.)

## THESE FIVE ELEMENTS INFLUENCE EACH OTHER IN THE FOLLOWING WAYS:

■ **Generation:** the elements are said to generate each other in this fashion.

# THE FIVE ELEMENTS

The Elements represent many different ideas, some of which are listed below:

| Wood | Fire | Earth | Metal | Water |
|------|------|-------|-------|-------|
| Spring | Summer | Last 18 days of each season | Fall | Winter |
| Green | Red | Yellow | White | Black |
| Liver | Heart | Spleen | Lungs | Kidneys |
| Gall bladder | Small intestine | Stomach | Large intestine | Urinary bladder |
| Wind | Heat | Dampness | Dryness | Cold |
| Sour | Bitter | Sweet | Pungent | Salty |
| East | South | Center | West | North |

■ **Control:** each Element "controls" another. Control was regarded as necessary to keep the Elements in balance.

■ **Over acting:** this follows the same course as the control sequence, but is a dis-ease cycle leading to a decrease in the overcontrolled Element.

■ **Insulting:** this sequence is in the opposite direction of the Control/Over act sequence. This is when one Element directly adversely affects another.

Thus Generation and Control deal with the normal balance of the Elements, whereas Overacting and Insulting are when the Elements become imbalanced.

■ **Substituting organs for elements**

We can start to see how in practice the relationships between the Elements can begin to affect our health. If, for example, we look at the overacting sequence we can see that the Liver "over acts" on the Spleen. This is very common and can mean that our emotions—stress, tension, irritability, etc.—can have a bad effect on our digestion, causing indigestion, pain, acidity and possibly ulcers.

If this (Liver over acting on Spleen) was the cause of the patient's stomach ache, the Chinese Herbalist would use Herbs not only to relieve the discomfort (the "Branch" of the disease) but also to soothe the Liver (the "Root" of the disease),

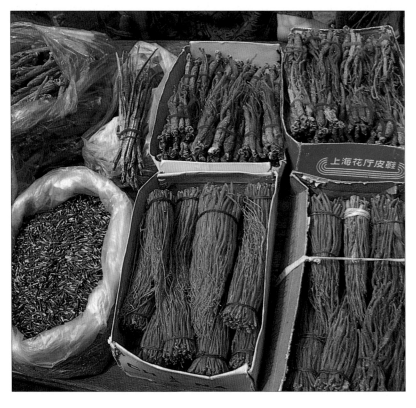

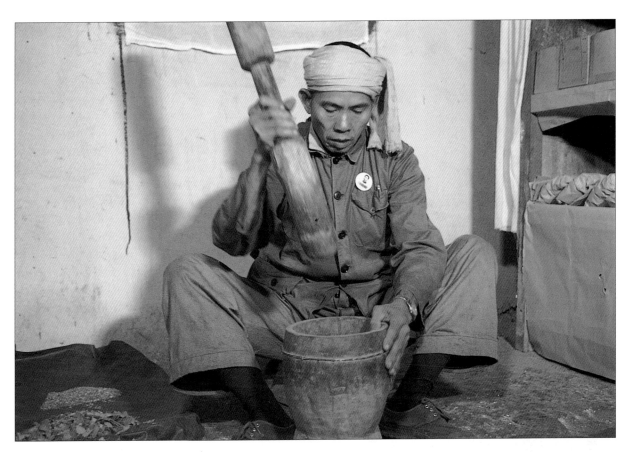

thus balancing the Elements and in so doing not only alleviating the symptoms, but also treating the underlying problem.

## 3 QI, BLOOD AND BODY FLUIDS

■ **Qi** is the basis of the universe—you, me, this table, my apartment, the Earth, mountains, rivers, plants. In fact, anything and everything is Qi. It is Substantial and/or Energetic at the same time, as is necessary. Qi transforms, transports, holds, raises, protects, and warms. In the body Qi manifests differently according to its environment and purpose. It tends to be more associated with Yang.

■ **Blood,** in the Chinese sense, is just a somewhat dense and slower moving form of Qi. "Qi is the commander of Blood. Blood is the Mother of Qi." Blood nourishes the body and moistens. It is the substantial basis for the mind—if we have problems sleeping it can be because the Spirit is not rooted properly in the blood of the Heart, so Herbs are used to nourish Heart blood, in this case promoting sleep.

■ **Body Fluids** come from the food and drink we consume. They help to moisten the skin and are transformed into waste fluids—sweat and urine—and a portion is expelled via the intestines.

■ **Essence** (Jing) is a special form of Qi which controls Birth, Growth, Development, and Reproduction.

**Note:** when talking about the Internal Organs (Zang Fu) the Liver Qi does not mean the more static Substantial "Qi of the Liver" but the more active Energetic aspect of the Liver function.

## 4 ZANG FU

■ **Zang** means "Yin internal organs" (the cold, dark, night aspect).

■ **Fu** means "Yang internal organs" (the warm, light, sunny aspect).

The organs are "paired" Yin-Yang as follows: Lungs/Large Intestine; Spleen/Stomach; the Heart/Small Intestine; Kidneys/Urinary Bladder; Pericardium/Triple Burner; Liver/Gall Bladder.

The internal organs are very important in health and disease as an imbalance will lead to symptoms manifesting. The Zang Fu do not necessarily carry out the same function as their counterparts in Western

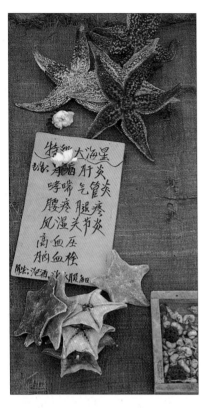

*Above: in China, traditional herbal medicines are on sale in many local markets as well as in pharmacists. They include herbs, pills, powders, decoctions and animal products, such as starfish.*

medicine. For instance, in Chinese medicine, the Spleen has the function of "Transforming and Transporting" fluids; thus if there is a case of edema (water retention), a herb to strengthen the Spleen may be used rather than a "Diuretic." In reality, with increasing analysis of Chinese Herbs, they do appear to work in an understandable fashion, but the terminology is different.

## 5 THE EIGHT PRINCIPLES
■ Hot/Cold; Full/Empty; Interior/Exterior; Yin/Yang.

These are said to be the "Eight Principles." They are used by the Herbalist to differentiate the disease and finely tune the Medicines given. This approach is unique to Chinese Herbal Medicine and allows for more precise diagnosis and therefore more accurate treatment.

### ■ DIAGNOSIS
Chinese diagnosis bases itself upon: Looking, Hearing, Asking, Feeling.

■ **Looking:** this involves not only looking at any external signs, such as skin conditions and facial appearance, but also at the general demeanor of the patient.

■ **Hearing:** Chinese Herbalists will not only listen to what you are telling them, but will also listen to the sound of your breathing, and digestion.

■ **Asking:** the most direct way of gaining information is by asking questions— you will be asked a lot.

■ **Feeling:** palpation, sensations of hot and cold, moisture levels, etc. are very important in reaching a correct diagnosis.

## VISITING A CHINESE HERBALIST

When you go to see a Chinese Herbalist, you will be asked many questions, some of which may not appear to be directly related to your specific complaint. For example, you may be asked if you prefer hot or cold drinks, and whether you prefer to gulp or sip them. Do you dream? Is it harder to go to sleep or stay asleep? Is the pain better for pressure or not? The color of bodily secretions may be asked. Yellow or green discharges tend to indicate heat, whereas white tends to be cold.

Do not be surprised if a number of highly personal questions are asked— for instance, menstruation, sex drive and bowel regularity are all areas that may need to be investigated.

Tongue and Pulse diagnosis are incredibly helpful, but Chinese Herbal Medicine is not a magic show; it is a two-way street. For herbalists to be able to use their abilities to the full, the patient must be as honest and helpful as possible. Healing comes from within the patient. To gain the most benefit from the plants that nature so abundantly provides, it is necessary for the questions to be answered candidly.

## DIET AND EXERCISE

Chinese Herbal Medicine is a Holistic subject. It is quite likely that you will receive certain dietary

## TONGUE AND PULSE DIAGNOSIS

These two techniques have been refined by the Chinese over many centuries. The Tongue is inspected for color, (a red tongue indicating Heat or Yin deficiency, a pale tongue indicating cold or Yang deficiency). Shape, moisture level and coating are some of the signs that the Herbalist will be looking for.

The Pulse is usually taken in three different positions at three different levels on both wrists, and there are a basic 28 different classifications of Pulse that can be felt. Obviously taking the Pulse is a subjective experience and one herbalist may be quite entitled to differ from a colleague.

advice, as well as possibly being asked to exercise sensibly and to think positively. In China it is not unusual to be prescribed Herbs, told to stop eating lamb and shellfish, advised to practice Qi Gong daily, and have a CAT scan. This Holistic approach is the most efficient and effective way to eliminate symptoms, bring the body back into balance, and strengthen the individual.

## CONDITIONS TREATED BY CHINESE HERBAL MEDICINE

Chinese Herbal Medicine is very effective in treating skin conditions, particularly eczema, psoriasis and acne. Digestive disturbances, ulcers, irritable bowel syndrome, indigestion and diverticulitis have all been helped with Chinese herbs as have problems of the respiratory system (coughs, colds, flu, bronchitis, asthma), the cardiovascular system (high blood pressure, angina, poor circulation) the nervous system (stress, anxiety, panic attacks, insomnia), and the reproductive system (amenorrhea, premenstrual syndrome, infertility, impotence) are just some of the areas that Chinese Herbal Medicine can benefit.

**Note:** it is imperative that you do not stop taking Western medication without consulting your herbalist and doctor. Sudden withdrawal of Western pharmaceutical medication is the best way to send your body, mind and emotions into turmoil, which can be potentially life threatening in some cases.

## COMMON HERBS

Thousands of herbs can be used in Chinese medicine but only a fraction of them are used regularly by herbalists. Below are some of the most commonly used herbs.

### GINSENG
(*Panax ginseng*)
There can't be many of us who have not heard of the legendary benefits of

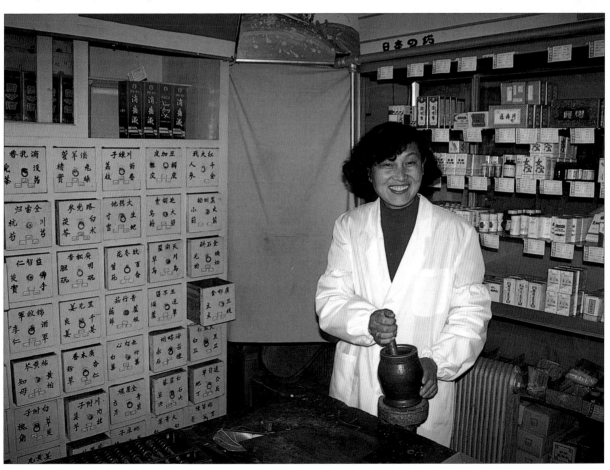

this Herb. But Ginseng is not applicable to all peoples of all ages at all times. It is a Qi tonic, and should not be taken within the first 48 to 72 hours of a cold/flu, as it will make the symptoms worse. It can also raise blood pressure. However, if taken at the correct time it will strengthen the Spleen (aid digestion, giving more energy, and stopping loose bowel motions), benefit the Heart (reducing palpitations), improve the Lungs (wheezing and shortness of breath), calm the spirit (for anxiety, insomnia and forgetfulness) and benefit the Yin.

### ▪ AMERICAN GINSENG
(*Panax quinquefolium*)
This species of ginseng is regarded as being "cooler" than other Ginseng. It is used more to nourish the Yin, especially of the Lungs. So for such conditions as T.B., types of pneumonia, and H.I.V./Aids syndrome, this herb has been used successfully.

### ▪ KOREAN GINSENG
This is the "Hottest" of the types of ginseng, and should be used very carefully if there are signs of heat manifesting itself in the body.

### ▪ DANG GUI
(*Angelica chinensis*)
Chinese angelica tones the blood and helps to regulate the menstrual cycle; it also invigorates and harmonizes the blood, and so is helpful in easing certain types of pain. It has been used to help fertility, and moves the bowels.

### ▪ HE SHOU WU
(*Polygonatum multiflorum*)
Literally this herb is called "Black Haired Mr. He." As the name implies, this herb has been used to keep the hair strong and to prevent greying; it also benefits the eyes, helps to stop skin irritation as well as moving the bowels.

### ▪ WU WEI ZI
(*Schizandra chinensis*)
This is known as "five flavored seed." If chewed, all five flavors emanate— Sweet, Sour, Salty, Bitter, and Pungent. This herb will help stop coughs and wheezing, astringes sweating, calms the spirit and is a reputed sex tonic.

**Note:** Chinese Herbs are usually combined into formulas which often have been used continuously for the same diagnosis for nigh on 2,000 years.

## THE FIVE TASTES

▪ **Earth** gives rise to sweetness, which tonifies, repairs harmonizes and nourishes. An excess can, amongst other things, cause muscle weakness.
▪ **Metal** gives rise to pungency, which disperses and moves Qi and blood. An excess scatters Qi, and should be avoided in Qi deficiency.
▪ **Water** gives rise to saltiness which softens hardness, dissolves,and disperses knottedness. An excess will dry the blood, and should be avoided in blood deficiency.
▪ **Wood** gives rise to sourness which astringes, contracts, gathers, firms and consolidates. An excess goes to the nerves and should be used sparingly if there is chronic pain.
▪ **Fire** gives rise to bitterness which descends, drains, clears heat, purges and dries damp. An excess will go to the bones—avoid an excess in bone disease.

## THE FOUR ENERGIES

These are Hot, Warm, Cool and Cold.
▪ In hot diseases the herbalist cools, and in cold disease he warms. Foods are also categorized in this manner.

| Hot or warm foods | Cold or cool foods |
|---|---|
| Beef | Almonds |
| Lamb | Chicken |
| Chocolate | Duck |
| Coffee | Green tea |
| Chillies | Most fish |
| Peanut butter | Broccoli |
| Deep fried food | Water melon |
| Pork | Cucumber |

# GLOSSARY

**ACUPRESSURE**
A combination of acupuncture and massage in which the thumbs and fingertips apply pressure massage on pressure points along the acupuncture meridians.

**ACUPUNCTURE**
Needles are inserted in the acupuncture points along the meridians running through the body to balance the flow of Qi.

**ALEXANDER TECHNIQUE**
A technique for improving posture in movement and using muscles efficiently with the minimum of effort.

**AROMATHERAPY**
The use of aromatic essential oils to treat many common illnesses and disorders.

**ART THERAPY**
A therapy that helps people to express themselves and gain relief through the art mediums of drawing, painting and modeling.

**AURA THERAPY**
The consideration of an individual's "aura" (a visible colored magnetic field) in order to make people more spiritually aware.

**AURICULAR THERAPY**
A form of acupuncture, using over 200 acupuncture points on the ear. These represent the different parts of the body and its structures.

**AUTOGENIC TRAINING AND THERAPY**
A means of self-healing to achieve relaxation and mental and physical harmony. Individuals are taught by the therapist how to use the therapy themselves.

**AYURVEDIC MEDICINES**
An ancient Indian system of holistic medicine, combining preventive and medicinal remedies with diet, meditation, breathing exercises and yoga.

**BACH FLOWER REMEDIES**
The 38 Bach remedies aim to correct health-threatening emotional imbalances, using infusions of different plants.

**BIOENERGETICS**
This Western form of yoga aims to understand the human personality through bodily energetic processes, including body movements and breathing exercises.

**BIOFEEDBACK THERAPY**
The practitioner uses sophisticated electrical instruments to monitor the patient's nervous system and emotional responses. It helps people become more aware of their physical, mental and emotional responses.

**CHIROPRACTIC**
A form of manipulation (literally "practice by hand") in which joints of the spine are manipulated by the practitioner, thereby alleviating problems in other parts of the body too as the spine is the main trunk of nerves to the body.

**COLOR THERAPY**
Devotees believe that color influences an individual's health and emotions, and that it can be used to treat a variety of emotional and physical conditions.

**CRANIAL OSTEOPATHY**
Also sometimes known as craniosacral therapy, this therapy uses a combination of gentle pressure and holding techniques on the patient's skull to release tension and to restore balance.

**CRYSTAL HEALING**
In this form of therapy, precious stones and gems may be immersed in water or worn to promote physical and spiritual healing. The gems are thought to emit healing vibrations.

**DANCE MOVEMENT THERAPY**
Dance forms and movements are used to help patients express themselves and to release emotions and tension. It is often used with physically handicapped and autistic children, and children with severe behavioral problems. Adults with communication and behavioral problems may benefit, too.

**DO-IN**
Commonly practiced in China and Japan, this self-help therapy is a complete program for personal health maintenance, including acupressure with massage and physical exercise.

## FELDENKRAIS

This system combines stretching, exercise and yoga to improve awareness of movement patterns and encourage proper body movement.

## FLOTATION THERAPY

This therapy involves sensory deprivation—the patient floats in an "isolation tank" filled with salt and mineral water, usually in complete darkness. Isolated from light and sound, the patient is cut off from any outside stimuli. The aim is to encourage a state of deep relaxation.

## GESTALT THERAPY

This is a holistic form of psychotherapy which aims to heighten an individual's self-awareness and perception of the moment, especially in terms of their relationships with other people and also with their environment.

## HERBAL MEDICINE

This is a complete holistic system of medicine which uses the healing properties of medicinal plants. Each patient is treated on an individual basis, according to his needs.

## HOMEOPATHY

This holistic approach is based on the principle that "like cures like." The homeopath uses minute amounts of diluted substances to treat a wide range of medical conditions. The patient's personality as well as his symptoms is assessed by the homeopathic doctor before prescribing a homeopathic remedy.

## HYDROTHERAPY

This ancient therapy advocates the therapeutic uses of water in treating many conditions, and in self-healing. Hot, cold and mineral baths, inhalation therapy, sitz baths, steam baths, hot and cold wrapping sheets, hot and cold compresses, and vapor baths and Turkish baths are all used.

## HYPNOTHERAPY

This form of therapy uses hypnotism to relax the conscious mind and induce a hypnotic trance. It can be used to bring the subconscious mind into alignment with the conscious mind to make positive suggestions. It is also used as a form of pain relief by some dentists and doctors.

## IRIDOLOGY

This is not a therapy in itself but a diagnostic tool which is used by some therapists to identify the underlying causes of disease. The markings and changes on the iris of the eye are studied for indications of any health problems.

## KINESIOLOGY

This uses muscle tests to locate specific weaknesses in muscles, which may be caused by food allergies, or vitamin and mineral deficiencies.

## MASSAGE

This "hands-on" ancient therapy takes many forms. The aims of therapeutic massage are to induce physical and mental relaxation, improve circulation and muscle tone, prevent soft tissue problems, aid the efficient functioning of the digestive system and encourage the elimination of toxins from the body.

## MEDITATION

A means of attaining spiritual enlightenment through personal growth. In addition to promoting relaxation and enabling a person to transcend their day-to-day anxieties, meditation is thought to have beneficial effects on the body, especially regarding high blood pressure and heart disease.

## MERIDIANS

In traditional Chinese medicine, the Meridians are the channels which run beneath the skin through which the "Qi" (the body's motivating energy) flows.

## METAMORPHIC TECHNIQUE

This form of reflexology uses circular finger movements on the feet, ankles, wrists, hands and head to balance the body's energies and help the patient discover their self-healing powers.

## MUSIC THERAPY

Music is used as a healing therapy to help patients express deep-set emotions, both positive and negative. It is thought to be successful in treating autism, mentally or emotionally disturbed children and adults, elderly and physically challenged people, and patients with schizophrenia, nervous disorders and stress.

## NATUROPATHY

This therapy stresses the body's natural vitality and its potential for self-healing and balancing. Holistic and preventive, it treats the whole person and emphasizes living a healthy, natural life. Eating a healthy diet of natural and organic foods, exercise, relaxation and hydrotherapy are all important aspects of naturopathy.

## OSTEOPATHY
This involves massage and the manipulation of joints, especially the vertebrae of the spine, to correct skeletal misalignment and encourage self-healing.

## POLARITY THERAPY
A therapy that aims to seek out and unblock any energy blockages in order to restore the balance of the body's vital energy. Therapists believe that illness is derived from blockages and imbalances in the body's energy system, and unblocking them will restore a patient's health and harmony.

## PSYCHOTHERAPY
A form of one-to-one or group therapy to enable people to break down their defenses and reveal and subsequently deal with repressed feelings and emotions and gain a better understanding of themselves. Humanistic psychotherapists treat the whole person, not just the mind in isolation from the body.

## QI
Pronounced "chee," in traditional Chinese medicine this is the vital motivating energy of the body.

## REFLEXOLOGY
This ancient therapy uses a method of foot massage, applying pressure to reflex zones mapped out on the feet. Reflexologists believe that the soles of the feet mirror the rest of the body and that by working on specific areas that correspond to other parts and organs of the body, a wide range of problems can be treated.

## ROGERIAN THERAPY
This form of "non-directive," person-centered psychotherapy was developed by Carl Rogers. It encourages self-reliance and self-responsibility in the client, and the ultimate aim is self-fulfillment.

## ROLFING
Sometimes known as structural integration, Rolfing aims to restore balance to the body and realign its structure. The Rolfing practitioner uses a form of gentle deep massage to work on the body's connective tissues and improve posture.

## SHAMANISM
This ancient method of healing was practiced by healers (shamans) in primitive tribes all over the world. Medicinal herbs and plants, prayers and ritual dance were all used by the shamans.

## SHIATSU
This "finger pressure" massage therapy originated in Japan. The practitioner applies pressure to specific points along the body's Meridians (energy channels), using the fingers, hands, elbows, knees and even feet. It is thought to be healing and energy-balancing and can be used to treat many common medical conditions.

## T'AI CHI CH'UAN
A Chinese system for preventing and treating disease which uses slow, smooth body movements to achieve a state of relaxation of body and mind.

## TRADITIONAL CHINESE MEDICINE
A complete system of medicine which has been practiced in China for over 2,000 years. It combines herbal medicine with acupuncture, manipulative therapy and food cures. It aims to restore harmony to the body and balance Yin and Yang.

## VISUALIZATION THERAPY
A form of therapy in which positive images are used for healing and to promote good health.

## YIN AND YANG
The equal and opposite qualities of Qi, the vital energy of the body.

## YOGA
An ancient holistic Indian system of exercises, postures, breathing, meditation and relaxation. It teaches self-control and a state of being at one with oneself, everything and everyone.

## ZEN THERAPY
A system of spiritual practises, including meditative exercises, which is based on Buddhist philosophy and beliefs. Its aim is to find self-enlightenment and integrate the body, mind and spirit in a state of total fulfillment.

## ZONE THERAPY
A form of reflexology or pressure point therapy in which pressure point massage is applied to the zones of the body to encourage self-healing.

# BIBLIOGRAPHY

ACUPRESSURE

**Hands-On Health Care Catalog** presents special healing books, acupressure charts, instructional videos, therapeutic music and self-care tools. For a free copy write to:
Acupressure Institute
1533 Shattuck Avenue
Berkeley CA 94709
USA

Hands-On Resources which are available from the Acupressure Institute at the above address are as follows:
Books by Michael Reed Gach
- *Acupressure's Potent Points*
- *Arthritis Relief at Your Fingertips*
- *Greater Energy at Your Fingertips*
- *Acu-Yoga Self-Help Techniques*
- *The Bum Back Book*

**Videos**
Instructional Hands-On vidoes
- *Fundamentals of Acupressure*
- *Releasing Shoulder & Neck Tension*
- *Zen Shiatsu: Instruction for Practitioners*
- *The Bum Back Video*

ACUPUNCTURE AND TRADITIONAL CHINESE MEDICINE

Auteroche, B. et al., *Acupuncture and Moxibustion, A Guide to Clinical Practice* (Churchill Livingstone, UK 1992)
Descartes, René, *Discourse on Method* (Hackett Publishing Company, Indianapolis, Indiana, USA 1980)
Fisch, Guido, *Die Traditionelle Chinesische Medizin* (Georg Wenderoth Verlag, Kassel, Germany 1994)
Fisch, Guido, *Chinesische Heilkunde in unsere Ernehiung* (Syntesis Verlag Essen, Germany 1982)
Helms, Joseph M., *Acupuncture Energetics. A Clinical Approach for Physicians* (Medical Acupuncture Publishers, Berkeley, California, USA 1995)
Lee-Kin and Tin Shen, *Handbook of Acupuncture Treatment for Dogs and Cats* (Medicine and Health Publishing Company, Hong Kong, China 1994)
Kewutgm G.T., *Moera Chinese Acupuncture* (Thorsons, HarperCollins Publishers, London, UK 1983)
Mann, Felix, *Acupuncture, Cure of Many Diseases* (2nd Edition, Butterworth-Heinemann Ltd., Oxford, UK 1994)
Molsberger, Albrecht, *Was Leistet die Akupunktur* (Hippokrates Ratgeber, Stuttgarta, Germany 1988)
Nguyen, Buc Hiep, *The Dictionary of Acupuncture of Moxibusion* (Thorsons HarperCollins Publishers, London, UK 1987)
Soulie de Morant, George, *Chinese Acupuncture* (Paradigm Publications, Brookline, Massachusetts, USA 1994)
Stux, Gabriel and Pomeranz, Bruce,
*Basics of Acupuncture* (Springer-Verlag, Berlin-Heidelberg-New York, Germany-US. 3rd Edition 1995)
Sussman, David. *Acupuntura. Ediciones Macchi* (Buenos Aires, Argentina 1967, original edition and Editorial Kier, SA, Buenos Aires, Argentina, reprint 1987)
Thorward, Juergen, *Science and Secrets of Early Medicine* (Thames and Hudson, London, UK.)
Hsu Pa-Chiun, *I-Hsueh Yuan Liu Lun of 1757*. Translated and annotated by Paul Unschuldas, *Forgotten Traditions of Ancient Chinese Medicine* (Paradigm Publications, Brookline, Massachusetts USA 1990)
Unschuld, Paul U., *Medicine in China, a History of Ideas* (University of California Press, Berkeley and Los Angeles, CA, USA 1985)
Van Alphen, Jan and Aris, Anthony, *Oriental Medicine. An Illustrative Guide to the Asian Arts of Healing.* (Shambhala Publications, Boston, Masachus Neolithic)
Williams, Tom, *Chinese Medicine, Acupuncture, Herbal Remedies, Nutrition, Qigong and Meditation for Total Health* (Element, Rockport, Massachusetts, USA 1966)
Wiseman, Nigel, and Boss, Ken, *Glossary of Chinese Medical Terms and Acupuncture Points* (Paradigm Publications, Brookline, Massachusetts USA 1990)
Yoo, Tae-Woo, Koryo Sooji Chim, *Koryo Hand Acupuncture*

(Volume 1, first printing in the English language. Eum Yang Mek Jin Publishing Company, Seoul, Korea 1988. Edited by Peter Eckman)

## AROMATHERAPY

Rose, Jeanne, *The Aromatherapy Book: Applications & Inhalations* (Berkeley: North Atlantic Books 1995)
*The Aromatherapy Studies Course* (San Francisco: The Herbal Studies Library 1995)
Price, Shirley, *Shirley Price's Aromatherapy Workbook* (Thorsons, HarperCollins Publishers, London, UK 1993)

## AUTOGENIC TRAINING

Kermani, Dr. Kai, *Autogenic Training; the effective holistic way to better health* (Pub. Souvenir Press, London 1996)

## CHINESE HERBAL MEDICINE

Maciocia, G., *The Foundations of Chinese Medicine.*
Bensky, D. and Gamble A., *Chinese Herbal Medicine Materia Medica.*

## COLOR HEALING

Gimbel, Theo, *Healing With Color and Light* (Gaia Books Ltd. London 1994)
Babey, Anna M., *Color Therapy* (Brooke, R. B. Amber Santa Barbara Press Inc. New York 1979)
Gerber, Richard, M.D.,*Vibrational Medicine* (Bear and Co., Santa Fe, New Mexico 1988)
Benz, Portmann et. al., *Color*

*Symbolism* (Spring Publications, Zurich 1977)
Brennan, Barbara, *Hands of Light, A Guide To Healing Through The Human Energy Field* (Bantam Books, New York 1988)
*Light: Medicine Of The Future: How We Can Use It To Heal Ourselves Now* (Bear and Co., New Mexico 1991)
Bruyere, Rosalyn, *Wheels of Light, Chakras, Auras, and the Healing Energy of the Body* (Fireside, Simon and Schuster, New York 1989)

## BACH FLOWER REMEDIES

Edward Bach, *Heal Thyself* (C.W. Daniel, Saffron Walden, UK 1931)
Edward Bach, *The Twelve Healers* (C.W. Daniel, Saffron Walden, UK 1933)
Barnard, Julian and Martine, *The Healing Herbs of Edward Bach* (Ashgrove Press, Bath, UK 1993)
Chancellor, Phillip M., *Handbook of the Bach Flower Remedies* (C.W. Daniel, Saffron Walden, UK 1971)
Gurudas, *Flower Essences and Vibrational Healing* (Cassandra Press, San Rafael, California 1983)
Scheffer, Mechthild, *Bach Flower Therapy* (Thorsons, HarperCollins Publishers, London 1993)
Vlamis, George, *Rescue Remedy* (Thorsons, HarperCollins Publishers, London 1994)

## CHIROPRACTIC

Courtenay, Anthea, *Chiropractic for Everyone* (Penguin Books, London 1987)
Howitt Wilson, Michael B., *Thorsons Introductory Guide to Chiropractic* (Thorsons, HarperCollins Publishers, London 1991)

## HERBAL MEDICINE

Griggs, Barbara, *Green Pharmacy* (1981)
Hoffmann, David, M.N.I.M.H., *The New Holistic Herbal* (Element Books)
Chevallier, Andrew B.A., *Herbal First Aid*
Corrigan, Desmond, B.Sc.(Pharms), M.A., PhD., F.L.S., F.P.S.I. *Indian Medicine for the Immune System— Echinacea* (Amberwood Publishing Ltd, Park Corner, East Horsley, Surrey KT24 56RZ)
Corrigan, Desmond, B.Sc.,(Pharms), M.A., Ph.D., F.L.S., F.P.S.I., *Ancient Medicine* and *Gingko biloba*, (Amberwood Publishing Ltd, Park Corner, East Horsley, Surrey KT24 56RZ)

## CRANIAL OSTEOPATHY

Sutherland, Ada Strand, *With Thinking Fingers* (The Cranial Academy, Indianapolis 1962)
Sutherland, William Garner, *The Cranial Bowl* (The Cranial Academy, Indianapolis 1939)

## HOMEOPATHY

### General
Panow, M.B., and Heimlich, J. *Homeopathic Medicine at Home*, 1980 (J.P. Tarcher, Inc., Los Angeles)
Vithoulkas, G. *The Science of Homeopathy* (1980, Grove Press, Inc., New York)
Ullman, D., *Discovering Homeopathy* (1991, North Atlantic Books, Berkeley, California.)
Hayfield, R., *Homeopathy for Common Ailments* (Frog Ltd and

Homeopathic Educational Services, Berkeley, California 1993)
Lockie, A, and Geddes, N. *Homeopathy: The Principles and Practice of Treatment* (1995, Dorling Kindersley Limited, London)
Jonas, W.B., and Jacobs, J., *Healing with Homeopathy* (Warner Books, New York, 1996)

**Scientific Research**
Reilly, D.T., Taylor, M.A., McSharry, C., Aitchison, T. *Is homoeopathy a placebo response? Controlled trial of homoeopathic potency, with pollen in hayfever as model.* (Lancet 1986ii881-5)
Fisher, P., Greenwood, A., Huskisson, E.C., Turner, P., Belon, P. *Effect of homoeopathic treatment on fibrositis (primary fibromyalgia).* (British Medical Journal, 1989;299:365-6.)
Ferley, J.P., Smirou, D., D'Adhemar, D., Balducci, F. *A controlled evaluation of a homoeopathic preparation in the treatment of influenza-like syndromes.* (Br J Clin Pharmacol 1989;27:329-35)
Kleijnen, J., Knipschild, P., ter Riet, G. *Clinical trials of homoeopathy.* (British Medical Journal 1991;302:316-23.)
Jacobs, J., Jimenez, L.M., Gloyd, S.S., Gale, J.L., Crothers, D. *Treatment of acute childhood diarrhea with homeopathic medicine: a randomized clinical trial in Nicaragua.* (Pediatrics 1994;93:719-25.)
Reilly, D.T., Taylor, M.A., Beattie, N.G.M., et al. *Is evidence of homoeopathy reproducible?* (Lancet 1994;344:1601-06

## HYPNOTHERAPY

Austin, Valerie, *Self-hypnosis* (Thorsons, HarperCollins Publishers, London 1994)
Karle, Helmut W.A., *Thorsons Introductory Guide to Hypnotherapy* (Thorsons, HarperCollins Publishers, London 1992)

## IRIDOLOGY

Jensen, Bernard, *Iridology Simplified* (B.Jensen, Escondido, California 1980)
Kriege, Theodore, *Disease Signs in the Iris* (L.N.Fowler & Co., Romford 1985)

## MUSIC THERAPY

Arnold Melville *Music Therapy in a Transactional Analysis setting* (Journal of Music Therapy Vol. 12 No 3, 1975)
Blatner, Adam, *Theoretical Principles Underlying Creative Arts Therapies* (Arts in Psychotherapy Pergamon Press Volume 18, No 5 1991)
Boxberger, Ruth *Historical Bases for the Use of Music in Therapy* (edited by E. H. Schneider Lawrence KS: National Association for Music Therapy Inc. 1962)
Bryant, David, R., *A Cognitive Approach to Therapy through Music* (Vol 24 No 1 1987)
Cassity, Michael & Julia, *Multimodal Psychiatric Music Therapy for Adults, Adolescents, and Children—A Clinical Manual* (MMB Music, Saint Louis, Missouri 1994)
Davis, William B., *Music Therapy in 19th Century America* (Journal of

Music Therapy Vol 24 N o 2, 1987)
David William, B., Gfeller, Kate E. and Thaut, Michael H. *An Introduction to Music Therapy— Theory and Practice* (Wm. C. Brown Publishers 1992)
DeWoskin, Kenneth J. *A Song For One or Two—Music and the Concept of Art in Early China* (Center for Chinese Studies—The University of Michigan, USA 1982. Ralph Spintge & Roland Droh, editors)
*Music Medicine* (MMB Music Inc 1992. Robert F. Unkefer, editor)
*Music Therapy Research— Quantitative and Qualitative Perspectives* (Barcelona Publishers 1995. Tony Wigram, Bruce Saperston and Robert West, editors)
*The Art and Science of Music Therapy: A Handbook* (Harwood Academic Publishers 1995. Cheryl D. Maranto, editor)
*Music Therapy: International Perspectives* (Jeffrey Books 1993. Paul Nordoff and Clive Robbins)
*Creative Music Therapy— Individualized Treatment for the Handicapped Child* (The John Day Company 1977)
Schalkwijk, F. W., *Music and People with Develomental Disabilities* (Jessica Kingsley Publishers 1994)
Sears, William W., *Processes in Music Therapy*, edited by E. Thayer Gaston (Macmillan Publishing Co Inc, 1969)
Wheeler, Barbara L. A., *Psychotherapeutic Classification of Music Therapy Practices. A continuum of procedures.* (Music Therapy Perspectives, Vol 1, No.2 1983)
**For further reading**
Bruscia, Kenneth E., *Case Studies in Music Therapy* (Barcelona Publishers 1991. Donald A. Hodges, editor)

*Handbook of Music Psychology*, (second edition. MMB Music, Saint Louis, Missouri, 1996)

Maranto, Cheryl D., *Applications of Music in Medicine* (National Association for Music Therapy 1991)

Priestley, Mary, *Essays on Analytical Music Therapy* (Barcelona Publishers 1994)

## NATUROPATHY

MacEoin, *Healthy by Nature* (Thorsons, HarperCollins Publishers, London 1994)

Turner, Roger Newman, *Naturopathic Medicine* (Thorsons, HarperCollins Publishers, London 1990)

## OSTEOPATHIC MEDICINE

Jones B., *The Difference a D.O. Makes (1978)* Times-Journal Publishing Co Oklahoma City OK)

Korr, I.M. (ed) *Research Workshop on Neurobiologic Mechanisms in Manipulative Therapy, The Neurobiologic Mechanisms in Manipulative Therapy (1978)* Plenum Press, New York NY)

Kuchera, M.L., Kuchera, W., *Osteopathic Considerations in Systemic Dysfunction*, (2nd edition—revised (1994). Greyden Press, Columbus OH)

Northup, G.W., *Osteopathic Medicine: An American Reformation, 2nd edition (1979)*. (American Osteopathic Association, Chicago IL)

Patterson, M.M., Powell, J.N. (eds): *The Central Connection: Somatovisceral/Viscerosomatic Interaction*, (1989 International Symposium of the American Academy of Osteopathy (1992). University Classics, Athens OH)

Postgraduate Institute of Osteopathic Medicine and Surgery: *The Physiological Basis of Osteopathic Medicine (1970)*. (Postgraduate Institute, New York NY)

Willard, F.H., Patterson, M.M. (eds): *Nociception and the Neuroendocrine-Immune Connection*, 1992 (International Symposium of the American Academy of Osteopathy (1994), University Classics, Athens OH)

## PSYCHOTHERAPY

*Self and Society* (The official journal of AHP—Britain)

*The Journal of Humanistic Psychology:* (The official journal of AHP, 1314 Westwood Boulevard, Suite 205, Los Angeles, California 90024)

*The Transpersonal Psychology Journal*, (345 California Street, Palo Alto, CA 94306)

*The Humanistic Psychologist*: The official journal of the Division of Humanistic Psychology of the American Psychological Association, (c/o Dr. D. Aanstoos, Department of Psychology, West Georgia College, Carolton, Georgia 30118)

*Self and Society* (Accesible articles on a range of personal growth and therapy subjects)

*The Family Therapy Networker* 8528 Bradford Road, Silver Spring, Maryland, 20901-9955, (An award winning non-technical magazine covering the whole spectrum of psychotherapy.)

*Common Boundary*, 4204 East-West Highway, Bethesda, Maryland 20814, (A non-technical magazine covering more psychospiritual concerns.)

## REFLEXOLOGY

Byers, Dwight C. *Better Health With Foot and Hand Reflexology, The Original Ingham Method* (Ingham Publishing Inc., St Petersburg, FL,1983)

The Original Works of Eunice D. Ingham, *Stories the Feet Can Tell Thru Reflexology* and *Stories the Feet Have Told Thru Reflexology* (Ingham Publishing Inc., St Petersburg, FL 1938 & 1951)

Dougans, Inge with Ellis, Suzanne, *The Art of Reflexology* (Element Books Ltd., 1992, & Barnes & Noble Books, NY 1995)

Fitzgerald, William H. and Bowers, Edwin F., *Zone Therapy* (Health Research, Mokelumne Hill, CA 1917)

Kunz, Devin & Barbara, *The Complete Guide to Foot Reflexology* (Prentice-Hall Inc., Englewood Cliffs, NJ 1982)

## SHIATSU

Jarmey, Chris, *Thorsons Introductory Guide to Shiatsu* (Thorsons, HarperCollins Publishers, London 1992)

Ridolfi, Ray, *Shiatsu* (Optima Alternative Health Series, 1990)

## TRADITIONAL CHINESE MEDICINE

Chuen, Lam Kam, *The Way of Energy* (Gaia Books, London, 1991)
McNamara, Sheila, *Traditional Chinese Medicine* (Hamish Hamilton, London 1995)
Porkert, M. and Ullman, C., *Chinese Medicine* (Morrow, New York, 1988)
*Basic Theory of Traditional Chinese Medicine* (Shanghai College of TCM Press, 1990)
*Diagnostics of Traditional Chinese Medicine* (Shanghai College of TCM Press, 1990)
*The Yellow Emperor's Classic of Internal Medicine* (University of California Press 1966)

## T'AI CHI CH'UAN

*T'ai Chi Magazine*, an international magazine published bi-monthly, contains articles by leading experts on T'ai chi Ch'uan and qigong as well as listings of videos and books. Both are available from Wayfarer Publications, PO Box 26156, Los Angeles, CA 90026. USA.
Tel. (213) 665-7773.
Fax (213) 665-7773.
E.mail: taichi@tai-chi.com. Web site: http://www.tai-chi.com.

## VISUALIZATION THERAPY

Kermani Dr. Kai, *Autogenic Training; the effective holistic way to better health* (Souvenir Press, London 1996)
Gawain, S, *Creative Visualization* (Bantam Books Inc., New York 1985)
Crysta, P., *Cutting the ties that bind* (Samuel Weisler Inc., Maine 1993)
Simonton, S. & O., *Getting well again* (Bantam Books Inc., New York 1988)

Le Shan, L., *How to Meditate* (Turnstone Press 1993)
McDonald, K., *How to Meditate* (Wisdom Publications 1984)
Achterberg, J., *Imagery in Healing* (Shambhala/Random House. Boston 1985)
Glouberman, D., *Life Choices & Life Changes Through Image Work* (Unwin Paperbacks 1989)
Fontana, D *The elements of meditation* (Element Books 1991)

## YOGA

*Yoga Journal* (800 334-8152) and *Yoga International* (800 822-4547) have teachers directories and many articles, advertising and listings of resources in the United States.

# USEFUL ADDRESSES

All the following information was correct at the time of going to press.

## ALTERNATIVE AND COMPLEMENTARY MEDICINE AND HOLISTIC HEALTH ORGANIZATIONS

### UNITED STATES

**Alliance/Foundation for Alternative Medicine**
160 NW Widmer Place
Albany,
OR 97321
Tel: (541) 926-4678

**American Holistic Nurses Association**
4101 Lake Boone Trail
Suite 201
Raleigh,
NC 27607
Tel: (800) 278-AHNA
Fax: (919) 787-4916

**American Holistic Veterinary Medical Association**
2214 Old Emmorton Road
Bel Air,
MD 21015
For information, send a self-addressed stamped envelope.

**American Preventive Medical Association**
459 Walker Road
Great Falls,
VA 22091
Tel: (800) 230-2762
Fax: (703) 759-6711

**American Holistic Health Association (AHHA)**
PO Box 17400
Anaheim,
CA 92817-7400
Tel: (714) 779 6152

**American Holistic Medical Association**
4101 Lake Boone Trail
Suite 201
Raleigh,
NC 27607
(919) 787-5181

**Association of Holistic Healing Centers**
109 Holly Crescent
Suite 201
Virginia Beach,
VA 23451
Tel: (804) 422-9033

**International Association of Holistic Health Practitioners**
21757 Devonshire
Chatsworth,
CA 91311
Tel: (702) 873-4542

**Holistic Dental Association**
PO Box 66609
Portland,
NV 89102
Tel: (702) 873-4542

### UNITED KINGDOM

For information on courses in most forms of Complementary Medicine, you should contact:

**The Institute for Complementary Medicine**
Unit 15
Tavern Quay
Commerical Centre
Rope Street
London
SE16 1TX
Tel: 0171 237 5165

For information on registered practitioners in most forms of Complementary Medicine, you should contact:

**The British Register of Complementary Practitioners**
PO Box 194
London
SE16 1QZ
Tel/Fax: 0171 237 5175

BRCP Divisions include: Aromatherapy, Chromotherapy, Colour, Chinese Medicine, Energy Medicine, Counseling, Healing Counselling, Herbal Medicine, Homeopathy, Medical Hypnotherapy and Psychotherapy, Indian Medicine, Japanese Medicine, Physical Medicine (Alexander Technique, Osteopathy, Chiropractic, Remedial Massage, Massage, Nutritional Medicine, Reflexology and others)
Diagnostic systems: Iridology, Kinesiology, Signalysis.
Professional techniques include: Heller Work, Rolfing, Bach Flower Remedies, Bates Eye Care.

**The Complementary Medical Practitioners' Union**
Freepost
London SW18 2BR

**British Holistic Medical Association**
179 Gloucester Place
London NW1 6DX
Tel: 0171 262 5299

## CANADA

**Canadian Holistic Medical Association (CHMA/OMC)**
491 Eglinton Avenue West
407 Toronto
Ontario M5N 1A8
Tel: (416) 485-3071

## AUSTRALIA

**Australasian College of Natural Therapies**
620 Harris Street
Ultimo
NSW 2007
Tel: 02 212 6699

## ACUPRESSURE

### UNITED STATES

**The Acupressure Institute**
1533 Shattuck Avenue
Berkeley, CA 94709
Tel: (510) 845-1059

**American Oriental Bodywork Association**
6801 Jericho Turnpike
Syosset,
NY 11791
Tel: (609) 782-1616
Fax: (516) 364-5559

## ACUPUNCTURE AND TRADITIONAL CHINESE MEDICINE

### UNITED STATES

**Acupuncture Research Institute**
313 W. Andrix Street
Monterey Park,
CA 91754
Tel: (213) 722-7353

**The American Academy of Medical Acupuncture**
5820 Wiltshire Boulevard
Suite 500
Los Angeles,
CA 90036
Tel: (213) 937-5514

**American Association of Acupuncture and Oriental Medicine (AAAOM)**
National Acupuncture Headquarters
1424 16th Street NW,
Suite 501
Washington, DC 20036

**American Foundation of Traditional Chinese Medicine**
505 Beach Street
San Francisco,
CA 94133
Tel: (415) 776-0502
Fax: (415) 776-9053

**The Center for Integrated Medicine**
3120 Southwest Freeway
Suite 41
Houston,
TX 77098
Tel: (713) 523-4181

**International Veterinary Acupuncture Society**
2140 Conestoga Road
Chester Springs,
PA 19425
Tel: (610) 827-7245

### UNITED KINGDOM

**Academy of Western Acupuncture**
112 Conway Road
Colwyn Bay
Clwyd LL29 7LL
Tel: 01492 534328

**Association of Chinese Acupuncture**
Prospect House
2 Grove Lane
Retford
Nottingham DN22 6NA
Tel: 01777 701509

**The British Acupuncture Council**
Park House
206 Latimer Road
London W10 6RE
Tel: 0181 964 0222

**The British Medical Acupuncture Society,**
Newton House
Newton Lane
Lower Whitley
Warrington
Cheshire WA4 4JA
Tel: 01925 73727

**The Council for Acupuncture**
179 Gloucester Road
London NW1 6DX
Tel: 0170 724 5756

**European Federation of
Modern Acupuncture**
59 Telford Crescent
Leigh
Lancashire
WN 5LY
Tel: 01942 678092

**The LIY Clinic of Traditional
Chinese Medicine**
13 Gunnersbury Avenue
Ealing Common
London W13
Tel: 0181 993 2549

**The Register of Chinese
Herbal Medicine**
PO Box 400
Wembley
Middlesex
HA9 9NZ
Tel: 0181 904 1357

**AUSTRALIA**

**Australia Acupuncture
Ethics and Standards
Organization**
PO Box 84
Merryland,
New South Wales 2160

**NEW ZEALAND**

**New Zealand Natural
Health Practitioners
Accreditation Board**
PO Box 37-491
Auckland
Tel: 96259966

**New Zealand Register
of Acupuncturists**
PO Box 9950
Wellington

# ALEXANDER TECHNIQUE

**UNITED STATES**
**North American Society of
Teachers of Alexander Technique**
PO Box 5536
Playa del Rey
CA 90296
Tel: (800) 473-0620

**UNITED KINGDOM**

**Alexander Teaching
Network**
PO Box 53
Kendal
Cumbria LA9 4UP

**Alexander Technique
International**
142 Thorpdale Rod
London
N4 3BS
Tel: 0171 281 7639

**The Society of Teachers of
Alexander Technique**
20 London House
266 Fulham Road
London
SW10 9EL
Tel: 0171 351 0828

# AROMATHERAPY

**UNITED STATES**

**Aromatherapy Institute
of Research**
PO Box 2354
Fair Oaks,
CA 95628
Tel: (916) 965-7546
Fax: (916) 962-3272

**National Association for
Holistic Aromatherapy**
219 Carl Street
San Francisco,
CA 94117 USA
Tel: (415) 564-6799

**UNITED KINGDOM**

**Aromatherapy Organizations
Council**
3 Latymer Close
Braybrooke
Market Harborough
Leicester
LE16 8LN
Tel: 01858 434242

**Aromatherapy & Allied
Practitioners' Association**
8 George Street
Croydon
Surrey
CR0 1PA
Tel: 0181-680 7761

**Aromatherapy Quarterly**
5 Ranelagh Avenue
London SW6 6RA

**Association of Medical
Aromatherapists**
Abergare
Rhu Point
Helensburgh
G84 8NF
Tel: 0141-332 4924

**International Federation of
Aromatherapists**
Stamford House
2-4 Chiswick High Road
London
W4 1TH
Tel: 0181 742 2605

## AUTOGENIC TRAINING

### UNITED KINGDOM

**British Association for Autogenic Training (BAFATT)**
Heath Cottage
Pitch Hill
Ewhurst
Nr. Cranleigh
Surrey
GU6 7NF

## CHIROPRACTIC

### UNITED STATES

**American Chiropractic Association**
1701 Clarendon Blvd
Arlington,
VA 22209
Tel: (703) 276-8800

**Federation of Straight Chiropractors and Organizations**
642 Broad Street
Clifton,
NJ 07013
Tel: (800) 423-4690

**International Chiropractors Association (ICA)**
1110 N. Glebe Road
Suite 1000
Arlington,
VA 22201
Tel: (703) 528-5000
(800) 423-4690
Fax: (703) 528-5023

**National Directory of Chiropractic**
PO Box 10056
Olathe,
KS 66051
Tel: (800) 888-7914
Fax: (913) 780-0658

**World Chiropractic Alliance**
2950 N. Dobson Road 1
Chander,
AZ 85224
Tel: (800) 347-1011

### UNITED KINGDOM

**British Chiropractic Association**
29 Whitley Street
Reading
Berks RG2 0EG
Tel: 01734 757557

**The British Association for Applied Chiropractic**
The Old Post Office
Cherry Street
Stratton Audley
Nr Bicester
Oxon OX6 9BA
Tel: 01869 277111

**McTimoney Chiropractic**
14 Park End Street
Oxford
OX1 1HH
Tel: 01865 246786

## COLOR THERAPY

### UNITED STATES

**California Institute for Integral Studies**
San Francisco, CA.
Tel: (415) 753-6100

**Omega Institute for Holistic Studies**
260 Lake Drive
Rhinebeck
NY, 12572
Tel (914) 266-4301

### UNITED KINGDOM

**Hygeia Studios and The Hygeia College of Color Therapy Ltd.**
Brook House
Avening
Tetbury GL8 8NS
Tel/Fax: 01453 832150

**The International Association of Color Therapists**
73 Elm Bank Gardens
London SW13 ONX

**College of Chromotherapy**
North London Tutorial College
228 Hendon Way
London NW4 3NE
Tel: 0181 202 7545

**Universal Color Healers Research (Chromotherapy)**
1 The Green
Nash
Milton Keynes MK17 0EN
Tel: 01908 501923

## CRANIAL OSTEOPATHY

### UNITED STATES

**Cranial Academy**
8606 Allisonville Road
Suite 130
Indianapolis,
IN 46250
Tel: (317) 594-0411

**Upledger Institute**
11211 Prosperity Farms Road
Palm Beach Gardens,
FL 33410
Tel: (407) 622-4706

### UNITED KINGDOM

**General Council and Register
of Osteopaths**
56 London Street
Reading
Berkshire RG1 4SQ

**Cranial Osteopathic Association**
478 Baker Street
Enfield
Middlesex EN1 3QS
Tel: 0181 367 5561

**Craniosacral Therapy Association**
8 Warren Road
Colliers Wood
London SW19 2HX

### AUSTRALIA

**The Sutherland Cranial
Teaching Foundation of
Australia and New Zealand**
2 Hillside Parade
Glen Iris 3146
Victoria, Australia

## DANCE THERAPY

### UNITED STATES

**American Dance Therapy
Association**
10632 Little Pateuxent Parkway
2000 Century Plaza
Suite 108
Columbia, MD 21044-3265
Tel: (410) 997-4040

## DIET THERAPIES

### UNITED STATES

**American Association of
Nutritional Consultants**
880 Canarios Court
Suite 210
Chula Vista,
CA 91910
Tel/Fax: (619) 482 8533

**American Academy of Nutrition**
*Send $5.00 for information and
member listing to AANP at*
2366 East Lake Ave.
Suite 322
Seattle,
WA 98102
Tel: (206) 323-7610

**Hospital Santa Monica**
Chula Vista,
CA 91910
Tel: (619) 482 8533
Fax: (619) 482 4485

**National Institute of
Nutritional Education**
1010 S. Joliet Street 107
Aurora,
CO 80012
Tel: (303) 340-2054

### UNITED KINGDOM
**Council for Nutrition
Education and Therapy**
34 Wadham Street
London SW15 2LR

**Society for the Promotion
of Nutrition Therapy**
PO Box 47
Hatfield
East Sussex  TN21 8ZX

## FLOWER ESSENCE
## THERAPY

### UNITED STATES

**Flower Essence Society**
PO Box 459
Nevada City,
CA 95959
Tel: (916) 265-9163

### UNITED KINGDOM

**The Dr Edward Bach Center**
Mount Vernon
Sotwell
Wallingford
Oxon
OX10 0PZ
Tel: 01491 834678

**Bach Flower Remedies
(Customer Enquiries)**
Broadheath House
83 Parkside
Wimbledon
London
SW19 5LP
Tel: 0181 780 4200

## HERBAL MEDICINE

### UNITED STATES

**American Botanical Council**
PO Box 201660
Austin,
TX 78720
Tel: (512) 331-8868

**American Herbalists Guild**
PO Box 1683
Sequel,
CA 95073
Tel: (408) 484-2441

**American Herb Association**
PO Box 1673
Nevada City,
CA 95959
Tel: (916) 265-9552

**Herb Research Foundation**
1007 Pearl Street, Suite 200
Boulder,
CO 80303
Tel: (303) 449-2265

## UNITED KINGDOM

**Healing Herbs Ltd**
PO Box 65
Hereford HR2 0UW
Tel: 01873 890 218

**National Institute of Medical Herbalists**
9 Palace Gate
Exeter EXZ1 1JA
Tel: 01392 426022

**The General Council and Register of Consultant Herbalists**
Grosvenor House
49 Seaway
Middleton-on-Sea
Sussex PO22 7SA
Tel: 01243 586012

## AUSTRALIA

**Australian Traditional Medicine Society**
120 Blaxland Road
Ryde NSW 2112
Tel: 808 2825

**National Herbalists Association of Australia**
14/249 Kingsgrove Road
Kingsgrove, NSW 2208

# HOMEOPATHY

## UNITED STATES

**American Institute of Homeopathy**
1585 Glencoe
Denver,
CO 80220
Tel: (303) 370-9164

**Homeopathic Academy of Naturopathic Physicians**
PO Box 69565
Portland,
OR 97201
Tel: (503) 795-0579

**Homeopathic Educational Services**
2124 Kittredge Street
Berkeley,
CA 94704

**International Foundation for Homeopathy**
2366 Eastlake Avenue, E, 329
Seattle,
WA 98102
Tel: (206) 776-4147

**The National Center for Homeopathy**
801 N. Fairfax
Suite 306
Alexandria, VA 22314
Tel: (703) 548-7790

## UNITED KINGDOM

**A. Nelson & Co., Ltd**
Broadheath House
83 Parkside
London SW19 5LP
Tel: 0181 780 4200

**British Association of Homeopathic Veterinary Surgeons**
Chinham House
Stanford-in-the-Vale
Faringdon
Oxon SN7 8NQ

**British Homeopathic Dental Association**
12 Wellington Road
Watford
Hertfordshire WD1 1QW

**British Institute of Homeopathy**
Victor House
Norris Road
Staines
Middlesex TW18 4DS
Tel: 01784 440467

**Faculty of Homeopathy**
Royal London Homeopathic Hospital
Great Ormond Street
London
WC1N 3HR
Tel: 0171 837 2495

**The Hahnemann Society**
Humane Education Center
Bounds Green Road
London N22 4EV
Tel: 0181 889 1595

**Society of Homeopaths**
2 Artizan Road
Northampton NN1 4HU
Tel: 01604 21400

**The United Kingdom Homeopathic Medical Association**
6 Livingstone Road
Gravesend
Kent DA12 5DZ
Tel: 01474 560336

CANADA

**S.P.H.Q. (Syndicat Professionnel des Homeopathes du Quebec)**
1600 De Lorimier
Local 295
Montreal
Qc H2K 3W5
Tel: (514)  525-2037
Fax: (514) 525-1299

**Vancouver Center for Homeopathy**
2246 Spruce Street
Vancouver, BC
V6H 2P3

AUSTRALIA

**Australian Federation of Homeopaths**
21 Bulah Close
Berowra Heights
NSW 2082
Australia
Tel: 02 456 3602

# HYPNOTHERAPY

UNITED STATES

**Academy of Scienfitic Hypnotherapy**
PO Box 12041
San Diego,
CA 92112
Tel: (619) 427-6225

**American Academy of Medical Hypnoanalysts**
1007 1/2 W. Jefferson St.
Joliet,
IL 60435
Tel: (800) 344-9766

**American Guild of Hypnotherapists**
2200 Veterans Boulevard
New Orleans (Kenner),
LA 70062

**American Institute of Hypnotherapy**
16842 Von Karman Avenue 475
Irvine,
CA 92714
Tel: (800) 872-9996

**International Medical and Dental Hypnotherapy Association**
4110 Edgeland, Suite 800
Royal Oaks,
MI 48073-2251
Tel: (810) 549-5594

**National Society of Hypnotherapists**
2175 NW 86th
Suite 6A
Des Moines,
IA 50325
Tel: (515) 255 8151

**The American Society of Clinical Hypnosis**
2200 East Devon Avenue
Suite 291
Des Plaines,
IL 60018

UNITED KINGDOM

**British Society of Medical and Dental Hypnosis**
73 Ware Road
Hartford
Herts
SG13 7ED
Tel: 0181 385 7575

**British Society of Hypnotherapists**
c/o 74 Halford Road
London
SW6 1JX
Tel: 0171 385 1166

**Central Register of Advanced Hypnotherapists**
28 Finsbury Park Road
London N4

**The National College of Hypnosis & Psychotherapy**
12 Cross Street
Nelson
Lancashire

**National Council of Psychotherapists & Hypnotherapy Register**
46 Oxhey Road
Oxhey
Watford
WD1 4QQ

**National Register of Hypnotherapists & Psychotherapists**
12 Cross Street
Nelson
Lancashire

# IRIDOLOGY

UNITED STATES

**National Iridology Research Association**
PO Box 1278
Glenneyre 153
Laguna Beach,
CA 92651

UNITED KINGDOM

**Guild of Naturopathic Iridologists (International)**
94 Grosvenor Road
London
SWlV 3LF
Tel/Fax: 0171 834 3579

**Holistic Health Consultancy & College**
94 Grosvenor Road
London
SW1V 3LF
Tel: 0171 834 3579

**International Association of Clinical Iridologists**
(with Canadian associates as well as British graduates)
12 Upper Station Road
Radlett
Herts
WD7 8BX
England
Tel/Fax: 01923 857670

# MASSAGE THERAPY

## UNITED STATES

**American Massage Therapy Association**
820 Davis Street, Suite 100
Evanston,
IL 60201-4444
Tel: (847) 864-0123

**Associated Bodywork and Massage Professionals**
28677 Buffalo Park Road
Evergreen,
CO 80439-7347
Tel: (303) 674-8478
(800) 458-2267

**The Feldenkrais Guild**
PO Box 489
Albany,
OR 97321
Tel: (541) 926-0981

**Body of Knowledge/Hellerwork**
406 Berry Street
Mt. Shasta,
CA 96067
Tel: (916) 926-2500
Fax: (916) 926-6839

**American International Reiki Association Inc**
2210 Wilshire Boulevard, 831
Santa Monica,
CA 90403

**Reiki Alliance**
PO Box 41
Cataldo,
ID 83810
Tel: (208) 682-3535

**Trager Institute**
33 Millwood Street
Mill Valley,
CA 94941
Tel: (415) 388-2688;

**North American Society of Teachers of the Alexander Technique**
PO Box 112484
Tacoma,
WA 98411
Tel: (206) 627-3766

**American Oriental Bodywork Therapy Association**
6801 Jericho Turnpike
Syosset,
MY 11791
Tel: (516) 364-5533

UNITED KINGDOM

**The Association of Massage Practitioners**
Flat 3
52 Redcliffe Square
London
SW10 9HQ
Tel: 0171 373 4697

**British Massage Therapy Council**
Greenbank House
65a Adelphi Street
Preston
PR1 7BH
Tel: 01772 881063

## AUSTRALIA

**Association of Massage Therapists**
19a Spit Road
Mosman
NSW 2088
Tel: 969 8445

**Association of Remedial Masseurs**
22 Stuart Street
Ryde
NSW 2112
Tel: 878 2159

# MEDITATION

## UNITED STATES

**Himalayan International Institute of Yoga Science and Philosophy of the U.S.A.**
RR 1
Box 400
Honesdale,
PA 18431
Tel: (717) 253-5551
Fax: (717) 253-9078

## UNITED KINGDOM

**Himalayan Institute of
Great Britain**
70 Claremont Road
West Ealing
London
W13 0DG
Tel: 0181 997 3544

## MUSIC THERAPY

### UNITED STATES

**American Association for
Music Therapy, Inc.**
1 Station Place
Ossining,
NY 10562
Tel: (914) 944-9260
Fax: (914) 944-9387

**American Association for
Music Therapy**
PO Box 80012
Valley Forge,
PA 19484
Tel: (610) 265-4006

**Certification Board for
Music Therapists**
1407 Huguenot Road
Midlothian,
VA 23113
Tel: (800) 765-2268

**National Association for Music
Therapy Inc.**
8455 Colesville Road
Suite 930
Silver Spring,
MA 20910, USA
Phone: (301) 589-3300
Fax: (301) 589-5175

### UNITED KINGDOM

**British Society for Music Therapy**
25 Rosslyn Avenue
East Barnet
Herts
EN4 8DH

## NATUROPATHY

### UNITED STATES

**The American Association of
Naturopathic Physicians**
2366 Eastlake Avenue East
Suite 322
Seattle, WA 98102
Tel: (206) 328-8510
For physician referrals:
Tel: (206) 323-7610

**American Naturopathic
Association**
1413 King Street
First Floor
Washington, DC 20005
Tel: (202) 682-7352
Fax: (202) 289-2027

**American Naturopathic
Medical Association**
PO Box 96273
Las Vegas,
NV 89193
Tel: (702) 897-7053

**Bastyr University of Natural
Health Sciences**
College of Naturopathic
Medicine
144 NE 54th
Seattle,
WA 98105
Tel: (206) 523-9585

**The National College of
Naturopathic Medicine**
11231 SE Market Street
Portland,
OR 97216
Tel: (503) 255-4860

**Southwest College of
Naturopathic Medicine
and Health Sciences**
6535 East Osborn Road,
Suite 703
Scottsdale,
AZ 85251
Tel: (602) 990-7424

### UNITED KINGDOM

**The British Naturopathic
Association**
c/o Roger Newman Turner, N.D.,
D.O., B.Ac
38 Weymouth Street
London W1

**General Council and
Register of Naturopaths**
Goswell House
2 Goswell Road
Street
Somerset BA16 0JG

**Incoporated Society of
Registered Naturopaths**
1 Albemarle Road
The Mount
York YO2 1EN

### CANADA

**Canadian College of
Naturopathic Medicine**
60 Berl Avenue
Toronto
ON M8Y 3C7

The Canadian Naturopathic
Association
P.O. Box 4520 T2T 5N3
Tel: (403) 244-4487

# OSTEOPATHY

## UNITED STATES

**The Cranial Academy**
8606 Allisonville Road,
130 Indianapolis,
IN 46250

**American Academy of
Osteopathy**
3500 DePauw Boulevard
Suite 1080
Indianapolis,
IN 46268
Tel: (317) 879-1881
Fax: (317) 879-0568

**American Osteopathic
Association**
142 East Ontario Street
Chicago,
IL 60611
Tel: (312) 280-5882

## UNITED KINGDOM

**The British School of
Osteopathy**
104 Suffolk Street
London
SW1Y 4HG
Tel: 01710930 9254
Fax: 0171-839 1098

**General Council and
Register of Osteopaths**
56 London Street
Reading
Berkshire RG1 4SQ

**Osteopathic Information Service**
PO Box 2074
Reading
Berks RG1 4YR
Tel: 01273 451 2051

## AUSTRALIA

**The Sutherland Cranial Teaching
Foundation of Australia and New
Zealand**
2 Hillside Parade
Glen Iris 3146
Victoria
Australia

# POLARITY THERAPY

## UNITED STATES

**American Polarity Therapy
Association**
2888 Bluff Street
Suite 149
Boulder,
CO 80301
Tel: (303) 545-2080
Fax: (303) 545-2161

## UNITED KINGDOM

**British Polarity Council**
Monomark House
27 Old Gloucester Street
London
WC1N 3XX

**British Complementary Medical
Association**
Mental Health Unit
St Charles' Hospital
Exmoor Street
London
W10 6DX
Tel: 0181 964 1205

**Polarity Therapy Association UK**
11 Willow Vale
Frome
Somerset BA11 1BG
Tel: 01373 452250

**Polarity Therapy Educational
Trust**
116 Ladysmith Road
Brighton
Sussex BN2 4EG
Tel: 01273 689215

# PSYCHOTHERAPY

## UNITED STATES

**Association for Humanistic
Psychology (International)**
45 Franklin Street
Suite 315
San Francisco,
CA 94102

**American Psychological
Association**
750 First Street NE
Washington,
DC 20002
Tel: (202) 336-5500

**Association for Transpersonal
Psychology**
345 California Street
Palo Alto,
CA 94306
Tel: (415) 327-2066

**International Transpersonal
Association**
20 Sunnyside Avenue
A-257
Mill Valley,
CA 94941
Tel: (415) 383-8819

**UNITED KINGDOM**

**Association of Child
Psychotherapists**
54 Gayton Road
London NW3
Tel: 0171 794 8881

**British Association for
Counseling**
1 Regent Place
Rugby
Warwickshire CV21 2PJ
Tel: 01788 578328

**College of Psychic Studies**
16 Queensbury Place
London SW7 3EB
Tel: 0171 589 3292

**Healer Practitioner Association
International**
1a Northcote Street
Cardiff
Tel: 01222 497837

**Institute of Dream Analysis**
8 Willow Road
London
NW3 1TJ
Tel: 0171 794 8717

**The Institute of Family
Therapy**
43 New Cavendish Street
London
W1M 7RG
Tel: 0171 935 1651

**The Institute of Group
Analysis**
1 Daleham Gardens
London
NW3 5BY
Tel: 0171 431 2693

# REFLEXOLOGY

**UNITED STATES**

**Foot Reflexology Awareness
Association**
PO Box 7622
Mission Hills, CA 91346
Tel: (818) 361-0528

**International Institute of
Reflexology**
PO Box 12642
St Petersburg,
FL 33733-2642
Tel: 813-343-4811

**Reflexology Association of
America**
4012 South Rainbow Boulevard
Box K-585
Las Vegas,
NV 89103-2059
Tel: 717-823-8750

**Reflexology Research**
PO Box 35820, Station D
Albuquerque,
NM 87176
Tel: (505) 344-9392
Fax: (505) 344-0246

**UNITED KINGDOM**

**Association of Reflexologists**
110 John Silkin Lane
London SE8 5BE

**The British Reflexology
Association**
Monk's Orchard
Whitbourne
Worcester
WR6 5RB
Tel: 01886 21207

**International Federation
of Reflexology**
51 Champion Close
Croydon
Surrey
CRO 5SN
Tel: 0181 680 9631

# ROLFING

**UNITED STATES**

**The Rolf Institute**
205 Canyon Boulevard
Boulder,
CO 80302

**UNITED KINGDOM**

**European Head Office**
European Rolfing Association
Ohmstrasse 9
80802 Munich,
Germany
Tel: 0049 89 39 6802

**UK representative**
J. Crewdson
Tel: 0171 834 1493

# SHIATSU

**UNITED STATES**

**The American Oriental
Bodywork Therapy
Association**
6801 Jericho Turnpike
Syosset,
NY 11791-4413
Tel: (516) 364-5533;
Fax: (516) 364-5559

**The School for Oriental Medicine**
The New Center for Wholistic
Health Education and Research
6801 Jericho Turnpike
Syosset,
NY 11791-4413
Tel: (516) 364-0808
Fax: (516) 364-0989

**UNITED KINGDOM**

**Faculty of Homeopathy**
Royal London Homoeopathic
Hospital
Great Ormond Street
London
WC1N 3HR
Tel: 0171 837 2495

**Shiatsu Society**
31 Pullman Lane
Godalming, Surrey GU7 1XY
Tel:01483860771

## TRANSCENDENTAL MEDITATION

**UNITED STATES**

**Maharishi University of
Management**
Fairfield,
IA 52557
Tel: (515) 472 7000

## VISUALIZATION THERAPY

**UNITED STATES**

**Academy for Guided Imagery**
PO Box 2070
Mill Valley,
CA 94942
Tel: (800) 726-2070

**UNITED KINGDOM**

**Dr. Kai Kermani**
Holistic Health and Healing Center
10 Connaught Hill
Loughton
Essex
IG10 4DU

## YOGA

**UNITED STATES**

**Ayurvedic Institute**
11311 Menaud NE, Suite A
Albuquerque,
NM 87112
Tel: (505) 291-9698

**College of Maharishi Ayurveda at
Maharishi International**
1603 North Fourth Street
PO Box 282
Fairfield, IA 52557
Tel: (515) 472-8477
**Integral Yoga Teachers'
Association**
Tel: (804) 969-3121

**Himalayan International
Institute of Yoga, Science and
Philosophy**
RRI, Box 400
Honesdale,
PA 18431
Tel: (800) 822-4547
(717) 253-5551

**The Meditation Center**
Tel: (612) 379-2386

**Mount Madonna Center**
Tel: (408) 847-0406
**Self-Realization Fellowship**
Tel: (213) 225-2471

**Sivananda Ashram**
Tel: (800) 783-YOGA

**The International Association of
Yoga Therapists**
109 Hillside Avenue
Mill Valley,
CA 94941
Tel: (415) 381-0876

**UNITED KINGDOM**

**British Wheel of Yoga**
1 Hamilton Place
Boston Road
Sleaford
Lincolnshire NG34 7ES
Tel: 01529 306851

**Yoga Biomedical Trust**
156 Cockerel Road
Cambridge
Tel: 01223 67301

# AMERICAN HOLISTIC HEALTH ASSOCIATION

The American Holistic Health Association (AHHA) is a national, nonprofit clearing house for resources that people can use to help themselves create wellness. AHHA is committed to providing practical quality information without affiliation with any product, service or method of healthcare delivery.

AHHA promotes a holistic approach to wellness, which encourages individuals to:
■ Balance and integrate their physical, mental, emotional and spiritual wellbeing.
■ Establish respectful, cooperative relationships with others and the environment.
■ Make wellness-oriented lifestyle choices.
■ Actively participate in their health decisions and healing process.

AAHA puts people in touch with the wealth of resources waiting to help them progress along the path to achieving wellness. AHHA has researched self-help resources—information, people and organizations—available in the United States, and offers this data free-of-charge as resource and networking lists. These lists and other AHHA educational materials are available by mail and on the Internet and enable people to:

■ Get involved—take responsibility for their health and wellbeing.
■ Become informed—learn how they can create wellness and identify the resources available to them.
■ Take action—make appropriate changes in their daily living to accomplish their personal wellness goals.

Deepak Chopra, M.D., Bernie Siegel, M.D., and other prestigious healthcare professionals endorse AHHA and act as advisors to the AHHA leadership. AHHA has been promoted as a valuable resource by the Institute of Noetic Sciences, the Omega Institute and the Office of Alternative Medicine/National Institutes of Health.

This non-profit organization is supported by tax-deductible contributions. To request lists or membership information, contact AHHA at:
American Holistic Health Association
P.O.Box 17400
Anaheim
California 92817-7400
Tel: (714) 779 6152
E-mail: ahha@healthy.net
Web site: http://www.healthy.net/ahha

# INDEX

# N

# O

# P

# PHOTOGRAPH CREDITS

**Hutchison Library:** pages 78, 90, 109, 164, 165 (Nick Haslam), 223 (Liba Taylor), 276 (Felix Greene), 281 (Felix Greene), 282 (Felix Greene), 283 (John Hatt), 285

**Frank Lane Picture Agency:** pages 13 (Eva Lindenburger), 28 (Fernand), 30 (L Bucci), 31 top (E & D Hosking), 33 (Silvestris), 34, 37 (B Borrell), 39 (W Wisniewski), 41 (D Allain), 51 (Eva Lindenburger), 68 (E & D Hosking), 73 top (E & D Hosking), 73 bottom left (A Whartom), 74 top (W Wisniewski), 74 bottom left (J Hutchings), 74 bottom right (E & D Hosking), 75 top right (E & D Hoskings), 92, 98, 100 (Eva Lindenburger), 102 (Moulu), 166, 186 (F Stock), 88 (F Stock), 190 (F Stock), 192 (Fernand), 206 ( Life Science Images), 284 (Roger Tidman), 286, 287 (Roger Tidman)

**Image Bank:** pages 26 (Pete Turner), 168 (Antony Edwards), 174 (A Boccaccio), 180 (David de Lossy), 253 (Garry Gay)

**Pictor International:**  page 42

**Science Photo Library:** pages 14 (Will & Dent McIntyre), 22 (John Mead), 24, 31 Bot (Charles D Winters, 36 (Dr. Morley Read), 38 (Dr. Jeremy Burgess), 48 (BSIP De Gennaro), 52 (Oscar Burriel), 64 (David Parker), 69 (BSIP Dequest), 71 (Michael Marten), 76 (Ricardo Arias), 79, 94 (Oscar Burriel), 97 (Paul Biddle), 99 (Hattie Young), 101 (Mehau Kulyk), 104 (Manfred Kage), 110 (James King-Holmes), 113 (Ron Sutherland), 118 (BSIP, Roux), 120 (Mehau Kulyk), 121 (David Gifford), 122 (John Bavosi), 124 (Hattie Young), 125 (Hattie Young), 127 bottom (Paul Biddle & Tim Malyon), 139 (John Greim), 146 (Bill Longcore), 148 (John Greim), 149 top (National Library of Medicine), 150 (John Greim), 151 (John Greim), 153 (John Greim), 154 (Larry Mulvehill), 156 (David Parker), 157 top (National Library of Medicine), 157 bottom (Jean-Loup Charmet), 158 (Sheila Terry), 159 Top (Phillippe Plailly), 159 Bot (Phillippe Plailly), 160 (Philippe Plailly), 161 (Francoise Sauze), 184 (Seth Joel), 189 (Doug Plummer), 191 (Paul Biddle), 193 (Francoise Sauze), 194 (Paul Biddle), 195 (Will & Deni McIntyre), 204 (Damien Lovegrove), 209 (Damien Lovegrove), 222 (Damien Lovegrove), 246 (Paul Biddle & Tim Malyon)

**Tony Stone Images:** pages 238 (Bruce Hands), 240 (Andy Whale), 247 (Zigy Kaluzny)

**Bruce Head:** pages 3, 5, 11, 52, 57, 72, 80, 83, 84, 85, 86, 87, 89, 91, 185, 197, 198, 199, 200, 201, 202, 203, 205, 207, 208, 210, 211, 212, 216, 217, 218, 219, 220, 221, 224, 225, 227, 229, 230, 231, 231, 233, 234, 235, 236, 237, 242, 256, 257, 259, 260, 265, 266, 270, 271, 272, 273, 274, 275

**A Nelson & Co Ltd:** pages 39, 40

**American Institute of Osteopathy:** pages 126, 127 top

**American Polarity Therapy Association:** page 49

**British Acupuncture Council:** page 245

**British School of Osteopathy:** pages 123, 128, 129 & 131 (John Tramper)

**Caroline Wheeler:** page 75

**Dorothee von Greiff:** page 149 bottom

**Dr. Edward Bach Center:** page 55

**Flower Essence Society:** pages 12, 54, 58, 59, 60, 61, 66

**Holistic Health College:** pages 44, 45, 46

**Julian Barnard,** Healing Herbs Ltd: page 59

**Paul Lam:** pages 277, 279, 280

**Rolfing Association:** pages 132, 134, 135

**SP:** pages 140, 142, 143, 144

**The Shiatsu Society:**  pages 254, 262

# ACKNOWLEDGEMENTS

The publishers would like to thank the following organizations for their assistance in preparing this book.

A. Nelson & Co. Ltd.

British Acupuncture Council

British School of Osteopathy

Flower Essence Society

Dr. Edward Bach Center

Holistic Health College

Institute of Complementary Medicine, London, UK

Jean Garron PR

Maureen Cropper PR

Office of Alternative Medicine, National Institutes of Health, Maryland

The Rolfing Institute
Jenny Crewdson, UK representative,

The Shiatsu Society

The Society of Teachers of the Alexander Technique

The Woodbridge Complementary Healing Center in Woodbridge, England, opened its doors on November 9 1992—the brainchild of Alice Strover, a homeopath with a vision, and her husband, John Strover, Practice Manager. The intervening three-and-a-half years have seen the center grow from strength to strength with a current complement of 12 practitioners offering 16 different disciplines. The committed and professional approach of the practitioners has benefited many people from many different walks of life. Open six days a week, the reception is manned Monday through Friday, 9.00am to 5.00pm. Free 15-minute consultations may be booked with any of the therapists.
Tel: (01394) 388234

Special thanks are extended to the following practitioners for their assistance in the special step-by-step photography:

Linda M Fell, Physiotherapist and Reflexologist, MCSP, SRP, MAR,

Maggie Kinnear, Aromatherapist and Reflexologist, MIFA, ITEC

Richard Graham, Acupuncturist and Shiatsu Practitioner, MTAS, MRSS Lic. Ac.

Thanks also to Lesley Ann Terry, Reflexologist and Aromatherapist, MAR, MISPA